Since its foundation in 1766, Addenbrooke's Hospital has strongly influenced both the development of medical practice and the social history of Cambridge. As one of Britain's first Voluntary Hospitals serving the needs of the sick, and as a centre of medical teaching, Addenbrooke's has always been a focal point in the community as well as a prestigious institute in the wider medical sphere.

This authoritative and absorbing account of the Hospital traces in detail its history and development, from its benefaction in 1719 by John Addenbrooke, through its early years of expansion, reforms and modernisation and over the period of the two World Wars. The final chapters bring the story up to date, with an account of the changes which have occurred in the Hospital since 1948, including the major reforms in the N.H.S. and the establishment of a Clinical School. The authors have a long and close association with Addenbrooke's and have written a book that reflects their unequalled knowledge and insight into the medical history of Cambridge. With the use of rare and previously unseen archive material, including the original Minutes, they have produced a careful, authoritative and fascinating account of the history and development of one of Britain's most famous hospitals: its buildings, staff, patients, policy and finances.

Embellished with evocative and often rare documentary illustrations, this book will be of the greatest interest and value to all those associated with Addenbrooke's, past and present – clinicians, nursing and administrative staff, students and patients, as well as to anyone with an interest in the social and medical history of Cambridge.

T0297328

The history of Addenbrooke's Hospital, Cambridge

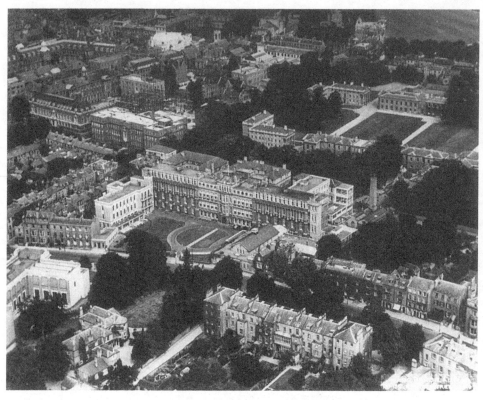

Addenbrooke's Hospital and environs, crossed in front by Trumpington Street, August 1937.
Photo by Aero Pictorial Ltd.

The history of Addenbrooke's Hospital, Cambridge

ARTHUR ROOK M.D., F.R.C.P.

MARGARET CARLTON M.Sc.
(London and Cantab) M.B., B.Chir
and

W. GRAHAM CANNON M.A., F.H.S.M.

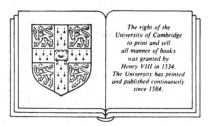

The right of the
University of Cambridge
to print and sell
all manner of books
was granted by
Henry VIII in 1534.
The University has printed
and published continuously
since 1584.

CAMBRIDGE UNIVERSITY PRESS
Cambridge
New York   Port Chester   Melbourne   Sydney

CAMBRIDGE UNIVERSITY PRESS
Cambridge, New York, Melbourne, Madrid, Cape Town, Singapore,
São Paulo, Delhi, Dubai, Tokyo

Cambridge University Press
The Edinburgh Building, Cambridge CB2 8RU, UK

Published in the United States of America by Cambridge University Press, New York

www.cambridge.org
Information on this title: www.cambridge.org/9780521142397

First published 1991
This digitally printed version 2010

A catalogue record for this publication is available from the British Library

Library of Congress Cataloguing in Publication data
Rook, Arthur.
The history of Addenbrooke's Hospital, Cambridge / Arthur Rook and
Margaret Carlton : epilogue, 1948 to 1974 by W. Graham Cannon.
p. cm.
Includes bibliographical references and index.
ISBN 0-521-40529-7
1. Addenbrooke's Hospital (Cambridge, England)–History.
2. Hospitals–England–Cambridge (Cambridgeshire)–History.
I. Carlton, Margaret. II. Title.
RA988.C8A347 1991
362.1'1'0942659–dc20
91–27793 CIP

ISBN 978-0-521-40529-4 Hardback
ISBN 978-0-521-14239-7 Paperback

Black & white cover illustration shows the Hospital in 1766.
Full colour cover photograph shows the Hospital in 1990.

Contents

CONTENTS

Foreword

I was greatly honoured by the invitation to write this foreword to such an impressive history of Addenbrooke's Hospital by Arthur Rook, Margaret Carlton and Graham Cannon.

May I touch first on the senior author, Arthur Rook. He has been one of the brightest stars in the Cambridge Clinical Medical firmament for over 30 years. He established himself as our dermatologist and built up a strong select school of contemplative colleagues. Between them under Rook's leadership they have made a wide range of clinical and research contributions to dermatology so giving this subject considerable status in the strong competitive atmosphere of scientific enquiry which abounds hereabouts. It is hardly surprising that Rook's *Textbook of Dermatology* was so widely acclaimed and is now in its fourth edition, and that his works have been translated and published abroad.

But alongside this invaluable clinical contribution Rook developed another side of his abilities and character. He patiently acquainted himself with and fostered an interest in the history of medicine in Cambridge. Indeed it was Rook who organised the Congress which formed the basis of *Cambridge and its contribution to Medicine*[1] which he edited and brought to publication in 1971. He also published a history of the Cambridge Medical Society 1880–1980.[2]

His many friends and admirers will now be delighted to have in this present volume the full fruits of his long-established historical scholarship and balanced wisdom, all brought to bear on the hospital which grew out of John Addenbrooke's will and his original benefaction for its establishment.

In all this Arthur Rook has been supported most admirably, first by Margaret Carlton, a medically qualified scientist who started her career as a writer. She must be accorded full and proper credit for participating in the detailed research behind the volume and for her writing where it is incorporated in the text. More recently Graham Cannon, who was House Governor of Addenbrooke's Hospital and Secretary to the Board of Governors until that body was abolished in 1974, has also made important contributions about the recent history of the Hospital; no one could have been in a better position to have done so than he.

This sort of collaboration is typical of Rook's style. Throughout his career he has always helped younger colleagues flourish and this is abundantly evident in the present venture. We, and historians of medicine everywhere, must be most grateful to all three of them for what they have achieved, as will be innumerable students of the Cambridge Medical School, both pre- and post-graduates, now and far into the future.

Cambridge 1990   John Butterfield

Preface

The writing of this History has been a labour of love and perhaps for this reason it has taken time to write. In 1956 the Board of Governors of the United Cambridge Hospitals agreed that Dr Arthur Rook should have access to all the papers of the Board and of its predecessor Authorities responsible for the administration of Addenbrooke's Hospital. Dr Rook was then a fairly newly appointed Consultant Dermatologist who was later to become a national and indeed international authority in his specialty.

Combining his clinical responsibilities at Addenbrooke's with his original work in dermatology, and the editorial activities that he accepted in his specialty, inevitably meant that his historical research proceeded slowly: notwithstanding the publication of a number of other medical historical works that he wrote during this time.

Dr Rook retired from Addenbrooke's in 1974 but this meant that he was able to devote more time to the History. Thanks to financial support from the Wellcome Institute for the History of Medicine it was possible to obtain the substantial help of Dr Margaret Carlton, herself a Cambridge medical graduate, and the work on the History was completed up to the year 1948 when the Hospital became the responsibility of the National Health Service.

Graham Cannon, who was House Governor of Addenbrooke's from 1962 until 1974 (when the Hospital came under the administration of the Area Health Authority (Teaching) of Cambridgeshire) is a History graduate of Emmanuel College Cambridge. Having assisted Dr Rook in some of the early stages of the work, it was natural that he should be asked to contribute a section on the history of the Hospital in more recent times.

None of the authors believe that contemporary 'history' can be written. This book concludes with an 'Epilogue' (Modern times) describing aspects of the development of Addenbrooke's with special emphasis on the building of a new Teaching Hospital at Hills Road, and the foundation of the Clinical School, the planning of which began as early as 1944. To bring the History up to date photographs of the Hospital and of the

Clinical School as they are at the time of going to press – 1990 – have been included. It will be for future historians to look at the period after 1948 in more detail; for the present it must suffice to say that the authors of this book have confidence that the benefaction of John Addenbrooke in 1719 will continue to benefit the citizens of Cambridge, and those far beyond, for many years to come.

September 1990

Dr Arthur Rook died on 30 July 1991. He had been seriously ill for some years, but his illness had not impaired his enthusiasm for *The history of Addenbrooke's Hospital* on which he continued to work until a few days before his death. He died having seen and approved the final page proofs, and in the knowledge that publication was assured.

August 1991   WGC

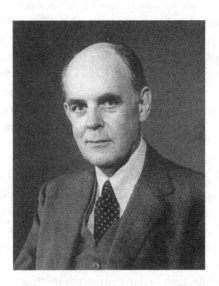

ARTHUR JAMES ROOK

1918–1991

Acknowledgements

In putting the final touches to this book after its gestation of more than 30 years, we would like to thank the many friends whose assistance and contributions have made it possible.

The project could never have been attempted without the kind cooperation of the present and past authorities at Addenbrooke's Hospital, whom we would like to thank.

The Wellcome Trust have generously given support for one of us through the Cambridge University Wellcome Unit for the History of Medicine, and further funds have come from the Trust Funds of the Cambridge Health Authority. We are indebted to the Trustees and administrators of these bodies and also to Dr Roger French and Ms Maureen Sauzier of the Wellcome Unit.

Mrs G.R. Cant, Archivist at Addenbrooke's Hospital, has been of great assistance over many years, as have also the staff at the Cambridge University Library, especially Dr D.M. Owen and Dr E.S. Leedham-Green. The material at the Cambridgeshire Collection, Cambridgeshire Libraries, has been invaluable and we would like to thank the staff there, particularly the Principal Librarian, Mr Michael J. Petty.

Thanks are due to Mrs Peggy Clarke for her secretarial and other contributions; to a member of the District Finance Department who advised when the finances of the Hospital were being studied; to Miss Anne Challice, secretary to the House Governor and to Ms Valerie Beamish, S.R.D. of the Cambridge Health Authority, who advised on dietetic matters.

Particular mention should be made of the help given over many years by Mr Leonard Beard, now in charge of the Department of Medical Photography at Hinchingbrooke Hospital, Huntingdon, but earlier Head of the Department of Medical Photography and Illustration at Addenbrooke's. He took many of the photographs of the earlier historical material and was always most generous of his time and energy. Similarly his successor at Addenbrooke's, Mr Martin Johns, has been particularly helpful with the illustrations and was good enough to supply some of them.

ACKNOWLEDGEMENTS

Grateful acknowledgement is given to the many bodies who have allowed us to use copyright material, particularly Cambridge University Press. Permission to quote from 'Cambridge and its Contribution to Medicine' was given by the Trustees of the Wellcome Trust, and to quote from the *Cambridge Chronicle* and the *Cambridge Daily News*, by the Cambridge Evening News. We are obliged for some set copy to the Syndics of the Cambridge University Library. We should especially wish to thank Mrs Jill Steinberg for help in preparing the index, and in proof reading.

Finally we should acknowledge the following for their ready agreement to include photographs owned by them: Lord Butterfield to whom we also owe a particular debt of gratitude for his prompt response to our request for a Foreword to the book; the Regius Professor of Physic, Professor Keith Peters; Sir Roy Calne; Miss M.M. Puddicombe O.B.E.; Lady Kathleen Lee; Dr A.S. Playfair; Sir Francis Pemberton, C.B.E., D.L.; Messrs Mowlem P.L.C. & B.A.A.; and the Master and Fellows of Darwin College for the photograph of Sir Frank Young.

The authors and the publishers have aimed to keep the cost of producing this book, and therefore its price, down to the minimum. To assist us the Hospital Trustees, and Trinity College, have made substantial grants and we wish publicly to acknowledge these and to thank them. In conclusion we would like to thank the members of staff, their relatives and many other interested people who have sent information, reminiscences, photographs or memorabilia, much of which unfortunately time and space have precluded us from using as we would have wished.

Introduction

Addenbrooke's Hospital at Cambridge admitted its first patients in October 1766. The founder of the Hospital, John Addenbrooke, died in 1719 and his wife, who enjoyed a life interest in his estate, died in 1720 only a few months later. In his will Addenbrooke left his quite modest fortune to erect and maintain a hospital for the poor. The trustees of his will were so dilatory in carrying out his instructions that the Hospital was not completed and equipped until 47 years after his death.

For centuries until the dissolution of the monasteries in the 1540s, many of the monasteries and other religious houses had provided care for the sick of their own order, and some of them also offered food, shelter and medical care to the destitute sick. After their disappearance there were few facilities to replace them. In London the Lord Mayor persuaded the King to re-establish the hospitals of St Thomas and Bartholomew, and also the hospital of St Mary of Bethlehem for the mentally ill. The authorities were very conscious of the threat to law and order from the thousands of destitute and unemployed, and introduced a succession of measures in an effort to alleviate it. These measures culminated in the Elizabethan Poor Law Act in 1601. This placed the responsibility for the relief of the poor on the individual parishes, and the overseers of the parishes were under heavy pressure to keep the poor rate as low as possible. Some parishes provided a workhouse for the able-bodied poor.

In placing on the parish the responsibility for providing relief the local magistrates at Quarter Sessions, who were obliged to enforce the provision of Poor Law relief, made every effort to prevent any settlement and in particular to prevent the birth of children, as these would become entitled to relief and thus become a charge on the parish.

This system, with occasional changes, remained in force until the Poor Law Reform Act of 1834. Under this Act the regime in the workhouses was made harsher and groups of neighbouring parishes were ordered to build a workhouse infirmary for each Union of parishes. Outdoor relief, that is to say the payment of money to those who remained in their homes, was forbidden and the poor were therefore compelled to seek admission to the Union infirmary.

In 1714 the Quaker, John Bellars, published 'An Essay towards the Improvement of Physic'. He advocated a hospital service supported by the State. Addenbrooke may well have seen this book; it certainly influenced other philanthropists to set up hospitals which were called voluntary because they were supported neither by the Church nor the State but by voluntary contributions. The Voluntary Hospital Movement which was to play such an important part in the development of medicine in England was initiated by Henry Hoare the banker and his associates who founded Westminster Hospital in 1719. Guy's Hospital was opened in 1725 and the London Hospital in 1740. If the trustees of Addenbrooke had acted more promptly his hospital would have been the first Voluntary Hospital outside London.

The histories of a great many of the voluntary hospitals of Britain have been written and inevitably they share many features in common. One of these features has been intense local pride in the hospital manifested as a sometimes ill-founded conviction of its superiority. The hospitals generally attracted the support of local notabilities and their evolution followed a consistent pattern differing only in details. However, in Cambridge, there were some special features which modified this pattern, the most important of these being the presence of the University which was numerically large in relation to the size of the town. There was, however, a long-standing tradition of hostility between the town and the University, both of which were represented among the governors.

Among the reforms made over the years was an attempt to introduce the 'new nursing'. The University supported the change which was opposed by the town. Also, in the 1880s, the University strongly supported the efforts of the medical staff to introduce and maintain a pathology service; this was opposed by representatives of the town who considered it an unnecessary expense.

By the last years of the nineteenth century, and largely on the advice of Sir Henry Burdett who had created for himself a position as the unchallenged authority on hospital administration, important changes were made which established a Board of Governors consisting of equal numbers of representatives of the Borough, the County, and the University.

Finally, during the tenure of the Regius Chair of Physic by John Ryle, the University approved the use of the Elmore funds to introduce reforms and improvements in practice and teaching.

The very active involvement of the University in the development of the Hospital has not been generally recognised.

The setting

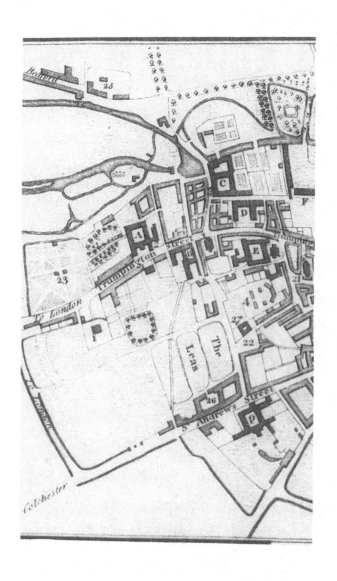

~ I ~

The background

During the seventeenth century the practice of medicine based on the careful and critical observation of the natural history of diseases began slowly to replace practice based on the theory of the humours as propounded by Galen and modified by generations of successors. Thomas Sydenham (1624–1689) and his followers were pioneers of the new medicine in England.

By the end of the eighteenth century the first medical journals had been established and new medical books were being published at a rate which contemporaries found bewildering. The flow from the presses of new journals and new books was to continue at a rapid rate and by the third or fourth decade of the following century it was already difficult for the keen practitioner to keep up to date.

As the eighteenth century drew to its close the medical practitioners of Britain were for historic reasons sharply divided into groups differing in their educational and social status, but with more in common in their interests and their methods of practice than these differences would suggest. Statistics of the profession before the publication of an unofficial medical register by Samuel Foart Simmons from 1779 to 1783 are hard to compile. Simmons' Register, however, while certainly incomplete, does serve as a useful guide.

According to him there were 4459 medical men in England and Wales in 1782. Most of those practising outside London and calling themselves physicians had degrees from Scottish or foreign universities. Of those practising as surgeons or apothecaries at least one in three had no qualification but this does not imply that in many cases they had not had as much training and experience as men who had obtained a diploma. Some had earned the right to practice as apothecaries by service in the Army or Navy.[1] Others may have seen little advantage in sitting an examination for a diploma they were under no obligation to possess.

Nevertheless there were doubtless many men in practice who had no training and little knowledge. Except in London and other large cities physicians, surgeons and apothecaries were in fact all in general practice.

Even in London there were very few who were pure physicians or pure surgeons. Sir Astley Cooper (1768–1841), the most eminent British surgeon of his day, saw twice as many medical as surgical patients.[2] The Apothecaries Act of 1815 was the fruit of some twenty years' campaigning by the qualified apothecaries to raise their status and eliminate the competition of their unqualified rivals including those chemists and druggists who practised.

The object of the Act was to restrict the practice of medicine to physicians and apothecaries, and the dispensing of physicians' prescriptions to apothecaries. An apprenticeship of five years was compulsory and all who entered practice from 1815 onward were obliged also to pass the examination of the Society of Apothecaries who had the right throughout England to prosecute those who practised without having done so. During part of the period of apprenticeship the student had to attend lectures and hospital practice.

The Act was undoubtedly an important advance and did much to stimulate the provision of better educational facilities in London and in provincial towns and to raise standards of practice; however, the Act did not go far enough. 'It left the practice of surgery and midwifery open to any unprincipled practitioner, and did not prevent the chemists and druggists from compounding physicians' prescriptions or from practising medicine.'[3]

The Act did nothing to diminish the privileges of the Universities of Oxford and Cambridge or of the Colleges of Physicians and Surgeons. Moreover the Society of Apothecaries never made full use of its powers in controlling unlicensed apothecaries. Langley,[4] writing in 1867, said that 'the Act seems never to have been rigidly put into force, and has of late years been practically abandoned'.

The lack of control of unqualified practice and the reactionary attitudes of the Royal Colleges were only two of the profession's many grievances during the first half of the nineteenth century. The Poor Law Amendment Act of 1834 was an important cause of justifiable anger and it is relevant also because it profoundly modified the pattern of medical practice.

Under the old Poor Law, parishes often called on the services of an apothecary or a surgeon to treat the sick poor, usually on the basis of a fee for each patient, but occasionally on a contract basis. Under the 1834 Act neighbouring parishes were grouped together to erect and maintain central workhouses. The local guardians divided their area into districts each of which often comprised several parishes. For each district they appointed a medical officer, usually choosing the man who would accept the lowest salary, and such a man was inevitably often totally unqualified. Where a reputable qualified practitioner took a Poor Law appointment, perhaps to exclude a potential rival, he might be forced by economic pressures to employ an unqualified assistant as his deputy. The workhouses (often referred to as Unions) were at first workhouses and no more but most took on increasingly the burden of caring for the chronic sick and some eventually functioned primarily as hospitals.*

The numerous grievances of the Poor Law medical officers led to insistent calls for medical reform but the profession was not united and there was so little agreement as to what shape or direction the reforms should take that a long series of abortive bills preceded the Medical Act of 1858.[5]

Largely through the activities of the Provincial Medical and Surgical Association which became the British Medical Association in 1855, some measure of agreement was achieved: there should be a single authority issuing a uniform qualification which entitled its holder to practise in any part of the country, and practice by the unqualified should be unlawful.

In the event the Medical Act did none of these things but it was a step in the right direction. It established the General Council of Medical Education and Registration (known since 1951 simply as the General Medical Council) to establish and ensure proper educational standards and to compile and publish a register.[6]

The first Register, which was published in July 1859, showed that only one in three practitioners was qualified. The unqualified were not forbidden to practice but were not allowed to claim to be qualified. Over many years, and by means of further Acts of Parliament and the decisions of the Courts, standards were raised and abuses eliminated.

The value of registration was greatly enhanced by the National

---

* The Cambridge Union Workhouse, to serve the Borough's 14 parishes, was erected in 1838 on Mill Road with accommodation for 250 persons. It was used as a general hospital under the Emergency Medical Service in 1939 and from 1948 became the local Maternity Hospital. The Chesterton Union Workhouse served 38 parishes covering an area of some 120 square miles. These parishes, which completely surrounded Cambridge, included Cottenham, Coton, Fulbourn, Grantchester, Harston, Histon, the Shelfords and Trumpington. After 1948 this workhouse was converted into a geriatric hospital. There were Union workhouses also at Caxton, Newmarket, Ely, Doddington, Whittlesey, Wisbech, Saffron Walden, Kedington and Huntingdon, all within the area now served by Addenbrooke's Hospital.

Insurance Act of 1911 under which only the registered practitioner could be employed and by subsequent legislation such as the Venereal Diseases Act of 1917 and the Dangerous Drugs Act of 1920.

The medical scene in 1880, the year in which the Cambridge Medical Society was founded, was strikingly different from that of today.[7] At the head of the profession there were still the pure physicians and the pure surgeons who were very few in number even in the largest towns. Even in London it was quite exceptional for a man to practise entirely as a consultant and the average physician or surgeon, including, in towns such as Cambridge, the Professors of Medicine, Surgery and Anatomy, were really engaged in what was called high-class general practice, with which they combined such consultant practice as came their way; they did not dispense.

Then there were the general practitioners in their several grades. First there were those with a private surgery, characteristic of the larger villages and smaller towns. They often dispensed and frequently employed an assistant, who was not necessarily qualified. Next there were the very numerous surgeon apothecaries, who kept shops with an open surgery and also dispensed, but did not run a retail business. Lowest in the professional and social scale were the surgeon–chemists, who kept shops with an open surgery, sometimes practised dentistry, and also sold 'anything that can be found at the shop of a regular chemist',[8] and this might include pickles, sauces, tobacco and cosmetics.

The conditions of employment in the Poor Law Medical Service remained in general deplorable. Salaries, including the supply of medicines, were still very low. 'The busy practitioner who has taken a district in order to make it a nidus, as it is called, for practice, cannot and does not give more than the merest fraction of his time.'[9] The Poor Law Medical Service was of course only for paupers: all other patients had to pay their doctors' fees. Only those who were unable to pay were entitled to attend the great majority of the numerous Voluntary Hospitals and Dispensaries, and then only with a letter of recommendation from a subscriber to the charity in question. Under these circumstances it is not surprising that the 'Club' system developed and remained an important feature of medical practice until the National Insurance Act of 1911 came into force, and by that date some six or seven million patients were covered by contract practice.[10]

Friendly Societies offering insurance against sickness, funeral expenses, and sometimes other benefits, can be traced back to the seventeenth century but began to increase rapidly in numbers after 1760.[11] In 1815 most of the Societies were local and in that year had 4739 members in Cambridgeshire, 2509 in Huntingdonshire, 20531 in Essex, and 13814 in Suffolk, and a total membership of about one million. Big national societies developed such as the Manchester Unity of Oddfellows and the Ancient Order of Foresters, with branches (known as lodges or courts) in most parts of the country. Some societies were run by their members. There were also numbers of county societies founded and run by gentry and clergy; a Cambridgeshire Society was founded in 1840. On a smaller scale were the 'Slate' and Public House Clubs usually started by a publican who acted as treasurer as well as president.[12]

There were other private clubs run by doctors themselves, and a few run for private profit. The tendency of most of these organisations was to exploit the medical profession by employing the lowest bidder, and as late as 1900 some doctors were accepting as little as two or three shillings per patient per year.[11] The better societies however made an effort to ensure a good standard of service for their members.

Provision for the hospital care of the mentally ill was restricted, with a few notable exceptions, to private homes often run by medical men. Even such small private establishments appear to have been very few in number in the Eastern Counties. The mentally sick poor were cared for quite inadequately by the workhouse. The Asylums Act of 1848 called on rate-levying authorities to provide Asylums.*

The organisation of medical practice was influenced and modified directly or indirectly by a number of other Acts of Parliament, many of which, such as the Midwives Act of 1902 and the Education Act of 1907, which established a statutory school medical service, aroused much controversy in the profession[13] and it would be interesting to study the impact of these and other Acts on the work of the medical practitioner. We must accept the generalisation that the pattern of practice was constantly changing and that sometimes legislation and sometimes scientific advances were responsible for such changes.

Of outstanding importance, however, was the National Health Insurance Act of 1911. This Act was opposed by most of the medical profession, because they feared they would suffer a drop in income, but also because many had fears, based on bitter experience, that the threatened increased power of Friendly Societies would be disastrous. The Act was in fact

---

* The County, the Isle of Ely and the Borough shared the cost of erecting the Fulbourn Asylum which received its first patients in 1858.

designed as the natural sequel to the Old Age Pension legislation of 1908 and set out to provide incomes for those who were at risk of pauperisation through ill health;[13] it did not set out to provide a National Health Service. The scheme was administered through the Friendly Societies and the big industrial insurance companies who were 'approved societies'. The medical opposition was, as usual, not united, and the great majority of doctors ultimately gave their cooperation.

From 1911 until 1948 this so called 'Panel' system was the dominant characteristic of a large section of medical practice in Britain. By 1945 24 million were covered by compulsory health service.[14] The scheme excluded all those earning more than a certain income (the limit was raised in 1942 from £250 to £420 per annum), all self-employed persons and all employed dependants of insured persons. The benefits provided were free general practice service, medicines, and a small cash payment during sickness.

For hospital services even the insured were still dependent on the Voluntary Hospitals or on the hospitals, some of them first class, which the Local Authorities were developing from the old workhouse infirmaries. The 'doctor's letter', traditionally demanded of patients attending hospital, except in emergency, originated soon after the National Insurance Act came into force. The hospitals, financially hard-pressed, were reluctant to accept the patients who could be cared for by their general practitioners. Subscribers' letters were, however, still usually required, but in most parts of the country Hospital Contributory schemes made such letters more readily available. Contributions, commonly at 2d. to 6d. weekly, were collected at the factory or office, or other place of work, and a subscribers' letter was obtained through the local organiser of the scheme.

By 1947 such schemes had ten million beneficiaries.[14] Despite this association, and the considerable sums some hospitals received from Local Authorities or central Government for treatment provided for certain special categories of patients, many hospitals were frequently in financial difficulties. Most Voluntary Hospitals had for some time found it necessary to make a small charge related to the patient's earnings as assessed by a social worker, who became known as a lady Almoner. Income from all these sources tended to fall behind expenditure; it was only the Emergency Medical Service, State financed, organised in preparation for the Second World War, which prolonged the life of the heterogeneous and cumbersome system which had evolved from such diverse origins.

The introduction of the National Health Service in July 1948 brought compulsory health insurance for the entire population, and brought all hospitals, except for a few small private hospitals, under the control of the Minister of Health. The medical profession had offered some opposition to the Bill but, as always, was not united and there were many doctors who welcomed it.

Changes in the pattern of practice in hospital and in primary care since 1948 have been immense, as the consequence of the interplay of social evolution, advances in medical science and Government legislation. In retrospect there are few who would deny that the Health Service, despite its shortcomings, has brought great benefits to the majority.

~ 2 ~

John Addenbrooke

John Addenbrooke was born in 1680 in the village of Kingswinford, Staffordshire, the only child of the Reverend Samuel Addenbrooke, Vicar of West Bromwich, and his wife Matilda Porry.[1] The date of his birth is unknown but the register of the parish church of West Bromwich records his baptism there on 13 June 1681. During his short life – he died in 1719 – he made no contribution to medical science and his career as a teacher and physician was not notably successful; had he not founded the hospital at Cambridge it is unlikely that he would have found his place, modest though it is, in the history of medicine.

The Addenbrooke family had been established around the borders of Worcestershire, Staffordshire and Shropshire for many centuries. The earliest record of the family refers to Richard, son of Richard de Adynbrok, who was sued for seven acres of land in Rowley Regis in 1271–1272.[2] From the sixteenth century onwards there are more numerous records of the family as small landowners. In the seventeenth and eighteenth centuries many entered the church. Thomas Addenbrooke of the Lye, Great Swinford, who died in 1550[3] was the direct ancestor of John Addenbrooke. Recent generations of the family have included some expert genealogists and the detailed pedigree of the Addenbrookes has been drawn up.[4]

The greatly simplified pedigree (Fig. 1) illustrates the descent of John Addenbrooke from Thomas and also the three lines of descent of the twentieth-century members of the family, many of them in the Church, medicine or law, and some now in the Commonwealth and in the United States. The arms[5] are described as follows: 'Quarterly, azure and argent, a fesse wavy or, between three crescents counterchanged. Mantling azure and argent. *Crest* on a wreath of the colours, on the bank side of a river proper, an otter passant per pale argent and sable, charged with two crescents counterchanged. Motto: "Nec temere nec timide"' (Neither rashly nor timidly).

This blazon comprises features seen in the arms of both the Addenbrooke and Homfray families. The 'fesse wavy between three crescents', is

THE FAMILY OF JOHN ADDENBROOKE

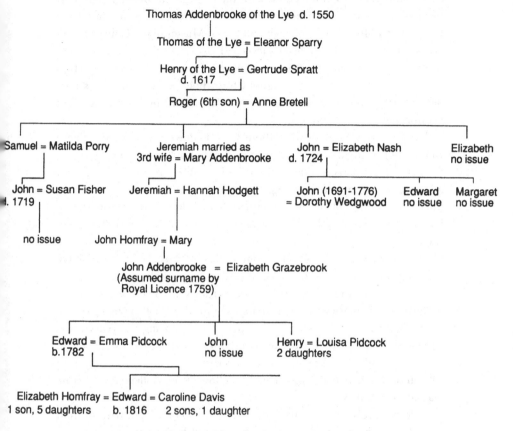

Fig. 1. The Addenbrooke family tree. Details kindly supplied by members of the Addenbrooke's family.

seen in the arms on John Addenbrooke's tombstone in St Catharine's College chapel, and the crest, showing 'an otter proper wounded in the sinister shoulder with a spear', is recorded by Burke for several Homfrays derived from Francis Homfray, Esquire, of Aston, County York, supposed to have been killed in the siege of Clonmel under Cromwell.

Early life and education.[6] Nothing is known of John Addenbrooke before his admission to Catharine Hall (later to become St Catharine's College) as a pensioner on 13 December 1697. At that time the majority of undergraduates were admitted as pensioners, paying for their tuition, board and lodging.

Samuel Addenbrooke no doubt chose to send John to Catharine Hall on account of family connections with the College; his brother John had been educated there and his brother's son was also to go to Catharine Hall. In 1697 John Eachard,[7] who had been Master of the College for 22 years, died and had just been succeeded by Sir William Dawes, Bart, when Addenbrooke entered the College. Dawes, a Tory and High Churchman, was Master throughout the whole of Addenbrooke's residence in the College. He was elected Archbishop of York in 1713 and left Cambridge the following year.

The College was small with about forty Fellows and students. There were only eleven admissions in 1697 and only four or five in each of the following four years although there had been an average of nineteen admissions a year between 1694 and 1696. Of the six Fellows only a minority holding College office retained their Fellowships for more than a few years; most resigned to marry and take livings, often those in the gift of the College.

In the first years of his Cambridge career Addenbrooke would have spent most of his time in his College taking the prescribed course for an Arts degree. For this he had to study classics, ethics, logic, metaphysics, divinity, mathematics and astronomy. He graduated B.A. in 1701. He held scholarships to the value of 30s per quarter during the years 1702, 1703 and 1704. The steward's account books for St Catharine's College[6] show that Addenbrooke continued in residence from 1697 until 1704, in March of which year he was elected a Fellow of the College. In 1704 he was admitted M.A.

It seems probable that like so many of his contemporaries he had intended to enter the Church; at what period he became interested in medicine is uncertain. He was the first member of his family to enter the medical profession and it seems probable therefore that his decision was reached as a result of Cambridge rather than home influences. Of students who matriculated at Cambridge during the decade 1690 to 1699, 71 eventually gained a medical qualification,[8] but only four of these men were members of St Catharine's College. Addenbrooke must have devoted himself seriously to medical studies from 1704 onwards. The Regius Professor of Physic from 1700 to 1741 was Christopher Green who appears to have undertaken little if any teaching.

William Stukeley,[9] the antiquary, who was about four years younger than Addenbrooke, studied medicine at Bene't College (Corpus Christi College) opposite St Catharine's College. He has left an account of his studies, which he began in 1704. He wrote: 'I contracted acquaintance with all the lads (and them only) in the University, that studied Physic'. He mentions nine of his fellow medical students by name, including Addenbrooke. At the request of Stukeley's tutor, Henry Plumptre of Queens' College acted as his director of studies and may have advised other medical students including John Addenbrooke. Plumptre had matriculated early in 1697, one month after Addenbrooke, and had been elected a Fellow of his College in February 1702/3. He proceeded M.A. in 1705. The fact that he was about the same seniority as most of those he was advising confirms the impression given by Stukeley that the enthusiastic group of medical students at Cambridge were largely self-educated. They went on botanical rambles in the countryside and they dissected a wide variety of animals. In Bene't College they watched the experiments of Waller, later the Professor of Chemistry, studied optics and microscopy, and watched physiological experiments with Stephen Hales. Although he had attended anatomical lectures, Stukeley had in 1706 not yet seen a human dissection so he attended George Rolfe's course in Chancery Lane in London. The following year Rolfe was dissecting as well as lecturing at Cambridge. Stukeley attended Vigani's course of chemistry lectures more than once and also his course on materia medica; he also 'visited the apothecary's shop to make myself perfect in the knowledge of drugs and official compositions'. He practised gratis 'among the poor people that depended upon the College and such lads as would trust themselves to my care'.

Clinical teaching in the modern sense did not exist for it was not customary to examine patients since only the grossest of physical signs were taken into consideration. Consultation by letter was therefore still a common and accepted practice. However, a few decades later, when William Heberden practised from his rooms in St John's College, he was sometimes accompanied by students.

Stukeley attended Mead's rounds at St Thomas' Hospital for seven months from September 1709; but once again there is no evidence that Addenbrooke did the same although it seems probable that the medical education, such as it was, of this group of young men followed a similar pattern. We have noted that Plumptre was acting director of studies in medicine before he took his degree. The steward's accounts of Catharine Hall show that Addenbrooke was teaching from 1705 although he did not proceed to the M.D. until 1710.

Addenbrooke's lectures were on the subject of materia medica and were based on the collection of drugs he had assembled which is still in the possession of his College. The collection is quite extensive,[10] and includes traditional drugs of plant or animal origin; more recent introductions such as quinine, julep, and balsam of Tolu; and chemicals such as antimony, arsenic, bismuth, mercury, lead and sulphur.

For one year from November 1709, Addenbrooke was Bursar of Catharine Hall. He had been closely associated with the building of the new chapel, commenced in 1704, and he lent considerable sums of money towards the building expenses.[11] During his seven years as a Fellow he was tutor to only seven students, two of them relatives, including his cousin John.

During his years at Cambridge, Addenbrooke had accumulated a considerable library. Books on anatomy and materia medica predominate. The books suggest a broad catholic approach to medicine; some obvious gaps in the collection may have been filled by books that Addenbrooke chose to take with him to London.

Addenbrooke was admitted as an extra-licentiate of the College of Physicians of London on 8 September 1706, which enabled him to practise medicine outside the seven mile limit around London. Addenbrooke did not take the examinations for either the Cambridge M.L. (University Licence to practise) or the M.B. degree, but proceeded directly to the M.D. in 1710. It was suggested by Langford[6] that this unusual course was possibly due to Addenbrooke's status as M.A. and Fellow of his College, which had exempted him from taking the lower examination, but we are unaware of any other examples. Nevertheless, Addenbrooke was certainly in a special position as a Fellow of Catharine Hall, upon which Jones[11] comments as follows: 'An interesting point in his career is that prior to 1860 he is the only Fellow to take the medical course at Cambridge. The founder permitted his Fellows to study (for a degree) only philosophy and sacred theology; the Edwardian Statutes added "the Arts" but not until 1860 was it strictly legal for a Fellow to study medicine. It is perhaps significant that Addenbrooke ceased to be a Fellow in the year following his taking of the degree of M.D.'

This comment, which was not available to Langford in 1934, is of great interest and may explain why Addenbrooke did not take the Cambridge M.L. or M.B. examinations but qualified to practise medicine by the relatively obscure license from the College of Physicians under his old home address. Thus he could legally practise medicine in Cambridge without the risk of infringing his Fellowship regulations by acquiring a

Cambridge degree. Also, perhaps when he married and would leave College in any case, he could resign his Fellowship at the same time as he took the M.D. degree.

His name does not appear in the College records after Michaelmas, 1711. He appears to have left Cambridge soon after this and about that time he presented his library and his Materia Medica Cabinet to the College. Before he left Cambridge he married Miss Fisher, niece of Sir William Dawes, Master of the College; her father was rector of Bennington in Hertfordshire.

Addenbrooke's life from 1711 to 1719 was for many years a matter of conjecture; it was assumed that he had practised medicine in Cambridge. The discovery of a letter[12] written in 1772 by Addenbrooke's cousin, John, Dean of Lichfield, to Charles Collignon, Professor of Anatomy and Physician at Addenbrooke's Hospital, established that Addenbrooke left Cambridge in 1711 or 1712 and settled in practice in London. How successfully he practised his profession is unknown. An undated letter was apparently written at this stage of his career in connection with a supposed breach of professional etiquette, but the style of the letter is so obscure that its meaning is far from clear. Whilst living in London he published in 1714 his only book, *An Essay on Free Thinking*. This is a forcefully written but obscurely phrased defence of the orthodox Anglican Christianity. This small tract of sixteen pages printed for Jonah Bower at the Rose in Ludgate Street, London, priced 3d., carries little conviction, for the thread of the argument is lost in a tangle of words.

At some time before 1719 Addenbrooke was forced by ill health to give up his London practice; he moved to Littlecourt, Buntingford, not far from his father-in-law's parish, and there he died on 7 June 1719. His wife moved back to London where she died some six months later. Addenbrooke was buried in the chapel of St Catharine's College (Fig. 3). Addenbrooke's cousin John recalled[12] that his portrait had been painted when he lived in Cambridge but as long ago as 1722 all trace of it had disappeared. There survived only a description of him by Mary Collis, one of his servants at Buntingford. This was in an undated letter, the writer of which is unknown, but it may have been addressed to Revd William Cole, the antiquary, as it appears in the Cole manuscripts.[13] Addenbrooke was said to have been tall and thin, of studious bearing and he wore a wig; he had many oddities and was at times supposed to be insane. Before his death he ordered and witnessed the burning of all his writings and manuscripts in the courtyard of his house, and one may be

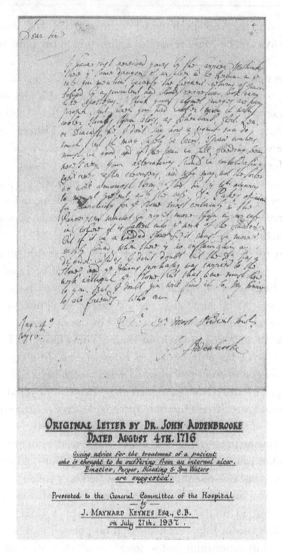

ORIGINAL LETTER BY DR. JOHN ADDENBROOKE
DATED AUGUST 4TH. 1716

*Giving advice for the treatment of a patient
who is thought to be suffering from an internal ulcer.
Emetics, Purges, Bleeding & Spa Waters
are suggested.*

Presented to the General Committee of the Hospital
— by —
J. MAYNARD KEYNES Esq., C.B.
on July 27th. 1937.

Fig. 2. Original letter by Dr John Addenbrooke

permitted to wonder if his portrait suffered the same fate. Being supposed
to be skilled in necromancy he foretold the day and hour of his death with
an accuracy which was fulfilled to within a few minutes.

He appears to have been of a retiring disposition, serious, earnest and
somewhat austere. He was not wealthy but had sufficient private income
to be independent of his practice earnings. He had inherited a one-third
share of the estate of his maternal uncle Humphrey Porry, but the

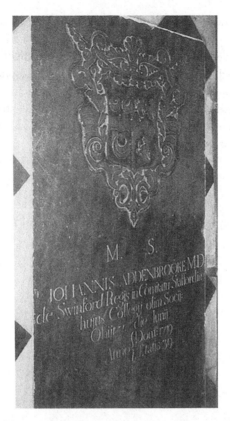

Fig. 3. Memorial plaque to John Addenbrooke in the floor of St
Catharine's College Chapel.

wording of his cousin's letter on the subject is ambiguous and the income
of £300 a year may have been Addenbrooke's one-third share or the total
from the whole estate. In his will he left his land to two of his relatives and
his money – about £4,500 – for the foundation of a hospital after a life
interest by his wife.[14] It may be surmised that his medical practice among
poor people had impressed him with the total inadequacy of parish relief
for the sick and prompted him to found a Voluntary Hospital, as was
already being done in London. The Master and Fellows of Catharine Hall
were thus charged as trustees 'to hire, fit-up, purchase or erect a building
fit for a small physicall hospital for poor people'. Those of any parish or
county should be admitted 'if there should be room and the revenue to
answer'.

Addenbrooke's Hospital was among the earliest Voluntary General

Hospitals to be opened in the provinces but had the trustees been less dilatory it might well have been the first. As it was, the first to open was in 1736 – some seventeen years after Addenbrooke's death – and other hospitals followed. The opening of Addenbrooke's Hospital forty-seven years after its founder's death, followed by the Radcliffe Infirmary at Oxford four years later on 18 October 1770 – no less than 56 years after the death of John Radcliffe – suggests that both Trustee bodies were guided by that academic axiom, *Festina Lente*.

~ 3 ~

Eighteenth-century Cambridge

In the last decades of the eighteenth century, when Addenbrooke's Hospital was opened, Cambridge was a market town with a population of under 10000, of whom about 800 were members of the University, and 120 were University or college servants.[1]

Between 1780 and 1801, when the first national census was taken, the population of England had increased by 20%. The greatest increase had occurred in London and in the industrial towns of the Midlands and North. The population of Cambridge, which a house to house enumeration in 1749 had shown to be 6131, excluding the University, had risen to about 9000 in 1794 and to 9276 in 1801.[2]

The comparative stagnation of Cambridge had many causes. There were no local industries of much importance, the wool trade had moved elsewhere, and Stourbridge Fair, once the largest in England, was a mere shadow of its former greatness. Many of the wealthy county gentry, good customers of Cambridge tradesmen, had left the county, and between 1780 and 1800 many old manor houses were pulled down. The fall in the number of students in the University which continued from 1700 almost to the end of the century, still further reduced the town's prosperity.

Although the increase in the population of Cambridge had been relatively small, it was proportionately very much greater than the increase in the number of inhabited houses; indeed, the built-up area in Cambridge was only slightly larger in 1766 than it had been two centuries earlier[3] and did not expand until after the Enclosure Acts of 1801 and 1807.

A map drawn in 1791[4] (Fig. 4) shows the Hospital at the southern edge of the town. On the same side of Trumpington Street a few houses reached almost to Spital End,* now the corner of Trumpington Street and Lensfield Road. Facing the Hospital were market gardens, and behind it were St Thomas' Leys (later the site of Downing College), and the Marsh

---

* Spital End was so called because the Hospital of St Anthony and St Eligius, founded in 1361, was situated at the corner of Trumpington Street and Lensfield Road.

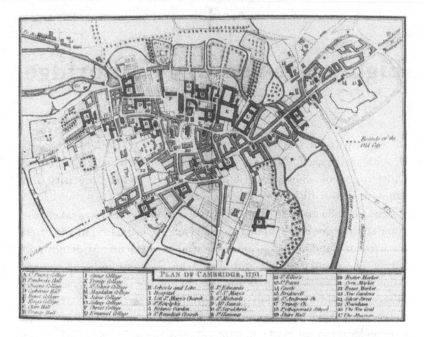

Fig. 4. Plan of Cambridge, 1791.

where Gunning remembered having seen undergraduates shooting snipe.[5] The New Plan of Cambridge made by William Custance in 1798 shows that on the Hills Road the inhabited area extended only to the near corner of Parker's Piece, and in Jesus Lane only as far as the Fellows' garden of Jesus College. There were a few cottages near Magdalene College, but they were separated from Chesterton village by open country. (West of the river there were only a few houses in Newnham village.)[6]

With few new houses to accommodate the growing population, existing houses were divided into three or four tenements and parts of the town were grossly overcrowded. Most houses were thatched. The streets were unpaved and dirty, with a central gutter, and visitors commented unfavourably on the mean and village-like appearance of the town, apart of course from the colleges.

The streets were too narrow for two carriages to pass, but there were few private carriages; Gunning recorded that in the 1790s there were only three.[7] (The owners of private carriages were the Bishop of Llandaff, Mr Ingle of Shelford, and of course Mr Mortlock, all of whom had a connection with the Hospital.) Ladies preferred a sedan chair for transport. The town was completely unlighted. The wretched state of the streets had long been a disgrace and an abortive attempt was made in 1769 to procure an Act for cleansing, lighting and paving the town. Eventually, in 1788, an Act created a body of Paving (later Improvement) Commissioners, who were empowered to pave, light and cleanse the town and to levy rates for these purposes.[8] In 1788 Petty Cury was paved with cobbles and lamps were attached to the walls of some houses and colleges. The paving of the town was completed by 1793.

Public health

The presence in Cambridgeshire of large areas of undrained fen ensured the persistence of malaria as a significant medical problem until well into the nineteenth century.

However, Cambridge's most serious public health problem arose from the flatness of the site, which made effective drainage difficult. Typhoid was endemic, and periodic, more extensive, outbreaks of 'Cambridge Fever' continued to provoke angry criticism of the Borough authorities until a new drainage system was installed in 1895. Defective sewerage was the cause of the greatest disaster in the history of the Hospital (see p. 224).

The River Cam was very heavily polluted, and sometimes visibly so. Most inhabitants obtained their water from the town pumps, from wells which were so shallow that they too were frequently polluted.[9] Among the projects to bring purer water to the town had been a scheme associated with the name of Hobson, the carrier, which was undertaken early in the seventeenth century, when a new water course was constructed to bring water from the springs near Trumpington, known as Nine Wells, to a Conduit Head near what is now Lensfield Road corner.[10] In 1769 negotiations were opened to secure for the Hospital a piped supply from this Head, but there were delays and difficulties and it was only after a Special Committee had been appointed in October 1772 that the Hospital's supply of good water was eventually secured.

Transport

The area effectively served by a hospital obviously depends on the quality and quantity of transport available. The coming of the railways (the world's first public locomotive railway, the Stockton and Darlington, opened in 1825) and later still of the motor car (1885 saw the first machine propelled by an internal combustion engine), each changed the catchment area of the Hospital. The balance between the Hospital's reputation and its accessibility, compared with other hospitals, determined the extent to which it was used.

In 1760[11] the fly, carrying four passengers daily at 12s. each, provided the most rapid service to London, which it reached in ten hours. Stage coaches cost only 10s. but the journey took longer. There were regular coaches to Norwich and Bury St Edmunds. The cheapest service, and the one used by those hospital patients who did not come on foot or in farm carts, was provided by carriers which plied once or twice a week to Huntingdon, St Ives, St Neots, Newmarket, Ipswich, Haverhill, Ely, Linton and Royston, and some more distant towns. Barge traffic from Kings Lynn and Wisbech to Cambridge was still considerable but there were also regular passenger services to these towns and to intermediate destinations, such as Ely and Downham Market.

By 1796,[12] travelling was more expensive, but if one chose to travel at night by the Royal Mail coach, the journey to London took only seven and a half hours, and cost 16s. The other services were more frequent but otherwise essentially similar to those available in 1760.

The University, the Borough and the County

Senior members of the University, acting as individuals and not in their official capacities, were the new Trustees and Governors appointed in 1758, who took the initiative in organising the completion and staffing of the Hospital. Members of the University, as individuals, were to continue to play a large part in the administration of the Hospital, and the University itself became increasingly involved in Hospital affairs in relation to the development of the Medical School. The formal relationship between the Hospital and University was at times cordial, but at times hostile, or tarnished by mutual suspicion, but even during the difficult decades which followed the death of Sir George Paget in 1892 members of the University were active on Hospital committees.

The division of responsibility between University, Borough and County for the government of the Hospital from its earliest days is well illustrated by the composition of the committee established on 26 May

1766 to draw up Rules and Orders of the Hospital. The University was represented by the Vice Chancellor and other Heads of Houses, the Borough by the Mayor and two other Aldermen, and the County by Lord Mountford and other noblemen and large landowners. The Lord Lieutenant for the time being was the President of the Hospital. The other 'perpetual governors' were[13] the Bishop of Ely, the High Sheriff of the County, the representatives in Parliament of the County, Town and University, the Vice Chancellor of the University, and the Mayor of Cambridge. The tripartite division of responsibility was more formally recognised when the method of election of members of the General Board was reformed in the 1900s (see p. 264) and the representation of the three interests was thereafter always evenly balanced. This system persisted until 1926/27, when six representatives of the bodies which collected or supplied funds to the Hospital joined the Board.[14]

The University

During the last 30 years of the eighteenth century the University was certainly small in numbers and low in reputation; the professors who failed to teach and the Fellows who failed to reside, and the eccentricities and extravagances of some of those who did reside have provided historians with the materials for a colourful story of lethargy, corruption and maladministration.[15] The general accuracy of their indictment is not disputed but it does less than justice to the many men who, eccentric or not, carried out their duties conscientiously and efficiently; many of these were actively involved in establishing and administering the Hospital. Before the end of the century the fortunes of the University had begun to recover and the number of students was rising.

At the weekly meetings of the Governors and at their Quarterly Courts, many members of the University attended with great regularity and, when important matters were on the agenda, large numbers attended.

Some of the ceremonies of the University year were turned to the Hospital's advantage. Cambridge was gayest and most crowded at the annual Commencement in July[16,17] at which most noblemen (who were not obliged to take an examination), Doctors and Masters, took their degrees. The degree ceremony was held on the Monday. On the preceding Sunday, Doctors wore their scarlet robes all day, and noblemen wore elaborate robes of any colour they chose (by 1785 they were uniformly purple). 'The College Walks were crowded' by the brilliantly

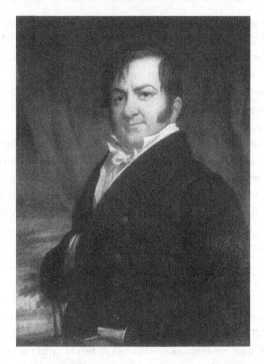

Fig. 5. William Mortlock (Governor), 1818.

robed academics, visiting ladies, and sightseers from neighbouring villages who did not venture onto the Walks. The ladies elected a Steward
from among the noblemen, who was responsible for organising on the
Saturday evening the Commencement Ball, the most important social
event of the year. The Steward was usually out of pocket. If the Ball made
any profit, this went to the Hospital. On the Thursday before Commencement the sermon for the benefit of the Hospital was preached to a crowded
church. 'The gentry and the clergy from the most distant parts of the
county and isle made a point of being present.'[18]

The Borough

The appointment of the Mayor of Cambridge for the time being
perpetuated the official association between the Corporation and the
Hospital. The complex history of the political manipulations at the local
level and in support of Parliamentary candidates has been well summarised.[19] Many Cambridge tradesmen were active in the affairs of the

Hospital, and many of those who devoted much time to local government also occupied prominent positions in the Hospital's committees.

Over a period of 35 years (1785–1820) the Mortlock family (Fig. 5) dominated Cambridge.[20] In 1785 John Mortlock was first elected Mayor, an office he held on thirteen occasions. In 1754 he had inherited a successful drapery business, some land and a large sum of money. After lending money unofficially for some years, he founded a bank. In 1784 he was elected a Member of Parliament for Cambridge. At Westminster he was not a success and in 1788 he resigned, but through his sons and his associates he controlled public affairs in Cambridge, including those of the Hospital of which he was treasurer, until his death in 1816. He was succeeded as treasurer by his son, J.C. Mortlock, who was Mayor nine times between 1804 and 1820.

The association between the Borough and the Hospital gradually changed its character when legislation imposed on the Local Authority the financial responsibility for providing certain medical services.

The County

The Lord Lieutenant of Cambridgeshire, as President of the Hospital, presided at the Quarterly Courts and lent social prestige to such fund-raising events as the Annual Sermon and the Commencement Ball which together made a considerable contribution to the Hospital's income.

The first President of the Hospital was Philip Yorke, second Earl of Hardwicke. When he died in 1790 he was succeeded by his nephew, Philip, the third earl. The Yorkes were one of a number of families owning a considerable acreage of land in the County, who subscribed generously to the Hospital funds and were active on Hospital committees, often in successive generations, and in a few instances from 1766 until the introduction of the National Health Service in 1948. Notable among these families were the Pembertons of Trumpington, the Adeanes of Babraham, the Townleys of Fulbourn, and the Cottons of Madingley.

The importance of the active interest in the Hospital taken by these families was considerable in the days when social stratification was rigid, for they made support of the Hospital a social virtue and encouraged the participation of the socially ambitious.

~4~

Building the Hospital

John Addenbrooke in his will, dated 1 May 1719, left the reversion of his fortune to setting up a hospital. His trustees were his executor, Edward Green, of the Middle Temple, Thomas Cross, Master of Catharine Hall, and Edmund Halfhyde and Edward Hubbard, Fellows of the same college.*

The legal difficulties began soon after Addenbrooke's death. On 19 November 1719, Cross and Halfhyde submitted to the Lord Chancellor a Bill of Complaint against Edward Green and John Addenbrooke (the cousin), concerning a marriage settlement entered into on 14 December 1716, by the late John Addenbrooke and the late Peter Fisher, his father-in-law. The former had agreed to pay £3,000 and the latter £1,500, to Sir William Dawes, Bishop of London, and Thomas Turner of the Middle Temple, as trustees of Susan Fisher (Addenbrooke) as her marriage portion.[2]

The Lord Chancellor referred the dispute to a Chancery Master to report on the value of the residue of the estate. Susan Addenbrooke died in London early in 1720. The Court declared the will proved, but £1,500 of the total legacy of £4,500 was consumed by legal costs, debts and legacies to the family. The Court ordered that 'the (will) ought to be established and the Trusts therein performed'. Despite this judgement Chancery proceedings continued intermittently until 1762.[3] By 1758 Edward Green was the sole survivor of the original trustees.

Some time between 1742 and 1745 Green was guilty of breach of trust, but it was not until 1757 that an interrogation by a Master in Chancery brought his offences to light. On 20 June 1758, Green was ordered to be removed from the Trust, and to surrender to new trustees to be appointed by Mr Burrough, one of the Masters of the High Court of Chancery, all the trusts vested in him and to convey to them 'all such messuages, lands,

---

* Thomas Cross, Master from 1719 to 1736, was an undistinguished and timid man. As Vice Chancellor in 1722 he laid the foundation stone of the present Senate House. Halfhyde (b. 1683) was a Fellow from 1707 to 1717. He was ordained in 1719 and from 1723 he was Rector of Girton. Hubbard, a Fellow since 1718, succeeded Cross as Master from 1736 to 1741. He is described as mild, placid, serene, modest and reserved.[1]

tenements and hereditaments as had been purchased in his name and of the said trust money'.

In pursuance of an order of 16 June 1757, Green passed over some £1,887 but he died before the end of the three years allowed for the transfer of the remaining £3,162.15s.9d. which was completely lost to the Hospital.

The original trustees had not been totally inactive; they had acquired much of the land on which the Hospital was to be erected and payments had been made to a number of building workers. However, after Hubbard's death in 1741 no further action was taken until the new trustees were appointed on 21 July 1758.

These trustees, or Trustees and Governors as they were called, were: John Green, D.D., Master of Bene't College; Roger Long, D.D., Master of Pembroke Hall; William Richardson, D.D., Master of Emmanuel College; John Sumner, D.D., Provost of King's College; Edmund Law, D.D., Master of St Peter's College; Thomas Chapman, D.D., Master of Magdalene College; Hugh Thomas, D.D., Master of Christ's College; Lynford Caryl, D.D., Master of Jesus College; Francis Sawyer Parris, D.D., Master of Sydney Sussex College; Kenrick Prescott, D.D., Master of Catharine Hall; James Burrough, M.A., Master of Caius College.*

On the evidence of their payments to builders, and confirmed by the description of the property conveyed to the new trustees as including the 'Physical Hospital or Edifice intended for an Hospital erected and built upon the said premises or some part thereof', the Hospital building had been started by the old trustees. The first recorded meeting of the new trustees took place on 5 January 1759, at the Lodge of Jesus College. Caryl, Long, Green, Law and Burrough were present and resolved to

---

* John Green (1706–1779) was Master of Bene't College, 1750–1763, and subsequently Bishop of Lincoln. He wrote on university reform. Roger Long, (1680–1770), F.R.S., was first Professor of Astronomy and Geometry 1750. William Richardson (1698–1779) was Master of Emmanuel College, 1736–1779, Vice Chancellor, 1737 and 1769, and Chaplain to George II and George III. John Sumner (d. 1772) was Headmaster of Eton, 1745–1754, and Provost of King's College, 1756–1772. Edmund Law (1703–1787) was Master of St Peter's College, 1756–1768, and Bishop of Carlisle, 1768–1787. Thomas Chapman (1717–1760) was Master of Madgalene, 1746–1768. Hugh Thomas (d. 1780) held many ecclesiastical offices and was Dean of Ely, 1758–1780. He was Master of Christ's College, 1754–1780. Lynford Caryl (d. 1781) was Registrary, 1751–1758, and Master of Jesus College, 1758–1781. Francis Sawyer Parris (d. 1760) was University Librarian, 1750–1760, and Master of Sidney Sussex College, 1746–1760. Kenrick Prescott (d. 1779) was Master of St Catharine's College, 1741–1779, and held many livings.

apply to the Court of Chancery for an Order 'for such sums of money as will be necessary for carrying on the further purposes of Dr Addenbrooke's Will by finishing the building erected, and purchasing two tenements situated between the said Hospital and the street, and repairing the garden wall'. They estimated they would need £1,072.6s.4d.

By October the two tenements in the Hospital grounds had been purchased and had been or were soon to be pulled down. In December two other tenements 'next the Hospital garden' were bought from Mr Canham for £70.

By April 1763, the building of the Hospital was at last virtually completed. The trustees met twice that month and were eager to open the Hospital to patients with as little delay as possible. On 2 April they asked Moxon, who had been their legal adviser since 1759, to apply to the Court of Chancery 'as soon as may be' . . . 'for so much money as will be necessary for the fitting of two wards and furnishing a room for the Trustees and such other parts of the Hospital as will be requisite for the taking in patients and proper Attendants for those two wards'.

The total expenditure for 1763 amounted to £84.13s.5½d. but after this the trustees were left with only £2.2s.4d. in hand. It was about a year before their next meeting on 29 October 1764, by which time a half-yearly dividend from the Accountant General made it possible to pay Moxon's bill, the first he had submitted, and to pay off other debts and current expenses. Sundry other costs continued to be met with, on the credit side, half-yearly dividends and a legacy of £100 from Burrough who had died. There were also miscellaneous receipts for the sale of rubble from the demolished tenements, and on 7 April 1765, the receipt of £160.3s.2d. was recorded, derived from the sale of 3% Annuities. The trustees seem personally to have supervised every practical detail relating to the setting up of the hospital.

More about the legal struggle which had raged since Addenbrooke's death is to be found in the archives of the Chancery Court.[3]

The appeal to the public

On 9 April 1766, the trustees felt that the time had come to lay before the public a statement of their affairs and a hundred copies were ordered to be printed and distributed. They reported:

	£	s	d
That the purchase of a Garden and of diverse tenements for the site of the Hospital amounted to	817	13	3
That there has been expended in the Building and about the Grounds and in Furniture	3,073	8	4½
	119	1	5
That by the foregoing Expenses some great Losses, Taxes and Law charges the Capital is now reduced to	1,804	16	4

That of the foregoing sum £1,600 is in the 3 per cents and meant to be continued there in the names of the Trustees and the yearly produce amounting to £48 to be laid out in Repairs and other necessaries for the Benefit of the Hospital.

And the remaining £204 16 4 is intended to be laid out in Furniture as it shall be wanted.

The Trustees now therefore offer the House and its Furniture to the Publick and hope that a sufficient number of voluntary subscriptions will be found to carry on so good a Design. And as to the Rules and Orders for the Government of the Hospital they refer all such points to be considered and settled by the subscribers themselves; desiring such Gentlemen as intend to be contributors to meet at the Hospital at 3 o'clock on Wednesday the 30th instant.

Whoever should be desirous of further satisfaction in the foregoing particulars may apply for that purpose to any of the Trustees, who are – The Bishop of Lincoln, Dr. Long, Dr. Richardson, Dr. Sumner, Dr. Law, Dr. Thomas, Dr. Prescott and Dr. Caryl.

This notice in a somewhat shortened version appeared in the *Cambridge Chronicle* on 12 April.

The meeting was very well attended by the gentlemen of the University, the County and Borough. The Vice Chancellor, W.S. Powell,* and the Mayor, William Weales, agreed to a proposal that they should jointly sign an appeal for subscriptions. This appeal was very successful. On 26 May at a General Meeting held at the Hospital, a Committee was appointed 'unanimously by the Nobility, Clergy and Gentry then present', to consider the Rules and Orders for the Hospital. The Committee was to consist of any five or more of the following: Lord Mountford, Sir Thomas Hatton, Sir John Hynde Cotton, the Vice Chancellor, William Greeves, Esquire, William Howell Ewin, Esquire, the Revd Dr Richardson, the Revd Dr Gooch, the Revd Dr Sharp, the Revd Dr Gordon, the Revd Mr Pemberton, the Worshipful the Mayor, Mr Alderman Gifford, Mr Alderman Norfolk and Mr John Hide.

* William Samuel Powell, D.D. (1717–1775), Master of St John's College.

At this meeting subscriptions were received,

	£	s	d
Towards an additional building	478	7	0
For general use	49	8	0
Annual subscriptions	269	18	0

The 83 subscribers were broadly representative of the local landowners, the University and the Town, and included large numbers of clergy and three surgeons who were later to be closely associated with the Hospital: Hayles, Hopkins and Thackeray.

At this meeting it was also agreed that William Howell Ewin* should be the treasurer and John Haggerstone the Secretary.

The Committee to consider the Rules and Orders met on 7 June and again on 19 June, with the Vice Chancellor in the Chair on both occasions. Having accomplished their task they resolved 'that 50 copyes of the Rules and Orders should be published and dispersed among the publick and subscribers against the next General Meeting' to be held on 2 July.

Meanwhile the trustees had met at Bene't College Lodge on 30 June and agreed that, 'a Lease of the said Hospital and the Ground thereunto belonging shall be made for the term of 99 years or any longer term to such Trustees as shall be nominated at the next General Meeting of the said Hospital, provided that we shall be advised by Counsell that we have power to do so'.

This agreement formed the most important business of the General Meeting which gave its approval and accepted a proposal that 'a Lease of the Hospital and the Ground thereunto belonging be made to the Earl of Hardwicke if Counsell so advise'.

Addenbrooke's was now for about a year in an anomalous situation. Legally it was a private hospital governed by its trustees, but financial difficulties had forced it to adopt the constitution of a public hospital controlled by governors elected by its subscribers. The new Governors,

---

* William Howell Ewin (d. 1804) the Hospital's first treasurer, perhaps owed his appointment to the fact that he was a pupil of W.S. Powell, the Vice Chancellor. Ewin, the son of a wealthy grocer and brewer, was B.A. St John's College, 1753, LL.D., 1760. He too was a brewer and a Justice of the Peace. The Dictionary of National Biography bluntly describes him as a 'usurer'. In 1778 he was suspended from his degrees by the University for lending money to undergraduates but was restored in 1779 as there was no University statute against his offence. He was precise, frugal or perhaps avaricious, and was generally unpopular. In 1781 he was deprived of his commission as a J.P.

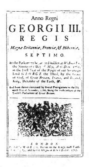

Fig. 6. First page of a book containing the Act of Parliament,
1766.

with the full support of the trustees, sought the opinion of counsel, Mr
Charles York of Lincoln's Inn. At a General Board held on 22 September
1766, with the Earl of Hardwicke* in the Chair, it was ordered that a copy
of York's report be sent to each trustee and that their concurrence be
obtained for an application to Parliament 'to enable them to make a
proper conveyance for the settling of the Public Infirmary'.

The trustees evidently concurred for at a meeting on 10 November the
Secretary was ordered to write to Lord Hardwicke 'to know whether Mr.
Points (sic) was the Gentleman he recommended for Drawing up the
Petition and Act of Parliament'. On 1 December the Secretary was
ordered to request Mr Poyntz to draw up the Petition.

The Bill was successfully presented to Parliament (Fig. 6). The
preamble summarised the terms of Addenbrooke's will and the various
proceedings in the Chancery Court which had led up to the public appeal
of May 1766. The Petition then went on to ask 'That from and after the
Twenty-fourth day of June in the Year of our Lord One thousand, seven
hundred and sixty-seven, there shall be a Corporation, to continue for
ever, for establishing and well Governing a General Hospital in the Town
of Cambridge, to be called Addenbrooke's Hospital'; and that the Lord
Lieutenant of the County of Cambridge, the Chancellor of the University
of Cambridge, the Bishop of Ely, the High Steward of the Corporation of
Cambridge, the High Sheriff for the County of Cambridge, the Representatives in Parliament for the County, University, and Town of Cambridge, the Vice Chancellor of the University of Cambridge, and the

---

* Philip Yorke of Wimpole Park was second Earl of Hardwicke, 1730–1790,
  M.P. for Cambridgeshire, 1747–1764, Lord Lieutenant, 1757, and High
  Steward of the University, 1764–1790.

Mayor of the Town of Cambridge, together with 'any Person who has paid or at any time hereafter shall pay into the hands of the Treasurer or Treasurers of the said Hospital for the time being, the sum of Twenty One Pounds or upwards at any one time for the use of the said Hospital, shall be and are appointed Governors of the said Hospital; and also every person who shall at any time hereafter pay into the hands of such Treasurer or Treasurers the yearly Sum of Two Guineas, or more, for the Use of the said Hospital, shall, during such Time as they shall respectively continue to pay the same, be respectively Governors of the said Hospital'; the Physicians and Surgeons appointed to the Hospital were also to act as Governors at all General Courts.

The Act also considered in detail other aspects of the administrative structure of the Hospital. No person gainfully employed by the Hospital or under contract to supply goods to the Hospital might qualify as a Governor. Lord Hardwicke (or his successor as Lord Lieutenant) was to be President of the Hospital and with eight or more Governors to constitute the General Court, the first meeting of which was to be held on 29 June 1767. The General Court was to meet at least four times every year, on the Monday next after 24 March, 24 June, 29 September and 25 December. Additional (Special) Courts might be held at the request of the Governors or any nine of them: at least 20 days notice of such meetings had to be given in the Cambridge newspapers and on the gate and in the boardroom of the Hospital. The General Court, with a quorum of nine, was to have full authority in the transaction of all the offices of the Hospital and to appoint such weekly or other meetings, with a quorum of five, as may be desirable for the speedy and effective management of the Hospital. The General Court was to make and enforce such bye-laws as seemed necessary and to invoke or modify these 'provided that the . . . Bye-laws . . . be not contrary or repugnant to the Statutes, Customs or Laws of this Kingdom'.

The Governors were to have effective power to ensure the honesty of their employees. Any employee who upon request failed to provide a written account, on oath, of his stewardship of the Hospital's funds, was to be brought before the Justices and upon conviction to be committed 'to the Common Gaol of the County of Cambridge, there to remain without Bail or Mainprize, until he or she shall have made a true and perfect Account and Payment as aforesaid'. As a further safeguard against peculation the Governors were to demand from the Treasurer such security as they thought appropriate.

The Act received the Royal Assent on 20 May 1767.

The trustees and the intended new Governors worked amicably together for the development of the Hospital and clearly took for granted the success of their Petition to Parliament.

The Governors' first objective was rapidly to complete the building of the Hospital and to open it to patients with the least possible delay. On 4 August 1766, two cottages adjoining the Hospital were bought for 40 guineas from Jacob Sims, a carpenter subsequently employed by the Hospital, and were converted into a kitchen. At the same meeting it was agreed that the East Room on the ground floor should be divided by partition to form an Apothecary's Shop and an Admissions Room.

GENERAL ACCOUNT[4]

From the death of Dr Addenbrook (sic) down to this 9th day of April 1766

CHARGE

	l.	s.	d.
Dr Addenbrook's personal Estate after Debts, Legacies, etc	4676	2	1¼
Interest of Ditto to Christmas 1764	5114	16	5
Sir James Burrough's Legacy	100	0	0
Rents received and Materials sold	189	9	5
Five Quarters Interest of 1600 *l.* 3 per cent due at Lady-day 1766	60	0	0
Total	10140	7	11¼

DISCHARGES

	l.	s.	d.
Taxes, Repairs, and allowed for trouble	158	11	3¾
Law-charges	568	3	8
Purchase of Garden and Tenements	817	13	3
Lost in buying and selling Stocks	435	17	9
The Building	3073	8	4½
Furniture	119	1	5
Lost by Edward Green, the Trustee	3162	15	9
Total	8335	11	6¼
Due to Ballance (sic)	1804	16	5
Viz. In 3 per Cents consol	1600	0	0
In the hands of Messrs Moxon and Brograve	160	3	2
In Dividends not yet received	60	0	0
	1820	3	2

It is proposed, on the 30th of this Month, at Three in the Afternoon, to have a Meeting of the Trustees, and such other Persons as are disposed to forward the Design of the Hospital, in order to consider of the properest Methods for that Purpose.

The Hospital
opens its doors

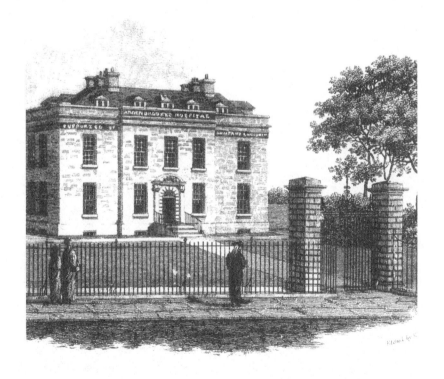

~ 5 ~

The opening preparations

The General Meeting of subscribers held at the Hospital on 2 July 1766, agreed that the Hospital should be opened to patients on Michaelmas day, with 20 beds or more. The Weekly Board met for the first time on Monday 7 July with the Vice Chancellor in the Chair, and made arrangements to advertise for 'an Apothecary, Matron and other servants'. Since, with the exception of Dr Collignon, the members of the Board were clergymen with no knowledge of hospitals, they followed the sensible course of writing to the Secretaries of the hospitals at Northampton and Shrewsbury asking for a priced inventory of their furniture and whether the hospitals or the surgeons themselves paid for surgical instruments.*

The Resident Apothecary

The General Board on 4 August considered applications for the post of Apothecary, agreed to reduce the candidates to two, and proceeded to elect Mr Lefebvre by ballot. It was agreed that his salary should be £25 and 'five pounds a year gratuity if he behaves well'.

The Resident Apothecary was a most important man for he combined the duties of resident medical officer and pharmacist and, in the absence of the non-resident Secretary, shared or disputed administrative resonsibilities with the Matron. It was usual to appoint a man with several years' experience after qualification.

The duties of the Apothecary were clearly defined in the Rules.[1] He had among other tasks, to fit two tickets on each patient's bed, one specifying the name of the patient together with that of his Physician or Surgeon or

---

* It appears that the surgeons were expected to provide their own instruments until 1780. At times concern was expressed about the borrowing of Hospital instruments and rules were proposed at the Weekly Meeting of 31 January 1900 at which the House Surgeon was authorised to lend an instrument to any qualified practitioner in the neighbourhood if he was satisfied that it was required 'for a case of urgent necessity'.

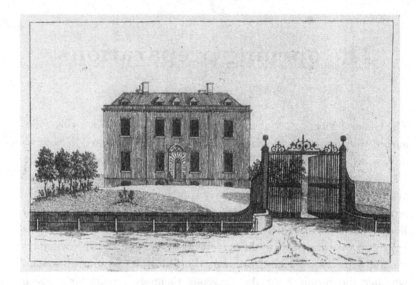

Fig. 7. Addenbrooke's Hospital, 1770.

both, and the other the diet according to the prescription of the Physician or Surgeon. He also had to give a list of these to the Matron each prescribing day.

He had to visit the wards every morning and be ready to report the state of the patients to the Physicians and Surgeons. He was not allowed to dispense medicines without the direction of the Physicians or Surgeons except in cases of necessity when they could not be consulted, and then he had to report to the Physician or Surgeon what he had done. He had to make a report to the Weekly Meeting of all patients received into the House in the foregoing week and deliver a list at every Board of such patients who had been in the House two months.

He was not allowed to practise as an apothecary out of the House or tend any other business except that of the Infirmary. The Rules also said 'That he never be absent from the Hospital at the time when the Physicians and Surgeons are to attend, or at any other time above two hours together; that he always give notice to the Matron and be within call; that he be at home at ten o'clock at farthest in the evening and do not lie out of the House without special leave from the Board or the House Visitors; and in such cases he appoint another apothecary who should be approved by the Physicians, to officiate in his place.'

In addition to regular supervision of his work by the visiting medical staff, the Resident Apothecary was subjected to visits to his Dispensary by such local apothecaries as were subscribers to the Hospital. They were desired to visit the Dispensary, by a monthly rotation, whenever they pleased, and to enter their observations in a book provided for this purpose.

The Secretary

John Haggerstone was elected Secretary at an annual salary of £10.[2] He was an attorney-at-law in practice in Cambridge, and his hospital appointment was intended to be a part-time one. However his duties were onerous.

He had to attend 'any Court and Meeting' to minute down and register all the proceedings, and he had always to be ready to produce the books and accounts. He had to register the names of in-patients and out-patients, the parish they belonged to, their age and 'distemper', when admitted, when discharged and in what state. He had to give notice in writing every Monday to the Physicians and Surgeons whose turn it was to take in patients; to the clergymen whose turn it was to visit; to the House Visitors who were appointed for the following week; and to the visiting apothecary every month before his turn began. He also had to transmit the minutes of any Quarterly Court to the President, regularly to write to the many individual and parish subscribers who failed to observe the Rules when referring patients, advertise for staff and tradesmen's tenders, and he often corresponded with the Secretaries of older hospitals to learn from the procedures they experienced.

He kept one of the two keys of the box containing the documents and great seal of the Hospital. He also kept one of the two keys of the Charities Box. He was also responsible for keeping an inventory of all furniture in the Hospital. It was the duty of the auditors to compile a new inventory at Michaelmas every year.

The routine correspondence must have been heavy; during the week preceding each anniversary it must have been overwhelming.

The Secretary was, of course, not formally forbidden to practise his profession at the same time and he may have done so, but he can have had little time to spare for it.

On 15 May a motion that the Secretary's salary should be increased or that he should be paid a gratuity, was referred to the General Board which decided that enquiries should first be made at other hospitals. The next Board refused an increase. Haggerstone can be forgiven for resigning in 1772.

The Matron and nurses

The advertisement for a Matron induced Ann Perry, spinster of Cambridge, and the widow Brand, to offer their services. But the Board[2] decided to advertise again, mentioning the fact that the salary would be £10 with a gratuity of £5 for good behaviour.

On 18 August Ann Perry was appointed Matron on these terms, and started work on 1 September, on which day she was ordered 'to make a list of such things as will be wanted in the Infirmary', and a week later she was ordered to buy 20 pairs of sheets and towels.

Nothing is known about Miss Perry; it is probable that like many of her successors she had been a housekeeper or other senior servant in a large household; certainly housekeeping, catering and the management of the staff were her principal responsibilities.

Her duties, as laid down in the Rules, were as follows:

That she take care of all the Household Goods and Furniture and be ready to give an account thereof when required.

That she keep a daily Account of the Provisions and other Necessaries that are brought into the House, and lay it before the Weekly Meeting every Monday.

That she take care that the Chambers, Beds, Clothes, Linen and all other things within the Hospital be kept clean.

That she keep a diet Book by which the number of patients on each diet may be known.

That she cause the Names of the Patients to be called over in each Ward every Morning and Evening and enter in the House Visitors Book the names of those who are absent.

That she take care of the Keys of the Doors and see that the outer gates be always locked at Eight in the evening from Michaelmas to Lady day and at Nine in the evening from Lady day to Michaelmas.

That she see that the Nurses, Servants and Patients do their duty and observe the Rules of the House and in case of misbehaviour or neglect acquaint the Weekly Meeting or House Visitors therewith.

The Matron, always referred to as Mrs Perry, although she was unmarried, was ordered[3] 'to look out for four maid servants, two for nurses and the others for kitchen servants, and a porter'.

On 29 September Ann Abbs and Sarah Brown were 'hired as nurses at £5 per annum'. The duties of the nurses are not considered in any detail in the Rules of 1766 or 1770. Only two refer specifically to them and were under the general heading of servants. They were to clean their wards by seven in summer and eight in winter, and they were to obey the Matron, 'behave with tenderness to the Patients', and respect to strangers.

Other Rules applied generally to the servants and nurses and such as related to their conduct were hung up in each ward and read publicly every Sunday morning. The most interesting of these Rules, and those most often broken, prohibited taking gratuities or rewards from patients or from any other person, and bringing food or drink into the Hospital for patients.

The careers of both Ann Abbs and Sarah Brown were brief; Sarah Brown was discharged for ill behaviour about six weeks later, and after a further week Ann Abbs left also. This was to set the pattern of the nursing staff for the early days of the Hospital.

The porters

The first porter to be appointed was Shand Newman, engaged on 29 September at £8 per annum. His duties were to attend carefully the gate, and suffer no in-patient to go out without leave, and to inform the Matron of any stranger that came in to the Infirmary. He had also to obey the orders of the Physicians, Surgeons and Apothecary; do the labouring work of the House, yard, or garden, when ordered by the Matron; and when he was to be absent upon any such business to give the Matron notice so that another could be appointed to attend the gate.

These Rules give no adequate impression of the real extent and importance of the Porter's duties. He was a man of all work, holding the patients down in the theatre, scrubbing the theatre, holding a candle for operations at night, running errands, even digging the patients' graves. It is not surprising that the post proved too much for many of its early occupants.

Stocking the Apothecary's Shop

The Governors now turned their attention to furnishing and stocking the dispensary, then usually referred to as the Apothecary's Shop. On 8 September a Committee was appointed for this purpose consisting of Plumptre, Glynn, Collignon, Hayles, Hopkins and Thackeray, together with the local apothecaries, Bond, Wall and Gray 'or any three of them, one being an apothecary . . . and that they be desired to go about it with all convenient speed'.[4] The physicians and surgeons named were elected to the staff of the Hospital two weeks after this Committee was appointed.

The Committee prepared a list of requirements and Mr Lefebvre was instructed to go to London to buy the goods, second-hand if possible, and, if not, to order them from 'shops of credit'. Unfortunately no records of the Apothecary's purchases have survived.

The purchase of medical equipment, instruments and appliances was normally the responsibility of the Weekly Meeting, which referred the more expensive items to the General Meeting of Governors at the Quarterly Court. The actual purchase was entrusted to the Apothecary, the Matron, the Secretary or sometimes to a Governor. The Court seems never to have refused to authorise any purchase recommended by the Physicians and Surgeons, but always took care to ensure that no money was wasted.

Provisions

The Governors left to the last moment the arrangements for the supply of provisions. On 6 October, only a week before the opening day, the Board ordered that an advertisement be inserted in the Cambridge papers 'for the Brewers to send in their proposals to serve the Infirmary'. Beer was the first commodity to be discussed because it was then an important constituent of the diet, and it was certainly a safer drink than Cambridge water which was so liable to be contaminated. The Board agreed that the under servants, that is to say the nurses and maids, should be allowed a pint of ale each day and small beer at Matron's discretion. Later, the daily ration of small beer was fixed at one quart.

The adjourned Weekly Board met on 8 October and arranged to advertise for tenders to supply the Hospital with bread, butter, milk, soap, candles, rice, sugar and oatmeal. Later, tenders were called for to supply other commodities, and were regularly renewed each quarter.

Final preparations

The minutes of the Weekly Board for the last few weeks before the Hospital opened on 13 October are brief and factual, but they nevertheless carry an impression of determination that the Hospital should indeed open on the appointed day, but also of a certain lack of forward planning, the result no doubt of inexperience.

Exactly a week before opening day the Board ordered that all the servants should be in the Hospital by Saturday, 11 October. At the same meeting a member of the Board must have drawn attention to the lack of heating in the Admissions Room for an order was given that a grate be installed there. The Board met again on Wednesday 8 October, and was once again occupied with such practical details as ordering the carpenter to put up the kitchen door and make one for the cellar. They felt sufficiently confident to order an advertisement to be inserted in the papers 'that the Hospital will be opened on Monday next for the reception of as many patients as can then be conveniently admitted'.

The Board met again at the Hospital on Saturday. They had once more to concern themselves with relative trivialities, ordering that the Apothecary's and Matron's beds be changed, that the servants have feather beds, and that servants who chose not to drink tea be allowed 10s.6d. each by the year instead of this.

The members of the Weekly Board who so consistently attended these frequent meetings included the Vice Chancellor, the Revd Mr Hubbard, the Revd Dr Sharp, the Revd Mr Ludlam, the Revd Dr Long, the Revd Dr Gordon, the Revd Dr Gooch, the Revd Mr Pemberton, Dr Ewin the Treasurer, and Dr Collignon. Long, Gooch, Gordon, Sharp and Collignon rarely missed a meeting. Roger Long, now in his eighty-sixth year, had been one of the most active of the new trustees appointed by the Chancery Court in 1758.

All the members of the Weekly Board were University men; all were in holy orders except the Treasurer and Collignon, who was the only medical member. Their efforts were successful and the Hospital opened its doors on the morning of 13 October 1766.

~ 6 ~

The first admissions

Admission procedures

No record has survived as to the number of patients who sought admission to the Hospital on Monday 13 October 1766. However, from the 'Rules of Admission'[1] and from the Minute Books it is not difficult to form a picture of the scene. The shortage of funds, which, except in a very few happy years, was the Hospital's permanent financial state, compelled the Secretary and the Governors at the Weekly Meetings to enforce the Rules very rigidly.

All admissions and discharges were the responsibility of the Governors at the Weekly Meeting, advised by the medical staff. No patients were admitted who were 'able to subsist themselves and pay for Medicines'.[2] A queue certainly formed outside the Admissions Room long before 11 a.m. Admissions took place, except in the case of emergencies, only between 11 a.m. and 12 noon. Patients arriving after 11 a.m. had to return the following week.

The Physicians and Surgeons had to ensure that the medical conditions for admission were met,

> That no woman big with child, no child under seven years of age (except in Extraordinary cases such as fractures, stone, or where couching, trepanning or amputation are necessary), no persons disordered in their senses, or subject to epileptic fits, suspected to have the Smallpox or other infectious distemper, having habitual ulcers, Cancers not admitting of operation, Consumptions or Dropsies in their last stages, in a dying condition or judged incurable, and for the present none in the venereal distemper, be admitted as In-patients, or if inadvertently admitted, be allowed to continue.

Once the medical eligibility of a patient had been established it was the Secretary's responsibility to ensure that the patient had brought a valid subscriber's recommendation. The Rules governing subscribers' recommendations were clearly defined: 'That for every guinea subscribed and for every Ten Guineas given as a Benefaction, the subscriber or benefactor shall have the right of recommending one In-patient in the year; but that no Contributor shall have more than one patient in the House at one time; that Out-patients be admitted by the recommendation of such subscriber or benefactor without any limitation of numbers'.[3]

No patient not residing in Cambridgeshire could be accepted unless recommended by a subscriber normally residing or having property in the county in question. Parishes and other corporate subscribers had the same rights of recommendation, with a subscription of half the value, as individual subscribers, but parish recommendations were acceptable only if the parish in question had been a subscriber for at least three months.[4]

It must have taken the Secretary some time to satisfy himself that a recommendation was acceptable; he had to consult his records to ascertain that the subscriber was not in arrears with his subscription and had not already used his permitted quota of recommendations. He had to remember that the members of the medical staff each had the right of recommendation of a subscriber of two guineas in addition to such rights as they enjoyed as subscribers[5] and that the Parish of St Benet's had the same privilege, 'whereas the Church-Yard of St. Bennet's Parish is the Burying Ground of the Hospital'.[6] If a prospective patient was a soldier he could not be admitted until 'His officer has engaged to pay his subsistence money to the Treasurer of the Hospital during such time as he shall continue there, except soldiers on furlough, when there is no officer at hand to engage for them'.[7]

Emergency admissions were frequently a cause of dissension. One bed in each ward was 'reserved as a provision for accidents that require immediate relief'.[8]

In cases of emergency a subscriber's letter was not essential. In such cases 'the Apothecary and Matron may receive patients, giving immediate notice to the Physician or Surgeon of the week'.[9]

The admission of patients who did not bring a subscriber's letter was a constant source of anxiety to the Governors, because a subscriber's responsibilities did not end when he handed the letter to a prospective patient. When a recommended patient attended the Weekly Meeting, a letter, signed by the Chairman, was sent to the subscriber informing him whether the patient had been admitted, postponed (i.e. put on the waiting list) or rejected as unsuitable for admission. A further letter was sent to the recommending subscriber when a patient was discharged.[10] If a patient's treatment required special measures involving additional expenditure the Secretary would approach the recommender. When the patient was ready for discharge the recommender, whether an individual or a parish, was expected to provide transport when this was needed.

The burial expenses of the totally indigent were a further source of anxiety to the Secretary. If a patient's prognosis appeared to be poor and he had not been recommended by a parish, which could be expected to accept responsibility, the Secretary would write to the recommending subscriber, as he did, for example, to Mrs Carney on 22 December 1766, asking her 'to remove Miss Patman or to give security for her burial fees'.

Hospital discipline

Many rules regulated the behaviour of patients in the Hospital, and they were very frequently broken. Any infringement was an 'irregularity' for which the penalty was discharge, immediate, or after a warning, according to the gravity of the offence. Swearing, cursing and 'rude or indecent behaviour' were common. Smoking was forbidden as was the playing 'at cards or dice or any other game'.[11] Patients who were capable of doing so were expected to help in nursing other patients, in cleaning the wards, in washing and ironing 'and any other business that the Matron shall require'.[12] No patient could remain in the Hospital for more than two months unless the Physicians and Surgeons would certify to the Weekly Meeting that there was 'a probability of their being cured or receiving considerable Relief'.[13]

It was expected that when patients returned home cured they would 'return public Thanks, in their respective place of divine Worship'.[14]

Patients' statistics

During the Hospital's first year 263 patients were treated, of whom 106 were in-patients. The figures for in-patients and out-patients are combined for the recording of cures and deaths. Of the total 263, 143 are recorded as cured, 5 as having received benefit, 26 as deceased, 11 as incurable and 27 as discharged for irregularity and non-attendance. This method of recording the statistics allows very little useful information to be extracted from them. No case records for the period are known to survive. The discharge of patients not responding to treatment, which was the regular policy, tended to increase the number in the 'incurable'

category and to reduce the mortality figures. The discharges 'for irregularity and non-attendance' of some 10% of the patients further reduces
the significance of the statistics. Patients so discharged were usually out-
patients living at a distance, who 'when they were cured forget or are
unwilling to return and give thanks; and so not appearing for two weeks
together, are agreeably to the Rules of the Hospital, entered in the books
as discharged for irregularity'.

The statistics are given in Appendix II. It has been claimed that
hospitals in the eighteenth century were 'gateways to death'. The early
statistics of Addenbrooke's Hospital provide no information on such
matters as the mortality after surgery or the incidence of fatal sepsis.
However, it is difficult to believe that the demand for subscriber's
recommendations would have increased so steadily had not patients and
their families been satisfied that admission would be to their advantage.

The loss of the early case records of the Hospital is particularly to be
regretted because in January 1767, at the instigation of Charles Collignon, the Governors ordered 'That in any doubtful case the Physicians and
Surgeons shall have power to open the body of any person dying in the
Infirmary without asking any Person leave.'[15] It was unusual for such
authority to carry out post mortem examinations to be granted, and the
regular performance of such examinations was exceptional until a century
later. It has not been possible to discover to what extent autopsies were in
fact carried out.

The burial of the dead

The Hospital is in the Parish of St Benet's and the Governors appear
originally to have believed that there would be few patients dying in the
Hospital for whom relatives, or the recommending parish or individual
subscribers, would not accept responsibility. These few would be buried in
the churchyard of St Benet's. The first such patient died in October 1766;
her coffin was made by Sims, the Hospital carpenter, and the Matron was
ordered to buy a shroud.[16]

The Hospital soon found that the number of patients, particularly
emergency admissions, for which it had to accept responsibility for the
burial expenses was larger than had been anticipated. For example, the
Hospital found itself obliged to pay the burial expenses of Daniel Eastick
in March, 1767, and ordered that he 'be buried as cheap as possible'.[17] In

April 1771, the Minister and Parish officers of Little St Mary's, a neighbouring parish, were asked if they would bury the dead of the Hospital in return for the same concessions allowed the Parish of St Benet's. It would seem that the officers of Little St Mary's Parish did not accept this offer, for in July the Bishop of Ely was asked if he would consecrate a piece of ground behind the Hospital. The Court of 30 September decided that such consecration was unnecessary as the Chapel of St Ann's had formerly stood on the site of the Hospital. In January 1772, it was ordered that all patients dying in the Hospital should be buried in the Hospital grounds and that the porter should dig the graves.

When the Rules of the Hospital were first drawn up in August 1766, the Governors had agreed 'that no security shall be taken for the burial of patients'.[18] Some hospitals demanded the payment of caution money and others expected the recommending subscriber to assume financial responsibility for burial. Addenbrooke's was obliged to adopt this policy, at least for patients coming from a distance, when the Rules were revised in 1778.

Income for the new Hospital

The influence of the clergy

The important part played by the clergy of the Church of England in the organisation of the Hospital has already been mentioned. This was due only in part to the fact that most Fellows of Colleges were in holy orders – most parish clergy were subscribers and many, subscribing two guineas or more, were Governors and were thus entitled to play an active part in the affairs of the Hospital.

In most parishes the incumbent accepted the care of the sick as his responsibility, often himself supplying the letter of recommendation for those who needed to attend the Hospital, or arranging for one of his wealthier parishioners or the parish itself to provide one. Some clergy had deliberately acquired a knowledge of medicine and some, in remote parishes, without a medical man in practice, prescribed for their parishioners in emergency or even ran a dispensary. The vicar's wife and daughters accepted visiting and home nursing as a duty.

If a vicar was dissatisfied with the treatment given a parishioner at the Hospital, he wrote on his behalf to the Secretary. On his return home from hospital the patient was expected publicly to give thanks in the parish church for his recovery. In addition to this direct involvement in their parishioners' physical and spiritual welfare, the clergy were indirectly involved in improving the Hospital's financial status by enrolling new subscribers, and, after 1802, in preaching an annual sermon in aid of the Hospital.

Even before the Evangelical movement was in full flower, and social work became much more closely connected with religious beliefs,[1] the patient in hospital was given no opportunity to neglect his responsibilities and duties as a Christian. In the early days of the Hospital, no chaplain was appointed, but a 'clergyman of the week' was nominated 'to visit the sick, to read prayers every day and to administer the Communion at proper times'. The nominations were made by an informal committee which included any of the visiting clergy who chose to attend its meetings.

As early as 1766[2] the Board bought 200 copies of 'Serious Advice to Persons who have been sick' to be given to patients. Five hundred more copies of this tract by Bishop Gibson were ordered in 1771 and yet more three years later. In 1769[3] 25 bibles and 25 copies of 'The Whole Duty of Man' were ordered for the use of the patients. Other tracts were from time to time presented and accepted for distribution.

In 1767[4] the Committee of Clergymen agreed upon a form of prayer for the use of the hospital. It was printed, and copies stitched in marble paper were provided for the Readers, and in blue paper wrappers for the patients.

The practice of nominating a visiting clergyman continued for many years. From 1774 his authority was considerably increased, when it was decided[5] that he should serve also as a House Visitor, that is to say he should on his daily visits record in a book provided for the purpose any complaints reported to him or any observations he cared to make.

Finance and fund raising

Addenbrooke's Hospital enjoyed no large endowments. In fact the balance received by the Governors from Addenbrooke's trustees in 1766 was only £62.9s.3d. The Hospital therefore depended solely on voluntary subscriptions and on funds raised by special appeals, sermons, collections or concerts.

The accounts for the year ending Michaelmas, 1767, are of interest for they already include almost all the principal sources of the Hospital's income for many years to come.

CHARGE

	£	s	d
Annual Subscriptions	521	9	0
Benefactions for additional building, or general use	867	11	0
Brought Forward	1,389	0	0
Ballance (sic) received from Dr Addenbrooke's trustees	62	9	3
Collection at church, 2nd July, 1767	161	6	4½
Cleared from the Oratorio, July 3rd	71	6	1
Charity Box	8	6	11
Half a year's rent of Mrs Cawthorne's land	2	6	6
	1,694	11	1½

The Subscribers

The annual subscribers were the main source of the Hospital's income, and gained by their subscription the right to recommend patients and the right to vote at the General Quarterly Courts. The names of subscribers and the amount of their subscriptions were printed in the Annual Report, which was widely circulated.

> BENEFACTORS of Twenty Guineas or upwards at one time, are Governors during life; they may attend the Board, and vote on all occasions.
> Benefactors of Ten Guineas or more, and less than Twenty Guineas, are not Governors, but may recommend Patients during life.
> Annual Subscribers of Two Guineas or more are Governors during payment.
> Annual Subscribers of One Guinea are not Governors, but may recommend Patients.
> Annual subscriptions become due on Michaelmas-day, to be paid in advance for the Year following.[6]

That charitable feeling motivated many subscribers need not be questioned, but there were also obvious material advantages to be gained. The subscriber's rights of patronage increased his standing in his local community, and the Quarterly Courts and other functions of the Hospital which he was entitled to attend gave him the opportunity of making himself known to the influential, and of furthering his own profession or business.

An analysis of any list of subscribers during the Hospital's early years shows to what a large extent the Hospital was dependent on the University and the clergy. In the year ending Michaelmas 1769, for example, there were 227 subscribers who gave a total of £613.13s.0d., an average of £2.14s. each. The largest individual subscribers, the Marquis of Granby, the Earl of Hardwicke, and Lord Mountford, each gave 20 guineas; the Bishop of Ely gave £20. The majority of subscribers gave one or two guineas.

No fewer than 78 subscribers were clergy. Of these, 38 were resident Fellows of Colleges, holding College and sometimes also University office; nine were Masters of Colleges. The total contribution of the clergy was £183.15s., which was approximately a third of the entire subscription income.

Twelve members of the nobility subscribed a total of £86.2s. The gentry, identified as Esquires, in contrast with the plain Mister of the tradesmen and small farmers, were also substantial subscribers. They ranged from large landowners like Charles Ollive of Swaffham and Christopher Anstey of Trumpington who each subscribed 5 guineas, to smaller proprietors and professional men. The list was personally drawn up by the Treasurer, William Howell Ewin, who described himself as Esquire; the Secretary was listed as *Mr* Haggerstone. The gentry, including six resident in College, subscribed £108.3s. Nine Aldermen of the Borough together subscribed ten guineas. Three physicians each subscribed four guineas, three surgeons each one guinea, and one apothecary two guineas. There were thirteen women subscribers who gave £25.4s., but it was not for many years that women enjoyed full Governors' privileges; they could vote in ballots, but by proxy.

The geographical distribution of individual subscribers is of interest, in that although Addenbrooke's Hospital was a general hospital, not restricting admission to residents of Cambridgeshire, all the subscribers but three were resident in this county or in the Isle of Ely, if the aristocrats with interests in many counties are excluded. Since a patient's letter of recommendation had to be provided by a subscriber resident in the same county as the patient, it seems likely that at this period few patients from other counties were treated.

The subscribing institutions deserve special mention as they were eventually to assume increasing importance. The University Chest subscribed 20 guineas. Four Cambridge parishes (All Saints, St Giles, St Mary the Great and St Michael's) subscribed two or three guineas, and six parishes in Cambridgeshire or the Isle of Ely (Balsham, Chesterton, Isleham, Over, Wicken, Willingham) subscribed from 2 to 4 guineas.

Benefactions

Benefactions were gifts and legacies which were treated as income if they were relatively small, but were invested if they were large, unless they were designated by the donor for some special purpose, or were needed to settle the Hospital's immediate debts.

The sermon and the oratorio

The University sermon was delivered each year in July, in Great St Mary's Church, after the Annual Meeting of the Governors at the

Hospital. The first Anniversary Sermon was preached by the Revd Dr Gordon on 2 July 1767. Handel's Te Deum, Jubilate and Coronation Anthem were performed during the service. The occasion was always elaborately organised and the arrangements were put in hand some three months before. The President and Governors walked in formal procession from the Hospital to the church. The collection taken at the church doors formed an important part of the Hospital's income. The sermon, preached by a man of some distinction, was usually printed and sold to raise further funds. Sermons praised the work of hospitals in general and of Addenbrooke's Hospital in particular, and emphasised not only the virtues of charity but the material benefits which support of the Hospital might bring to the charitable.

The day after the Sermon a concert was held, also in Great St Mary's Church. In 1767 Handel's Messiah was performed. Admission was by ticket, price 5s., available from the Treasurer or the Secretary. The £71.6s.1d. entered in the accounts was the profit after all expenses had been paid.

These annual functions increased steadily in importance. It was the practice to nominate prominent citizens of Town or University to take the collection at the church doors, no doubt to encourage generosity. The Hospital was prepared for a considerable financial outlay to ensure the success of two days' activities. In 1769 'Music Expenses' amounted to £176.13s.10d. but the collection at the church doors took £225.12s.8d. and the sale of tickets for the Oratorio brought in £405.8s.6d. In 1771 a concert was arranged in the evening, after the Oratorio, and by 1775 there were evening concerts on both days.

Charity box
This box in the Hospital invited contributions from patients and their friends and visitors. The money collected varied around £10 a year.

Land and investments
Initially the Hospital owned only Mrs Cawthorne's land at Barnwell, which brought in a small rent. Later, other property was purchased and was rented until it was required for the Hospital's own use. Early in 1768 there was sufficient cash in hand for the investment of £1,600 in 3%

~ 55 ~

Consols and it was possible to increase this investment by a further £600 in 1769. Nevertheless investment income accounted in 1770 for no more than about 3% of the Hospital's total income.

Other sources of income

The organisers of Balls or concerts often agreed to give the Hospital a proportion of their profits. 'A Ball at the Red Lion' brought in £63 in 1768/9 but only 5 guineas the following year.

~ 8 ~

The medical staff

The visiting medical staff

The Physicians and Surgeons to the Hospital were elected by the General Board on 22 September 1766, only three weeks before the Hospital opened. The Board thanked them 'for the kind offer of assistance' and there is no mention of other candidates or of a ballot. The lack of a ballot is surprising as future appointments were hotly contested.

The system, which gave all annual subscribers to the Hospital funds of two guineas or more, the right to act as Governors, and therefore to vote at the General Courts of the Governors, ensured the lively participation of interested subscribers in the affairs of the Hospital, and often introduced political influences, local or national, into contested elections. Cambridge medical practitioners could, and did, attend Governors' meetings as subscribers and there can be no doubt that diligent participation in the Hospital's affairs was often inspired by the hope, sometimes realised, that election to the staff would follow when a vacancy occurred.

The lack of involvement of local medical men in the planning and organisation of the Hospital during its early days is notable. The Surgeons Hayles, Hopkins and Thackeray, were present at the meeting held on 20 May 1766, to appoint a committee to draw up the Rules and Orders, but were not appointed to the Committee. Plumptre, Hayles, Glynn and Hopkins, occasionally attended the General or Weekly Board, but only Collignon was a regular attendant.

The original staff of the Hospital consisted of three Physicians, Plumptre, Glynn and Collignon, and three Surgeons, Hayles, Hopkins and Thackeray. The Rules and Orders concerning the method of election of Physicians and Surgeons were as follows.

For the election of Physicians or Surgeons, a Weekly Board, at which not fewer than seven Governors were present, was to call a Special General Court unless a Quarterly Court was to be held at about the appropriate date. Twenty days notice was to be given of any elections and all elections were to be by ballot. If on the first sounding no candidate had a clear majority, then a second and if necessary a third ballot was to be held, leaving out on each occasion the name of the candidate with the fewest votes.

The duties of Physicians and Surgeons were clearly defined:

> That the Physicians and Surgeons, one of each, attend in their turns every Monday at 11 of the clock to examine those who should be recommended for patients; to certify their opinions of their cases to the Court or Weekly Meeting, and to prescribe for such as shall be admitted.[1]
>
> That the Physicians and Surgeons must attend at the Hospital every Wednesday and Friday at 11 of the clock to visit their In-patients and consult upon difficult cases; that on every Friday they do likewise prescribe for the Out-patients then on the book, and minute down what patient could properly be discharged the following Monday.[2]
>
> That all patients during their continuance be under the care of the Physicians or Surgeons (and in mixed cases of both) whose turn it was to attend when they were admitted.[3]
>
> That each Physician and Surgeon visit his respective In-patients at other times as often as he shall find it necessary, or shall have notice of any sudden emergency from the Apothecary.[4]
>
> That each Physician or Surgeon whose business or indisposition shall oblige him to be absent, engage some other Physician or Surgeon of the Hospital to attend for him.[5]

All the newly elected staff were already resident and practising in Cambridge and, necessarily so, since the Hospital appointments were Honorary. The Surgeons were, in fact, in general practice, for the limited range of surgical procedures made strict specialisation in surgery an uneconomic proposition, except in very large cities, and even in these most surgeons made the majority of their income from consultations in what we should now call medical conditions. The Physicians, though at that time their education differed widely from that of the Surgeons, were also in general practice, though the more eminent saw many referred patients in consultation. Their fees were higher than those of the Surgeons and their practice tended to be 'better class'. Fellows of Colleges often practised from their rooms and continued to do so until late in the nineteenth century.

Russell Plumptre (1709–1793) was the son of Henry Plumptre, President of the Royal College of Physicians, who had probably helped the young John Addenbrooke make the best use of the limited medical teaching available at Cambridge early in the century. Educated at Eton and at Queen's College, he had been elected Regius Professor of Physic in 1741.

He held the Chair for over 50 years but was not active as a teacher, nor, after 1767, in his duties at the Hospital.

Robert Glynn (1719–1800) was a Cornishman who came to King's College from Eton, and as a medical student was a pupil of William Heberden of St John's College. From 1749 to 1800 Glynn practised as a physician from his rooms in Gibbs Building, King's College. He was witty and eccentric and had a considerable reputation as a physician. He was very actively involved in the Chatterton controversy. He took little interest in the administration of Addenbrooke's Hospital but there is no reason to believe that he did not carry out his duties conscientiously. He was an impetuous and outspoken man, but amicable and popular. His quick temper may explain his quarrel with the Resident Apothecary. In 1773 he resigned from the Hospital staff on the grounds that his health did not permit him to continue, yet he remained in active practice until his death 27 years later.[6]

Charles Collignon (1725–1785) was a member of Trinity College and a pupil of William Heberden, who, with Plumptre, examined him for the M.B. in 1748.[7] He was later at Edinburgh and at Leyden. While still a student at Cambridge he visited France and studied in London.[8] In 1753 he was elected Professor of Anatomy at Cambridge and from 1754 he lectured regularly on the Edinburgh pattern, incorporating comparative anatomy and pathology and much clinical information and general medicine into his anatomy courses. His lectures were attended by theology students as well as by medical students. He attended the Weekly Board with great regularity and, as well as being responsible for the regulation regarding post-mortem examinations, he expressed enlightened views on the principles on which patients should be selected for admission to hospital.

The Revd William Cole left an entertaining account of his eccentricities, chief of which appears to have been a failure to conform to the grossly self-indulgent habits of his contemporaries. His qualities were fully appreciated by his colleagues on the Weekly Board, even if Plumptre and Glynn achieved greater success in fashionable practice.[7]

Richard Hayles (1714–1781) took a house in Trumpington Street in 1737. From 1739 onwards his name appears frequently in the records of almost all Cambridge parishes. In 1751 he took Thomas Thackeray as his apprentice at a premium of £150, which suggests that he enjoyed a considerable reputation. He resigned as Surgeon to the Hospital in 1775.[9]

Allan Hopkins (d. 1777). Nothing is known of his early life and apprentice-ship. From 1751 onwards he had patients in many parishes. In 1759 he was in court for body-snatching. By 1776 he was a very sick man and he took T.V. Okes into partnership. In February 1777 he died, in debt, and was buried in St Michael's Church.[9]

Thomas Thackeray (1736–1806) was the most successful of the original surgeons. He was the fourth son of Archdeacon Thackeray and was educated at Eton. At the age of 15 he was apprenticed to Richard Hayles, whose partner he became. His name appears frequently with those of Plumptre and Glynn in consultations on the local gentry. With Glynn he attended Mr Panton of Newmarket; Glynn's fee was £80, Thackeray's was £50 – enormous sums in terms of the value of money in the late eighteenth century.[10] He was a tall handsome man with an impressive manner. 'If he were consulted by a Student for any bodily imfirmity, he never missed the opportunity of improving the mind too.' In 1765 a patient left him a large house in St Andrew's Street, which remained the family home for two medical generations.[11] He was Surgeon to the Hospital 1766–1796.

Later Physicians

Edward Waring (1734–1798) who succeeded Plumptre as Physician to the Hospital in 1768, was Lucasian Professor of Mathematics. He was M.D. 1767. He was a most reluctant physician and it is said he sometimes paid his patients to go elsewhere. It is unlikely that he practised after he resigned from the Hospital in 1775.

Isaac Pennington (1745–1817) who was Regius Professor from 1794 to 1817, was Physician to the Hospital from 1773, in which year he obtained from the University the licence to practise, until 1816. He was a bachelor and lived in St John's College.

Henry Ainslie (1760–1834) of Pembroke College, graduated A.B. in 1781 and was Senior Wrangler of his year. He was elected Physician to the Hospital in 1786, before he received the licence to practise. He resigned after two years and moved to London where he was elected as Physician to St Thomas' Hospital in 1795.

Busick Harwood (1745–1814) succeeded Collignon in 1785 as Professor of Anatomy and as Physician to the Hospital, and in 1800 became also Downing Professor of Medicine.

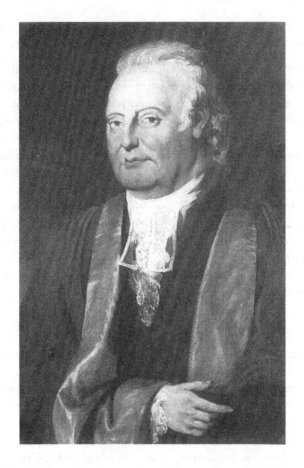

Fig. 8. Edward Waring, 1734–1798. By courtesy of the Master and
Fellows of Magdalene College.

Robert Stockdale (1761–1831) was elected a Medical Fellow of Pembroke College in 1785, and Physician to the Hospital in 1790, the year
before he was granted the University Licence to practise. He resigned in
1809.

Thomas Ingle (1765–1838) was elected a Fellow of Peterhouse in 1788.
He was elected Physician to the Hospital in 1793, the year before he was
licensed to practise medicine.

Martin Davy (1763–1839) was also Physician in 1793. He had graduated M.B. from Caius College in 1792, but he was not licensed to
practise medicine until 1794. He became Master of his College in 1803, in

which year he resigned from the Hospital, but he practised medicine with considerable success both before and after his election as Master.

These seven, with Plumptre, Glynn and Collignon, are the only physicians who are known to have practised in Cambridge during the years 1750–1800. There were four who occupied Chairs of Anatomy or of Medicine, already in practice in the town at the time of their election to these Chairs. All ten were already in practice before they were elected Physicians to Addenbrooke's Hospital, although three of them did not find it necessary to obtain the University's licence to practise until after their election. The fact that the Hospital and University offices were always filled by men already in practice avoided clashes of interests, which were later to become disruptive. It is interesting that Plumptre, Glynn and Davy, who were notably successful in practice, soon resigned from the Hospital staff. The very early age at which Stockdale, Ingle and Davy were elected to the staff suggests that the appointment was at that time not greatly sought after.

Later Surgeons

Surgeons were not University graduates and biographical information concerning them must be compiled from the Overseers' Accounts of the Cambridge parishes (overseers were parish officers responsible for the care of the sick poor), from the Apprenticeship records in the Public Record Office, and from their wills.[9]

Thomas Bond (1740–1821) was the son of John Bond the apothecary. A Thomas Bond who qualified at the Company of Surgeons on 16 October 1760, is probably the same man. He was a member of All Saints Parish from 1765, living opposite Jesus Lane. In 1777, when he moved to his late father's house, near Magdalene Bridge, he described himself as surgeon and man-midwife. From 1765 he was employed by various parishes. From 1779 to 1813 he was Surgeon to the Hospital. He was very active in civic affairs and was Mayor in 1783.

John Griffies (d. 1784) apprenticed to Thackeray in 1770, was elected Surgeon to the Hospital in 1780. He died only four years later. His name appeared only once in Overseers' Accounts, which suggests that he was incapacitated by illness for some years before his death.

Thomas Verney Okes (1755–1828). Where Okes served his apprenticeship is not known. He received the diploma of the Surgeons' Company on 30 March 1766. He came to Cambridge later that year as partner to

Hopkins. In May 1777, he married Ann, daughter of Mrs Ann Gray, a well-known Cambridge apothecary. From his house in Trinity Street he carried on a general practice which soon became very large. His family of 18 children included Francis, who qualified in medicine but soon entered the Church, John, who joined his father in practice, and Richard, who became Provost of King's College. On his bills Okes described himself as surgeon until about 1800, after which he was surgeon and apothecary. The practice of the surgeon and the apothecary had indeed become essentially the same. The parishes employed Okes frequently, some times as a surgeon, and at others as an apothecary. He was Surgeon to the Hospital from 1779 to 1817.

James Farish settled in practice in Trumpington Street before 1784 and for many years was employed as a surgeon by most of the Cambridge parishes. In 1784 he was elected Surgeon to the Hospital, but he resigned in 1787. He was in partnership with A.M. Fawcett for a time between 1829 and 1832.

Frederic Thackeray (1774–1852) succeeded his father as Surgeon to the Hospital in 1796. He had previously worked as a pupil at the Hospital, and also in London and in Paris. He was extremely successful in practice, but as early as 1800 took steps to qualify as a physician, but was prevented for some years from graduating by the efforts of rival physicians (see p. 100).

These five surgeons, together with Hayles, Hopkins and Thomas Thackeray, and a William Lunn (c. 1700–1769), are the only surgeons known to have practised in Cambridge between 1750 and 1800. All but Lunn, who was already too old when the Hospital opened, served for a time as Surgeons to the Hospital. Many were very young when they were elected to the staff, and some, such as Hopkins, resigned when their reputations and practice permitted it. Farish's term of office was shortened by professional rivalries and political pressures.

The surgeons differed little, if at all, from the physicians in their social origins, but they were not members of the University. Many of them earned a considerable income from private patients to whom the physicians were very rarely called, but in private practice physicians charged higher fees than surgeons. Frederic Thackeray's transfer from the surgical to the medical staff of the Hospital in 1827 is an indication of the relatively small difference between the work of two threads of the profession in a small town in pre-anaesthetic days, just as Okes' career, and the interchangeability of surgeon and apothecary in parish and other appointments indicate that the work of these branches had come, by the end of the century, to vary by very little.

The Resident Apothecary

The Minute Books contain few references to the activities of Lefebvre, the first Resident Apothecary: the implication is that he carried out his duties adequately and was on reasonable terms with his chiefs and with the Matron. In 1768 he offered his resignation, but later withdrew it, apologising for 'angrily giving warning to leave the Hospital upon being reprimanded'.[12] Each year he was awarded his gratuity of £5 for good behaviour, although in January 1769, with this episode in mind, the Weekly Meeting saw fit to refer the matter to the General Court, which approved the payment.

The Apothecary's responsibilities were gradually increasing. He was, of course, already entrusted with the admission of emergencies. From May 1769,[13] he was authorised to deputise for the Physicians and Surgeons when an admission day coincided with Monday of Commencement Week, an Oratorio, or Christmas Day.

Lefebvre resigned on Lady Day, 1770, and at a Special General Court held on 29 January 1770, John Debraz (also spelt Debraw) was elected his successor; there were other candidates but their names were not recorded. Debraz was one of the most remarkable men ever associated with the Hospital. Nothing is known of his early career. He was certainly widely read in chemistry and in biology. In 1777, whilst he was still working at the Hospital, he read to the Royal Society a paper on the fertilisation of bees.[14] After he left Cambridge he crossed the path of Jeremy Bentham, probably early in 1785, when Bentham was looking for a man to help his brother Samuel at Krichev in Russia. Debraz arrived at Riga early in 1786 as a speculative venture, for he had made no agreement with Samuel. Samuel Bentham, who had hoped that Debraz would be able to help him with his various industrial enterprises found him too cantankerous. Early in 1787 Debraz left Krichev and rapidly established a considerable professional reputation for himself in southern Russia. In 1788 he was appointed First Physician of the Russian Armies, but he died before the patent of his appointment reached him.[15]

Debraz's career at the Hospital appears at first to have been uneventful, and although he was once reprimanded for swearing,[16] he was regularly awarded his gratuity; indeed, in December 1771, he was allowed an additional £2 'for his trouble in the laboratory'. This work was probably the preparation of medicines of plant origin, for the following year 'a press for squeezing herbs' was ordered to be made for him. In 1775 he applied successfully for an increase in his salary, which was raised to £40, but without a gratuity.[17]

Debraz's difficulties began in 1776 when a local newspaper published an anonymous letter from a subscriber to the Hospital.[18] He was, he wrote, 'alarmed at the enormous expense of the Apothecary's shop and housekeeping, when I compared the said expenses and the number of patients, In and Out, in 1772 with those of 1775'. In the latter year there were 234 fewer patients than in 1772, yet the expenditure was nearly £120 more; over £64 of this additional sum was in the running cost of the Apothecary's shop. The subscriber then went on to say (totally dishonestly), 'as to the Apothecary's drugs, I am not acquainted with their value', but with increased expenditure on fewer patients, 'surely there is some mismanagement'.

The author of this letter was John Hoffman, a local chemist, druggist and apothecary,[19] who as a subscriber and Governor, was actually present at the Quarterly Court on 25 March, at which the charges were discussed.

A lengthy reply, refuting the charges, was drafted by Collignon. In this reply it was admitted that 'some abuses will creep into any house and easily may into an Hospital . . . House Visitors are appointed to examine into abuses and our present Apothecary is always kindly assisting and has more than once by his diligence detected beginning mismanagements'. Hoffman failed to produce evidence in support of his allegations, and an action against him for defamation was considered.

The Hoffman affair must have aroused much indignation for it was debated in the local press for some weeks. Hoffman continued his vigorously worded accusations and personal attacks on Debraz. The significant feature of the whole affair is that Hoffman, as a Governor who was also a practising apothecary, had the right to visit and supervise the Hospital Apothecary's Shop. If its affairs were mismanaged this was partly Hoffman's responsibility. From what we know of both men it seems likely that a clash of two aggressive personalities was the origin of the conflict.

Two years later, in October 1778, the Matron submitted her resignation and made allegations against Debraz. In the same month[20] Robert Glynn, the Senior Physician, wrote that he had long had his 'suspicions in regard to our Apothecary, and has long been of opinion that he was a very improper man for the office and that his whole conduct should be enquired into'. Committees composed of very senior Governors were set up to enquire into both sets of allegations. The quarrel between Matron and Apothecary had evidently been a petty and sordid affair of precedence and status.[21] It was considered that 'the Apothecary had interferred improperly in the department of the Matron'. The correspondence which has passed between them was ordered to be burned. The second Committee found that 'Mr Debraz has in some instances been too inattentive to his business, but that of late years he has in general approved himself as a diligent and able officer in his capacity as Apothecary'. Debraz was reprimanded but continued to hold his appointment until December 1781, without again incurring the recorded displeasure of Governors or staff.

Debraz's successor was John Cotton (1751–1793), the son of William, a Cambridge apothecary. He was the only applicant for the post.[22]

He resigned in 1784 and two years later became the partner of Peter Kelty, a successful Cambridge apothecary. Of his work at the Hospital nothing of interest is recorded. He was succeeded by Joseph Gray, the son of Robert Gray, also a Cambridge apothecary.

Joseph Gray was born in 1761. His father died in 1765, but his mother carried on the business. His sister Ann married in 1777 Thomas Verney Okes who in 1779 had been elected Surgeon to the Hospital. This family connection may have helped Joseph to secure a very large majority (44 to 16) of the votes in the ballot for the appointment of an Apothecary to the Hospital;[23] there was one other applicant, Montague Sterling. But even if his relationship to Okes favoured him, he was undoubtedly the ideal man for the job. He was Apothecary for 23 years, yet his name rarely appeared in the Minute Books, and then only in the record of tributes to his efficiency and his friendly personality. In 1794 his salary was raised from £40 to £50 'in consideration of his particular attention to the duties of his office for near ten years'.[24] It is surprising that he was able to devote so much time to the Hospital after his marriage in 1786, but he continued to do so and in 1802 his services were again recognised, this time by the presentation of a piece of silver plate, inscribed to record 'his meritorious Conduct in the discharge of that important and arduous office which he has so long filled with Skill, Attention, Humanity and Honor'.[25]

Gray continued as Apothecary until his death on 12 March 1808. The nature of his illness is not recorded, but the bill for drugs ordered for his treatment amounted to the enormous sum of £69.12s.10d. The Governors erected a tablet to his memory in St Clement's Church: 'a numerous body of the governors, wishing to shew their regard for his memory, assembled themselves at Addenbrooke's Hospital and followed him in procession to the grave'.[26]

The careers of Debraz and of Gray have been considered in some detail because of the importance of the Resident Apothecary in the Hospital hierarchy of the eighteenth and early nineteenth centuries. The Apothecary was, in fact, resident medical superintendent and chief pharmacist. The reputation of a hospital, and in particular, the relationship between staff and patients, depended to a large extent on his example.

Other practitioners

There were perhaps 30–40 apothecaries practising in Cambridge between 1750 and 1800. Although the Physicians and Surgeons to the Hospital were appointed from amongst men already in practice in the town, the first two Resident Apothecaries to the Hospital were not local men. The leading local apothecaries had been asked to advise on their selection and may have preferred to recommend an outsider, as the local firms were in competition for the supply of drugs to the Hospital. The third apothecary to be appointed, John Cotton, was probably a local man; he certainly joined a successful local firm after spending three years at the Hospital. Joseph Gray, Resident Apothecary from 1784 to 1808, was local, and also the brother-in-law of T.V. Okes, the Surgeon.

Apothecaries at that time differed very widely in their social and financial status. Some of the more successful competed with the physicians as general practitioners to the local gentry. Most were in direct competition with the surgeons both for private practice and for parish work. It is probable that they all kept shops for the sale of medicines and also of cosmetics, tobacco and groceries, but it was largely the less successful in practice who advertised a wide range of goods for sale.

The fees of even the most humble apothecaries were high in relation to average wages and there can be no doubt that many of the large number of poor who were not yet destitute, and 'on the parish', resorted frequently to the very large number of herbalists and quacks who advertised their wares so freely in the local press.

~ 9 ~

The early years: patients, nursing and administration

Patients

During the Hospital's first year 106 in-patients and 157 out-patients were treated. The numbers increased slowly and irregularly (see Appendix II). The average bed occupancy in the eighteenth century was about 24, but fluctuated widely, sometimes rising in the winter months to over 30.[1]

The statistics show that although the men's wards were frequently full and sometimes overcrowded, the number of women in-patients seldom exceeded 10, and as the upper women's ward could accommodate 12, the lower women's ward was often closed. The minutes were seldom detailed and the evidence that the lower ward was closed is provided by the order that it be opened on 3 February 1783, and again on 27 October.

The figures suggest that the Hospital as originally designed was for its first two decades large enough to accommodate those patients who were medically and financially eligible to avail themselves of its services. Towards the end of 1767 a Committee was appointed 'to examine the Underground Floor'. James Essex (1722–1784), a builder and architect who had been employed in the building of the Hospital, was consulted and the plans he prepared were accepted. The basement was divided up to accommodate the 'kitchen, coal house, pantry, cellars, Elaboratory, Wash house, bath room, Matron's store room and lumbar (sic) room'. The Committee optimistically predicted that 'the Execution of this Plan will, for some time at least, make all additional buildings needless'. The alterations planned by Essex were apparently carried out for in March 1769 the house adjoining the Hospital, which had been used as the kitchen, was ordered to be demolished. The Governors' optimism proved to be justified for no further building was undertaken for over 20 years.

In 1783 the Governors agreed that the words 'Addenbrooke's Hospital' should be put in front of the Hospital.

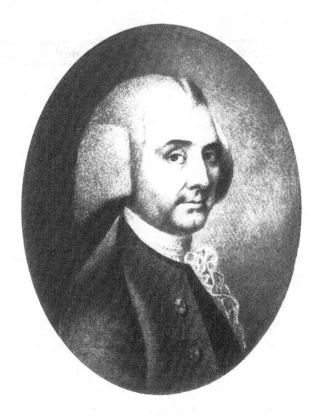

Fig. 9. James Essex, architect.

Patients coming from a distance increased in numbers, as indicated by the changing distribution of subscribing parishes (see Table 1). Such patients presented the Hospital with special problems. Patients who had made a journey taking several hours might prove to be ineligible or unsuitable for admission. In 1771[2] a notice was printed and put over the Hospital gate: 'No Horse or Cart bringing a patient to the Hospital shall return home until it is known whether the patient can be admitted or not.' Contact between the Governors and subscribers in other counties was less easy to maintain than with local parishes. Hence the ruling of the Board in May 1772 that[3] 'all Persons admitted from a distance into this Hospital bring with them clean Apparel, a change of Linnen, Money to pay for the Washing their Linnen and likewise some person to engage to pay the funeral Expenses of any Person who shall happen to die'.

~ 69 ~

Table 1. *Subscribing parishes*

	Cambridge	Cambridgeshire	Huntingdonshire.	Essex	Hertfordshire	Norfolk
1767	3					
1768	3	4				
1769	4	6				
1770	5	12				
1771	5	12				
1772	9	13				
1773	9	16				
1774	9	16				
1775	11	13			1	
1776						
1777						
1778						
1779	12	16	2		2	
1780	11	17	2		1	
1781	11	16	1		1	
1782	11	16	2	1	1	
1783	11	19	2	1	1	
1784	11	21	3	1	1	
1785	11	27	4	1	1	1
1786	11	29	5	1	1	1
1787	11	30	6	1	1	1
1788	11	29	5	1	1	1
1789	11	28	5	1	1	1
1790	12	27	2			1
1791	12	30	2			
1792	12	30	2			
1793	10	30	2			
1794	12	31	1			
1795	12	34	1			
1796	12	37	2			
1797	11	39	2			
1798	11	39	2			
1799	11	39	7			
1800	11	39	7			
1801	11	40	7			

In 1771 Glynn arranged to see his out-patients on Saturdays, so that they might take advantage of the better transport facilities on a market day.[4]

The distribution of subscribing parishes gives the best indication of the area principally served by the Hospital. It was not until 1779 that all the town parishes were subscribing; there were so many private subscribers in

Cambridge, and the University Chest regularly subscribed 20 guineas from 1768, therefore patients living in the town are unlikely to have had much difficulty in securing a letter of recommendation. Rural patients in Cambridgeshire seem at first to have relied on the local incumbent and the local gentry, but gradually more parishes found it in their interest to subscribe. Whilst many continued to subscribe regularly, others allowed their subscriptions to lapse after a year or two. The more or less steady increase in the numbers shown in the table conceals frequent minor changes from year to year. For example, in 1782 the sixteen subscribing parishes included Littleport and Chatteris for the first time and omitted Burwell and Landbeach, both in arrears. The first parish outside the county to subscribe was Elmdon in Essex in 1775. Parishes in the eastern parts of Huntingdonshire made increasing use of the Hospital. Ashwell in Hertfordshire subscribed for a few years. Newmarket, now in Suffolk, but then partly in Cambridgeshire, subscribed for 1792 (All Saints) and 1793 (St Mary's). The only subscribing parish in Norfolk was Methwold.

Neither the Governors nor the officers they employed had had any experience of Hospital administration. It is therefore not surprising that frequent difficulties arose concerning administrative procedure, the precise definition of each employee's duties and the relationship of employees to each other. It was not long before the inadequacy of the original Rules and Orders became apparent. The Secretary was ordered to write to the Dean of Salisbury for copies of the local hospital's Rules[5] and a Committee was appointed[6] 'to Inspect the Rules and Orders of this Hospital and to see if any Improvements can be made from the Rules and Practice of other Hospitals'. The changes made in the rules were not extensive, but they described each employee's duties with greater clarity and precision.

The elaborate arrangements for the admission and discharge of patients were unchanged in principle but in practice they were changing. Five Governors were required to be present on these occasions, but if 'from the Badness of the weather or from any other causes' the necessary number failed to attend, then the Physician and Surgeon of the week were authorised to admit or discharge patients 'with the consent of as many Governors as may happen to be present'.[7] In time, the admission and discharge of patients came to be left entirely to the medical staff. During the 1780s and 1790s Weekly Meetings were often poorly attended or were not held. Conscious of the need to economise, the Governors continued to apply to the referring subscriber if a patient required any special treatment or applicance. In July 1768, the Secretary wrote to a subscriber informing him that the patient he had recommended 'is admitted an Out-patient, but that he cannot receive any benefit, without a truss, which the Hospital does not possess'.[8] The following year the Matron was ordered to provide trusses for patients when required.[9]

Parishes or individuals failing to meet their obligations found it impossible to admit further patients. On 21 March 1768, the Overseers of Chesterton were informed that two girls they had recommended were to be refused because they had not paid the expenses incurred on behalf of a girl they had referred the previous year, who had developed smallpox whilst in Hospital. Three years later[10] the officers of the same parish were informed that Mary Howard could not be admitted 'till they have first provided for the care of her child and also have furnished her with some necessary cloathes'.

During the first two decades in particular the Governors had to devote much effort to persuade the patients to conform to the rules. At first nurses and porters had frequently to be dismissed for being continually drunk or for selling drink to the patients. Whilst such offences by the staff became less frequent, patients were sometimes admonished or discharged for going into the town and returning 'very much in liquor'. Discharge for this offence, or 'for ill behaviour to the Matron'[11] or for any other 'irregularity', made a patient ineligible for further treatment, and in February 1771 the Secretary was ordered to keep a list of patients so discharged. In 1774[12] the Quarterly Court ordered that a book be provided in which to record the names of such patients and also the names 'of such persons who do not appear to return thanks for the care and benefit they receive in this Hospital'.

Despite the penalities some patients continued to go into the town and to return intoxicated. In an attempt to prevent them doing so a new rule was introduced in 1781:[13] 'In-patients who shall be detected hereafter in walking out of the Hospital gates without an express leave of their Physicians or Surgeons shall be discharged for irregularity'.

There can be no doubt that some of the offences committed by patients called for strict discipline, in the interests of the majority. However, some of the orders seem harshly oppressive, such as the order made in 1781[14] that any patient refusing or complaining about the food should be immediately discharged and never readmitted. It is difficult, too, to see the justification for a rule made in 1783[15] that all out-patients must attend every week or be discharged for non-attendance. This must have imposed unnecessary hardship and expense on those patients living at a distance from the Hospital.

During the late 1780s and the 1790s there were far fewer records of discharge of patients for disciplinary reasons but whether this reflects a decline in the frequency of the offences or laxity in keeping the Minutes is not clear. Certainly a more humane and tolerant attitude towards the sick was shown in January 1798: William Satchell was discharged for an unspecified 'irregularity' but immediately readmitted when Mr Okes protested that his discharge 'would render his cure improbable'.[16]

In that same month the fourteen Governors present at a Weekly Meeting inspected the wards, because a rumour had been circulated that the patients were neglected; they found the rumour to be 'without the least foundation'.[17]

Matron and nurses

During the Hospital's early years only two nurses were regularly employed, but extra nurses were taken on for short periods during the illness of one of the regular staff. This arrangement soon proved inadequate and in October 1770 Mrs Perry was ordered 'to look out for an Occasional nurse, and to make the best arrangement she can, not exceeding 4s. per week.' Soon afterwards[18] the Governors agreed that the number of patients in the men's ward was too great for one nurse, and the Matron was ordered to engage an additional nurse as a helper.

The difficulty of recruiting women who would make satisfactory nurses in the days before there was universal elementary education, or any system of nursing training, led to the practice of engaging nurses 'on trial for a month'. There was no shortage of applicants, but the turnover was rapid. Some nurses resigned, usually on health grounds, but most were dismissed, sometimes for petty 'irregularities' but often for more serious offences, which throw some light on the problems confronting the Matron.

Nurse Davies was dismissed in 1770[19] 'for taking a man to lodge in the Hospital', and turning out a patient to provide a bed for him. The common offences were being drunk on duty, selling alcohol to the patients or taking money from them. On more than one occasion a porter and a nurse were discharged simultaneously; in 1774, after the discharge of William Hall and Lettie Martin,[20] an advertisement asked for applicants 'whose ages are not to be under 40'. It is possible that by 1779 it had become more difficult to obtain nurses. Nurse Sarah Puntsby[21] was merely admonished by the Governors for 'getting intoxicated with liquor and for other irregularities'. Ten years earlier she would have been instantly dismissed for such offences. Two years later she was admonished for repeatedly accepting money from the patients. In 1787 she was again admonished for getting intoxicated and for bringing beer in for the patients. Nurse Puntsby must have had exceptional qualities, for in 1788 another nurse was discharged for intoxication, although this was her first recorded offence.

In the 1790s the Weekly Meetings were poorly attended; sometimes not even the Secretary was present, and the Minutes were very uninformative. The few references to the nurses suggest, however, that standards of conduct were improving; the infrequency of advertisements in the local papers for new nurses tends to confirm that the lack of references in the Minutes to nurses' misdemeanors is not merely a reflection of the Secretary's inefficiency. In December 1793, Nurse Pearson, not fit enough 'for the whole business of a nurse', was allowed to continue to live in the Hospital as 'an occasional nurse' at $5\frac{1}{2}$ guineas per annum, in recognition of her past services. This became a common practice when nurses retired through age or ill health. The ward nurses slept in rooms off their own wards. Accommodation in the hospital was very restricted, and it seems likely that pensioners slept in the women's ward, which was seldom full. In 1794 the wages of the nurses were raised to £8 and 'in consideration of their good Behaviour it shall be at the discretion of Mrs Williams the Matron to make them any further advance not exceeding 40 Shillings each'.[22]

The health of the Matron, Mrs Perry, began to fail in 1774 and she was given leave, the first since her appointment nearly eight years before. Mrs Perry did not recover and she died some time in December. In January 1775, Mrs Dorothy Spencer was elected her successor;[23] no other candidates are mentioned in the Minutes, but Jane Mathan, an unsuccessful candidate, expressed her grateful thanks to her supporters and hoped for their support and interest in the next vacancy.[24] Mrs Spencer resigned in December 1776. Her successor, Mrs Barnes, one of two candidates, held office only for one year, from March 1777. She died in February 1778, 'lamented by all who knew her unaffected piety and unusual benevolence'.[25] The advertisement for her successor carried a revealing footnote: 'The importance of the station to be filled up renders it a matter of great moment that the selection be made with the strictest attendance to the merits of the candidates.' Miss Ann Edwards, age 35, one of three candidates, resigned after only six months; she had quarrelled with Debraz, the Apothecary, whose uncongenial temperament may well have been responsible for the earlier resignation of two of her predecessors.

Mrs Mary Hopkins, one of four candidates, was elected to the position,[26] but was taken seriously ill in January 1779. Her deputy, Mrs Wilson of Histon, was one of three candidates for the post in February 1779, but Mrs Ann Fletcher was elected by a substantial majority. She died in December 1786.

The frequent changes of Matron must have had an unsettling effect on the nursing and domestic staff. Of Mrs Fletcher and her five predecessors nothing is known. However, Mrs Fletcher appears to have improved the status, though not the emoluments, of the appointment, since there were no fewer than seven applicants in January 1787.[27] Mrs Mary Williams was elected, having obtained 55 of the 70 votes cast. She was immediately successful and, as early as January 1790, was awarded an additional gratuity of 10 guineas 'in appreciation of her care and attention to the business of the Hospital'. This was awarded again annually from 1791 to 1794, and in 1795 her salary was increased to £40 per annum. She appears to have been popular and efficient and must be given credit for the improvement in the conduct of the nurses during her years in office. Her career ended sadly, when in 1802 she was accused of entering on the Hospital account goods purchased for her own use. She confessed and was suspended. In June she was discharged.[28]

General administration

John Bones succeeded Haggerstone as Secretary in 1772. The Minutes continued to be well kept and usually patients' statistics were added. However, Bones resigned after only three years, because the Governors would not raise his salary. They still expected a man of good education to undertake what must have been almost a full-time occupation, for a ridiculously small salary. His successor, Robert Gee, took up his appointment on 2 October 1775. In 1779 he applied for an increase in salary and the Quarterly Court of 29 March granted him an annual gratuity of £5: he later received further increases and he remained Secretary until his death in 1817.

The Hospital's cumbersome administrative system served it well in its early years, thanks to the initial enthusiasm of the Governors. However, as this enthusiasm waned, and the attendance of Governors at meetings declined, the inadequacies of the system became apparent. Between 1790 and 1801 the attendance at Weekly Meetings was very poor; sometimes only the Secretary was present; occasionally he too failed to attend. In 1801 'no business' was recorded in the Minutes for weeks on end, and in the Annual Report for the year ending Michaelmas 1801 the expenses significantly exceeded the receipts for the first time and the deficit of £310.5s.0d. was large enough to cause alarm, since it amounted to more than a quarter of the total expenditure of £1,188.10s.5d.

On 10 May 1802, a Committee was set up to examine the accounts and management of the Hospital. The Hospital's second phase dates from the acceptance of the report of the Committee on 14 June 1802.

A period
of expansion

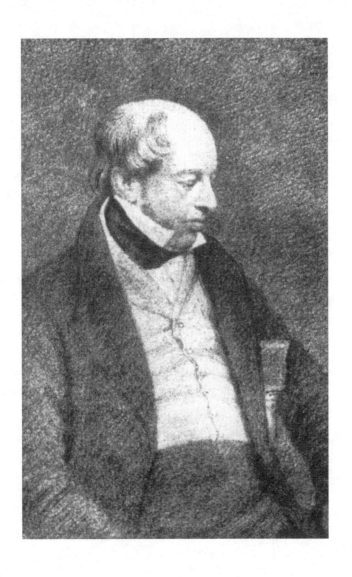

~ 10 ~

A turning point

Finance

It was during the early months of 1802 that the Governors became aware of the serious financial situation of the Hospital. Over the past seven years all legacies and benefactions (donations other than subscriptions) had been used to meet the deficiency in regular income, yet each year the balance remaining in the Treasurer's hands grew smaller. In the year ending Michaelmas 1801 expenditure exceeded income by £310.5s. and, even after the receipt of a timely legacy of £300, the Treasurer was left with a deficit.

On the instructions of the Weekly Meeting of 12 April 1802, the Secretary informed the public of the Hospital's plight[1] and, in the same notice, announced that a Special General Court of the Governors would be held on 10 May. 'An Inhabitant of Cambridge' suggested in a letter to the *Cambridge Chronicle*[2] that a subscription to the Hospital would be a better way of celebrating the Proclamation of the Peace than wasting money on illuminations. The Special General Court,[3] which was well attended, ordered that the figures be made public, and that an appeal be launched. The Governors explained that it was important that all maintenance expenses should be covered by income from investments and subscriptions so that benefactions and legacies could be employed to increase capital investment.

By Michaelmas 1802,[4] benefactions had enabled the Treasurer to purchase such additional Government stock as would increase the investment income by £36. The principal benefactors on this occasion had been the Duke of Rutland and Sir Henry Peyton, each of whom gave 100 guineas, the Bishop of Ely and Lord Charles Manners, who gave 50 guineas, and Charles Yorke who gave £50. A collection taken in most of the parish churches of the county brought in a total of £1,012.11s.3¼d.

By the end of 1802,[5] the crisis was over, but the Treasurer emphasised the need for more regular subscribers and the more active participation of Governors at the Weekly Board; 'the late difficulties must in great

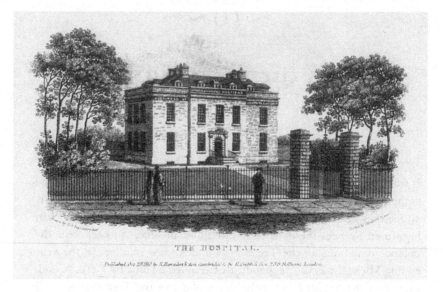

Fig. 10. Addenbrooke's Hospital, 1810. View of the hospital
frontage and grounds from Trumpington Street.

measure be attributed to their non-attendance'. The problems had not,
however, been completely overcome. In 1803 expenses exceeded income
by over £100, but there had been heavy expenditure on repairs and
furniture and with legacies and donations it had been possible to buy more
stock to increase the annual investment income by £84.[6] In their
'Observations on the State of the Hospital' for 1803,[7] the auditors
expressed their satisfaction with the progress made. They praised Alderman Newling for the accuracy and neatness with which he had kept the
accounts for over 30 years. They thanked everyone who had helped the
Hospital, but expressed their particular obligation to the clergy of the
County, who, with the encouragement of the Bishop of Ely, 'have
laudably exerted themselves in behalf of the charity'. They appealed for
more subscribers and hoped that, with their support, 'the Hospital will
continue to do that credit to the County which its unrivalled excellence
and cleanliness so justly deserve'. Subscribers were invited to visit the
Hospital; many did so after the Anniversary sermon in July 1804,[8] and
'expressed their astonishment at seeing such an extraordinary specimen of
cleanliness and convenience'.

The people of Cambridgeshire were beginning to take a pride in their
Hospital and subscription income increased so that from 1804 to 1808

receipts comfortably exceeded expenditure. An addition to the traditional sources of income – subscriptions, church collections, dividends – was the cash paid by the public for the use of the baths. This brought in £11.13s. in 1805, and more in the following years. Legacies and donations, no longer needed to meet current expenses, were regularly invested in the Public Funds. In 1806 the subscription income was the highest in the history of the Hospital. Some legacies and donations were designated for specific purposes. Mr Merrill's legacy of £300 in 1806 provided the Hospital with 'handsome stone piers and an iron pallisade towards the street'. The Paving Commissioners gave £40 to complete the work. In the same year 'R.W.' gave £20 to establish a Samaritan fund to help patients financially when they were ready for discharge from Hospital.

There had been an increasingly humane approach to patients' social problems. In 1805, for example,[9] the Board ordered the discharge of William Richards 'because medical assistance can be of no use to him'. A week later,[10] the Board ordered 'that he be moved upstairs for the present and that letters be written to the parish of his mother'. The Matron and Apothecary were asked to find suitable lodgings for him in the town and to move him to them if his Physician, Dr Ingle, approved. Richards was moved to lodgings and the Board[11] approved the payment of 15s. a week for maintenance and lodgings.

It was no doubt this and similar episodes which prompted 'R.W.' to make his gift. The Governors were reluctant to approve the scheme as they feared it might divert donations from the general fund.[12] However, they were clearly in favour in principle of the proposed fund, since they suggested, as an alternative, an independent Samaritan's Society to relieve 'distressed objects discharged from the Hospital, the gaols or the Spinning House'. They eventually agreed that the interest on R.W.'s donation be applied as he had requested, and that donations and subscriptions to augment the fund might be received under the same general conditions. They further agreed that a Visitor or Visitors be appointed for enquiring into the merits of any case proposals for relief, and to report the same to the Weekly Board. These recommendations were adopted by the next Quarterly Court, and the Minutes of subsequent Weekly Meetings occasionally refer to patients who were assisted – 'a distressed Irishman' in 1813[13] and another in 1814[14] were each given £1, and in 1818 'a Waterloo man' 10s.[15] Some patients were considered 'not a proper object of charity'.[16]

In 1809 Hospital expenses were over £82 in excess of income, but the auditors were not unduly concerned;[17] the druggist's bill of over £240 was

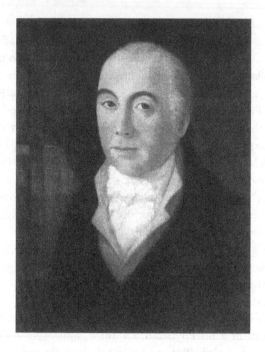

Fig. 11. John Bowtell, bookbinder of Cambridge. Benefactor, 1809.

more than £130 higher than in the previous year. This was due to the increased prevalence of ague (malaria), and over £100 had been spent on bark alone (quinine). The Treasurer was able to continue to increase the Hospital's investment in the Public Funds, and he did so again in 1810 when the deficit on the current account was over £90.

During the next ten years the current account was only twice in the red (in 1812 and 1813) and by 1820 the Hospital's investment in Public Funds was £25,400.[18] This sound investment policy made the Hospital relatively less dependent on other sources of income, but the financial situation had become by 1817 sufficiently secure to justify planning a programme of reconstruction and expansion, only as a result of the Bowtell bequest.

John Bowtell (1753–1813) was a bookbinder and bookseller, in business at 32 Trinity Street. He was also an antiquary, whose valuable collection of manuscripts is now the property of Downing College. In 1809 he gave the Hospital 3% Consols to the value of £100, and, by his will in 1814, further shares to the value of £7,000, about half of his estate.[19] This bequest marked a turning point in the development of the Hospital.

Visiting medical staff

Reference has already been made to the very poor attendance of Governors at Weekly Meetings, particularly between 1790 and 1802. The same Committee, which during May and June 1802 examined the Hospital's financial affairs, attempted also to reform the system of management. The change they introduced was the principle of Select Governors,[20] who were to be appointed annually. These eighteen Governors agreed to attend the Weekly Board in rotation.

Robert Gee, who had been appointed Secretary in 1802, continued in this office until his death in 1817. The very heavy increase in his work as a result of the fund-raising activities, was recognised in 1809, when his annual salary was increased to 20 guineas.

The changes introduced by the 1802 Committee covered also the medical staff[21] and restricted the number of Physicians and Surgeons to three of each. When Martin Davy resigned as Physician in 1803 he was therefore not replaced, nor was Gregory, the Surgeon, when he left Cambridge later in the same year. The Rule was again invoked in 1805 when Dr Richard Sill's offer of his services as a Physician was declined. However, Harwood's repeated absenteeism was clearly still resented, for the same Court[22] ordered that the routine printed reminder be sent to Harwood 'when it shall be his turn to attend at the Hospital and examine the patients previous to their admission'. Harwood took the hint, for later in the year his name reappeared in rotation as Physician of the week. Harwood was, in his lifetime, and remains today, a controversial character. In 1813 the Governors present[23] unanimously carried a vote of thanks to Sir Busick Harwood 'for his kind and unwearied attention to the best interests of the charity for the period of thirty years'. The same meeting carried a vote of thanks to Dr Ingle 'for his kind assistance on many occasions when Sir Busick was unable to attend in his own person'.

Harwood's death in November 1814 created a vacancy for a Physician. There were two candidates, both local men. Although John Haviland was proposed by Pennington, he was defeated in the ballot by 105 votes to 67, by Woodhouse of Caius College.[24] John Thomas Woodhouse (1780–1845)[25] was born at Norwich, the son of a woollen draper. He entered Caius College as a pensioner in December, 1798. He was admitted M.B. in 1804 and proceeded M.D. in 1810. He was a Fellow of Caius College from 1804 until his death and held at various times the offices of steward,

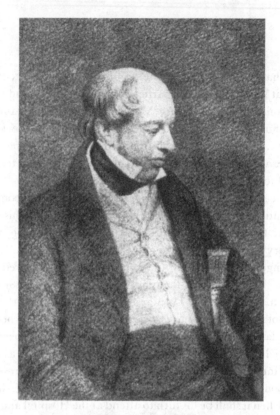

Fig. 12. John Haviland, Regius Professor of Physic, 1817–1851.
From a print in the Wellcome Institute of the History of Medicine.
By courtesy of 'The Wellcome Trustees'.

registrar, bursar, Greek lecturer, and Hebrew lecturer. He remained a
bachelor and lived in college, but he was also in practice as a physician. In
1841 he published 'An Essay on Single Vision'. He was a talented artist
and had been a pupil of Opie of Norwich. He is said to have been of
eccentric habits and to have had a special taste for cock-fighting. His elder
brother, Robert, of the same college, was a distinguished mathematician.
John Woodhouse appears to have attended the Hospital regularly but to
have been otherwise little involved in the affairs of the Hospital. He
resigned in February 1828.

It is difficult to understand why the Governors preferred Woodhouse to
Haviland, but Haviland did not have long to wait as Pennington's death
in January 1817 created another vacancy for a Physician. The two
candidates were Cornwallis Hewitt and John Haviland.

Cornwallis Hewitt (1787–1841), of Downing College, had received the University licence to practise medicine (M.L.) in 1814 in which year he was elected Downing Professor of Medicine. He is notable as the only holder of that Chair not to be a Physician to Addenbrooke's Hospital. He practised in London and in Cambridge and was from 1825 Physician to St George's Hospital. If the editor of *The Lancet* is to be believed, Addenbrooke's had a fortunate escape. *The Lancet* published many scurrilous attacks on Hewitt's professional competence, particularly in obstetrics. A report of one of his cases[26] was introduced as a case 'which could scarce do credit to the most stupid apothecary's apprentice in the Kingdom'.

Haviland (1785–1851) was elected by 115 votes to 44.[27] He was a man of a very different stamp and both the Cambridge Medical School and the Hospital owe a great deal to his work to reform the teaching curriculum and to improve and expand the facilities of the Hospital. He was born in Bridgewater, Somerset, the only son of John Haviland, surgeon, and was at school at Winchester. In 1803 he entered Caius College, but the following year migrated to St John's College. He graduated B.A. in 1807 and spent two years at Edinburgh, and then three at St Bartholomew's Hospital. He had been elected a Fellow of St John's College in 1810, when he proceeded M.A. In 1812 he was granted the University licence to practise medicine and he soon acquired a large and lucrative practice. In 1814 he was appointed Professor of Anatomy but resigned this Chair in 1817 when he was elected Regius Professor of Physic. He was a man of great earnestness and high character, an excellent physician of sound judgement.[28] His contributions to the development of medical teaching are considered elsewhere (see p. 235). He resigned as Physician to the Hospital in 1839, for reasons of health, and in that year he also gave up his private practice, but he continued as Regius Professor until his death in 1851. He was buried at Fen Ditton, where he had acquired considerable property.

The changes in the surgical staff during this period were less significant, but aroused more local controversy. Bond resigned in March 1813. There were three applicants for the appointment: Abbott, Lestourgeon and Headley. An unsuccessful attempt was made to rescind the Rule limiting the number of Surgeons to three.[29] Abbott and Headley would not accept a ballot and Lestourgeon was therefore elected.

Charles Lestourgeon (1779–1853) was perhaps not the ideal surgeon for a hospital with growing scientific pretensions. He had been apprenticed to a surgeon in Westminster and had then served for some years as an assistant surgeon to the 1st Regiment of the Dragoons. He resigned his commission as he lacked the influence at headquarters to secure his promotion. By 1807 he was in practice in Edmonton. In 1808 or 1809 he moved to Cambridge in partnership with Thomas Verney Okes. He had a genial manner and enjoyed a reputation as a gynaecologist.[30]

In May 1817, T.V. Okes and Frederic Thackeray sent in their resignations. Okes was retiring after nearly 40 years as a surgeon in the hope that his son would succeed him – 'if my son should be thought worthy of the same confidence, it will be one of the greatest consolations I can receive during the end of a life which has been and always will be devoted to the public service'.[31] Thackeray resigned because he had recently been granted the University licence to practise medicine; he asked that he should be considered if a vacancy should occur 'in the medical department'.

No fewer than 215 Governors attended the Special General Court on 30 May, and 60 ladies voted by proxy. As there were two vacancies to fill, each Governor could vote for two of the three candidates. John Okes received 222 votes, Alexander Scott Abbott 148; the unfortunate Charles Headley, with 130 votes, was again defeated.

John Okes (1793–1870) was apprenticed to his father, but without formal indentures, and in 1818 joined his father and Lestourgeon as a partner. In 1826, while continuing in practice, he entered Sidney Sussex College as a Fellow Commoner, and in 1832 was M.B. In 1842 he became M.R.C.S. and was admitted F.R.C.S. the following year. He was very successful in practice, and for many years lived at Cherry Hinton Hall.

Alexander Scott Abbott (c. 1790–1843) was a son of William Abbott, surgeon, of Needham Market. He was a pupil of John Abernethy at St Bartholomew's Hospital and was admitted M.R.C.S. in December 1810. He started to practise at Cambridge very soon after this. He was actively involved in municipal affairs and was Mayor of Cambridge in 1823 and 1829. He gave evidence in 1833 to the Commissioners appointed to enquire into the state of the Corporation. He admitted that there were abuses and proved that he had attempted to remedy some of these; it seems that his own hands were clean.

The last Resident Apothecaries

As we have seen, the work of the Resident Apothecary combined the duties of house surgeon and pharmacist. As a result of the increase in the

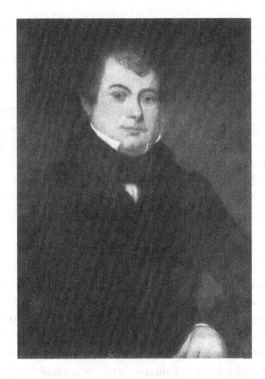

Fig. 13. Alexander Scott Abbott. Surgeon to Addenbrooke's.
1817–1843.

number of patients attending the Hospital, and the evolution and progressive separation of the two professions in the country generally, Charles Yorke in 1816 was the last man to be described simply as Resident Apothecary. His successor was Apothecary and House Surgeon and from 1840 the two appointments were separated.

In 1802, Joseph Gray was still Apothecary and he continued to hold the office until his death in 1808. During Gray's last illness, and for a few weeks after his death, a Mr Gill acted as Apothecary. On 2 May 1808, Samuel Brown Stevens was elected Apothecary. He resigned five years later because the Physicians were dissatisfied with him. The post was advertised and seven applications were received; three of these were considered by the General Quarterly Court in October. As was usual when the agenda included an election to the staff, the Court was well attended, and the President of the Hospital, the Earl of Hardwicke, was in the Chair. Isaiah Dick of Bury, favoured by the medical staff, was proposed by Pennington and seconded by Harwood, but Thomas Bell of Newport, proposed by Hardwicke himself, was elected by a majority of ten votes. About three years later Bell resigned and the meeting to elect his successor followed a similar pattern.

Charles Dancer Yorke was elected. He was proposed by the very influential Sir John Mortlock. Yorke was the family name of the Earls of Hardwicke, but a relationship has not been established. Yorke was admitted L.S.A. in May 1816, shortly before he was appointed. He was Apothecary to the Hospital until 1830. He died in 1838 and is described in his will as 'surgeon'.

Matron and nurses

The unfortunate Mrs Williams was succeeded as Matron by Miss Charlotte Whybrow. She gained 46 of the 87 votes cast for the seven candidates; her nearest rival only 15. Mrs (Miss) Whybrow proved to be a conscientious and efficient Matron. On several occasions she was thanked by the Governors for 'her general good conduct and economy in the management of the affairs of the Hospital'. She regularly received her gratuity, and in October, 1810, this was increased to £20 a year.

The scanty references to her activities emphasise that she was, above all, the housekeeper. In March, 1818, for example, she was ordered to arrange that 'such white washing be done in the House as may be necessary' and many similar duties concerning furnishing and maintenance were her responsibility. When she retired in 1834 she was given an annuity of £60 for life 'on account of the length of her service and the exemplary manner in which, according to the unanimous opinion of the Governors and the Medical Officers of the Institution, she has invariably discharged the duties of her office'.

Until 1824 there were still only four nurses, one for each ward.[32] In January, 1814, their wages were increased to £9 a year. The Minutes are free from criticisms of their conduct, and most continued to serve the Hospital until they retired. On retiring some nurses chose to continue to live in the Hospital, receiving a pension of 1 guinea a year. Others left the Hospital and received 2 guineas a quarter for life.

In addition to the nurses there were nightwatchers, who were engaged as required.

Table 2. *Subscribing parishes, 1802–1825*

	Cambridge	Cambridgeshire	Huntingdonshire	Essex	Hertfordshire	Suffolk
1802	12	45	3			
1805	12	46	4	1	1	1
1810	12	49	5			1
1815	12	60	9			3
1820	12	58	11		1	3
1825	13	54	9		1	3

Patients

The first quarter of the nineteenth century saw a gradual improvement in the Hospital's financial position, and an increased demand for its services, as reflected in the growing number of subscribers, parishes and individuals, from an expanding area which soon included many parishes in Huntingdonshire, some in Suffolk, and some in Hertfordshire (see Table 2). The average bed occupancy was 25 when this figure was first recorded in 1803; it first exceeded 30 in 1810 and was 46 in 1820. However, as in its earlier decades, the men's wards were almost always more crowded than the women's wards. In 1805 the Hospital warned subscribers[33] that no more men could be admitted until some had been discharged. The pressure on beds had become even heavier since 1817, in which year the Court[34] appointed a Committee to 'enquire into the necessity of enlarging the Hospital and the most proper means of effecting the same, if thought requisite'. This Committee set in motion the planning and negotiations which were to result, after many legal impediments, in the extensive reconstruction and enlargement of the Hospital, completed seven years later.

Diet

A copy of early nineteenth-century diet in the Hospital (see the Table of Diets, pp. 90–1) has been found among the records[35] and the nutrient values appear[36] to be surprisingly close to those recommended today, so far as can be determined.

1802

THE TABLE OF DIETS[35]

Subject to the occasional alteration of the Physicians, or Surgeons

MILK DIET	FULL DIET
SUNDAY	**SUNDAY**
Breakfast, a pint of milk-pottage,	Breakfast, a pint of milk-pottage,
Dinner, flour pudding, with half an ounce of butter.	Dinner, half a pound of boiled mutton, or beef,
Supper, a pint of milk-pottage, milk-gruel, or broth.	Supper, a pint of broth, milk-pottage or gruel.
MONDAY,	**MONDAY,**
Breakfast, a pint of water-gruel, with half an ounce of butter,	Breakfast, a pint of water-gruel, with half an ounce of butter,
Dinner, rice pudding,	Dinner, half a pound of mutton or beef,
Supper, a pint of milk-pottage, milk-gruel, or broth.	Supper, a pint of milk-pottage, gruel, or broth.
TUESDAY,	**TUESDAY,**
Breakfast, Dinner, Supper, } The same as on Sunday.	Breakfast, Dinner, Supper, } The same as on Sunday.
WEDNESDAY,	**WEDNESDAY**
Breakfast, a pint of milk-pottage, or milk-gruel,	Breakfast, a pint of milk-pottage, or milk-gruel,
Dinner, rice pudding,	Dinner, rice pudding,
Supper, two ounces of cheese,	Supper, two ounces of cheese.
THURSDAY,	**THURSDAY**
Breakfast, Dinner, Supper, } The same as on Sunday.	Breakfast, Dinner, Supper, } The same as on Sunday.

FRIDAY,

Breakfast, a pint of water-gruel, and half an ounce of butter,
Dinner, rice-milk, or rice-pudding,
Supper, one ounce of butter,

FRIDAY,

Breakfast, a pint of water-gruel, with half an ounce of butter,
Dinner, rice-pudding,
Supper, one ounce of butter.

SATURDAY

Breakfast,
Dinner, } The same as on Sunday.
Supper,
　Vegetables every day at Dinner,
A loaf a head every day weighing 14 ounces.
Small-beer, a pint a day.

SATURDAY,

Breakfast,
Dinner, } The same as on Sunday.
Supper,
　Vegetables every day at Dinner,
A loaf every day to each weighing as do.
Small-beer, a quart.

A single Patient consumes in a Week:

on MILK DIET				on FULL DIET			
Meat,	—	—	none	Meat,	—	—	2½ pound
Bread,	—	—	98 ounces	Bread,	—	—	98 ounces
Butter,	—	—	4 ounces	Butter,	—	—	2 ounces
Milk,	—	—	8 pints	Milk,	—	—	4 pints
Cheese,	—	—	2 ounces	Cheese,	—	—	2 ounces.

The allowances to the Porter, Nurses, and to each of the other Servants kept in the House, is as follows:

One pound of meat to each every day.
Fourteen ounces of bread, or a common patient's loaf.
Ten ounces of butter per week.
Eleven ounces of cheese per do.
Vegetables every day at dinner.
Porter and Nurses, a pint and a half of ale every day.
Other Servants, half a pint every day.

Each Servant consumes in a Week,			
Meat,	—	—	7 pounds
Bread,	—	—	98 ounces
Butter,	—	—	10 ounces
Cheese,	—	—	11 ounces

By modern standards a good daily intake for a moderately active healthy male aged 35–64[37] would be:

Energy   2,750 kilocalories
Protein   69 g
Calcium   500 mg
Iron   10 mg

On the Full Diet in 1802 a patient would obtain:

Energy   2,272 kilocalories
Protein   118.9 g
Calcium   1,048 mg
Iron   17 mg;

and on the Milk Diet:

Energy   1,930 kilocalories
Protein   75.7 g
Calcium   1,340 mg
Iron   12.5 mg

therefore the patients would probably be better fed in hospital at that time than they were at home and the good food and the rest may well have made a major contribution to recovery.

The daily intake for porters and nurses on the information available has been worked out[36] as:

Energy   2,780 kilocalories
Protein   199.7 g
Calcium   627 mg
Iron   25.2 mg,

which was generous particularly with regard to protein intake. The fat content of this diet would also be high. The actual nutrient intake would probably be in excess of levels quoted above as no indication is given of what cereals or milk were consumed.

The vitamin content of all the diets is difficult to assess as insufficient detail about the vegetables and fruits consumed is available.

Expansion: the new wings

The Committee appointed in June 1817, to consider the need to enlarge the Hospital and the means of doing so, consisted of P.S. Kelty, the Revd James Hicks, Mr Milner, and the Revd Mr Chapman. This Committee, with Hicks as Chairman, co-opted members of the medical staff, Mr

Humfrey the architect, S.P. Beales and John Finch. They presented their report to the Quarterly Court in October.[38]

They were of the opinion that it was necessary to enlarge the Hospital to provide in particular 'a room for operations to be performed in, more accommodation for patients, more accommodation for Physicians and Surgeons when they receive and examine the patients', and also a room for religious worship. The Committee believed that the Bowtell legacy could be applied to these purposes and had optimistically requested Humfrey to prepare a plan. The Court approved a proposal that an application be made to the Chancery Court to establish whether the legacy could indeed be so applied, and ordered that the plan be deposited in the Hospital Chest 'till wanted'.

The negotiations with the Chancery Court were protracted. The Master in Chancery did not approve a proposal that the Governors should be allowed to apply the legacy as if it had been bequeathed without restrictions. The Master's report was read to a Special Court in January 1820.[39] A large committee was appointed to consider plans to be submitted for Counsel's opinion.

The Committee reported back about a year later.[40] Of their proposals the Court agreed that the following should be submitted to the Chancery Court by their Counsel, Mr Bell:

1st. Surgical Cases as distinguished from Medical Cases.
2nd. Building a Ward for the reception of patients applying for vaccination.
3rd. Building a Ward for the reception of Persons labouring under personal deformity and capable of being relieved by machinery or other means.
4th. Building a Ward for the reception of contagious cutaneous patients.
5th. Building a Ward for convalescents.

It was further agreed that, should the Court of Chancery reject all these proposals, Mr Bell was 'to suggest to the Court the propriety of a Lunatic Asylum to be erected upon ground belonging to the Hospital; but at a short distance from the same'.

Mr Pemberton, who had accepted financial responsibility for the application to the Court of Chancery,[41] was requested to obtain for presentation to that Court, affidavits showing the objections to the admission of women in labour for delivery in the Hospital. Bowtell's will had left £7,000 worth of stock to Addenbrooke's 'to be by them applied in enlarging the said Hospital, if necessary, for the purpose of receiving

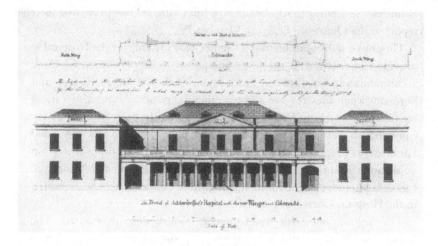

Fig. 14. Suggestion for the alteration of the front of the hospital.
Architect's drawing, October 1823.

persons of other descriptions than those of sick patients, such as poor
married women during their confinement, or otherwise, as they shall see
fit and advisable'.[42]

By April[43] 1823, the Master in Chancery's report, confirmed by the
Court of Chancery, was finally received. The report approved the first,
second, third and fifth proposals, but defined the fifth more precisely as 'a
Ward for Convalescents who under the present regulations of the Hospital
are discharged when cured, but from weakness are disabled from maintaining themselves and are thereby exposed to the danger of a relapse'.

A committee was appointed to consider the best means of applying the
legacy within the terms of the Chancery report. This Committee reported
the following month.[44] They recommended that wings two storeys high,
measuring 40 feet by 31 feet, should be erected on the north and south
sides of the existing Hospital, to provide four new wards. The report and
Mr Charles Humfrey's plans were adopted provided the cost of erecting
the building did not exceed £3,150. The Committee was 'reappointed to
carry their report into execution'. This Committee wasted no time. In
June[45] they reported that they had accepted the estimate of Messrs
William Bell, Charles Asby and Thomas Jonson of Cambridge, amounting to £2,785.5s.0d. The Governors gave their approval and requested
Humfrey to prepare a plan of a colonnade to be erected in front of the
Hospital (Fig. 14). His plan was accepted;[46] the cost of the portico was to

be covered by 'such part of the Volunteers' Subscription Fund as may be given to the Hospital'.

There are few references to the progress of the new buildings. It is possible that the Minutes of the Committee supervising the erection of the new wings were recorded in a separate volume which has not survived. The Committee's long report to the Governors in November 1824[47] indicated that they had met frequently. Additional expenses had been incurred, partly because changes had been made in the internal plan and partly because structural defects in the original building had come to light, and repairs to the existing drains and sewers were found necessary. On the advice of the medical staff, six rather than two water closets had been installed and a laboratory had been constructed. The total expenditure, excluding the colonnade, had been £4,155.16s.7½d.

The cost of the new wings, the laboratory and the water closets were paid out of Bowtell's bequest, as was the cost of furnishing the new wings. The extra expenses were paid out of the General Fund, except for the cost of the colonnade. The subscriptions received from the Volunteer Fund amounted to £469. The Governors decided that the rest of the £666.4s.8½d. for the colonnade should be raised by public subscription.

Amongst the defects discovered in the old building was the poor state of the roof. When the roof was repaired in 1825[48] some structural alterations were made which must have changed the appearance of the Hospital. Slate replaced tiles and the roof was lowered to avoid reducing the height of the upper rooms, and the chimneys were ordered to be removed or lowered.

There were no other structural changes until the next decade, but the Governors, with an eye to further developments, lost no opportunity of acquiring adjacent properties, which they let on favourable terms if they were not immediately required for Hospital purposes.

~ I I ~

Humphry and Paget join the medical staff

The resident medical staff

In 1824 the extensions to the Hospital made it possible to provide the Apothecary with a new and larger pharmacy. Later that year it was agreed[1] that 'in consequence of the increase in Business falling on the Apothecary' he should be allowed to take an apprentice. Accommodation would be provided for the apprentice by partitioning off a room in the attic.[2] He would pay a premium of £50 a year for five years, of which £20 would cover the cost of board and lodging. His father should covenant 'to find him clothing apparel and washing'.[3]

The first apprentice, Arthur Wellington Thurnall, served a term of six years and formally wrote his thanks to the Governors and the Medical Gentlemen.

Charles Yorke resigned as Apothecary in June 1830. The salary of the House Surgeon and Apothecary was increased from £50 to £80 and the post was advertised. Three of five candidates attended for interview, and George Johnson of Cambridge was appointed. He had recently qualified L.S.A. from St Bartholomew's Hospital. Johnson held the combined post for ten years, and continued as House Surgeon only for a further four years after the posts of House Surgeon and Dispenser were separated in 1840. The year before he left the Hospital he took the additional qualification of M.R.C.S. and set up as a general practitioner in St Andrew's Street, Cambridge.

In 1831, William Paley, son of the Revd Edmund Paley of Easingworth, Yorkshire, was appointed as Johnson's apprentice on the same terms as Thurnall, but the Hospital's annual share of the premium was increased to £30. Johnson was allowed to take a second apprentice in 1835 and Edmund, the son of the Revd W. Metcalf of Fowlmere, was accepted on the same general terms. In June 1836, Master William Clarence was taken on to replace Paley whose term would soon expire. It appears that this overlapping of apprentices was arranged, at least in the case of Clarence,[4] to allow the apprentice to attend lectures in London during his final year. This may indeed have been the regular practice. In 1838,[5] after the acceptance of Henry Mitchell as an apprentice, it appears that there may have been for a time as many as three apprentices.

When the posts of House Surgeon and Dispenser were finally separated in 1840, it was ordered[6] that in future the House Surgeon should not take more than one apprentice at one time. The annual premium would be raised to £80, of which half would be paid to the Hospital. A committee was appointed to review the applications for the apprenticeship, the duties of the apprentice and the advisability of establishing a new post of Dispensing Assistant.

Johnson Kaye Baines was accepted as apprentice. The rules and regulations for the House Apprentice were approved in October.[7] He was not to be allowed to have or to use a key to any of the gates of the Hospital, and he was not to leave the Hospital without the consent of the House Surgeon. 'If at any time he should be in a state of intoxication in the Hospital he should be reported to the Weekly Board, and if such conduct be persisted in, be liable to be dismissed'.

Henry Mitchell was elected House Surgeon in 1844. He was the first of several former apprentices to hold this appointment. The rules regulating the duties of the House Surgeon were amended.[8] It is interesting that although a Dispenser was now employed, the House Surgeon was still responsible for dispensing the medicines 'with the assistance of the Dispenser', and that he had to keep a daily account of all goods delivered for the use of the dispensary.

The next apprentice, William Swann Daniel, appointed in 1846, was, like three of his predecessors, a parson's son. We hear of him again in April 1847, 'when a complaint of inattention was laid against him', but a week later[9] Dr Bond complained on behalf of the medical staff that the House Surgeon and Dispenser had been negligent generally in performing their duties. They were called before the Governors and warned by the Chairman, Lord Godolphin, that the matter would be brought up again in a month unless there had been a considerable improvement. Presumably this improvement took place for we next hear of Mitchell on 14 July, when he complained that the porter had three times refused to pump up water into the surgery. The porter was suspended for one week and was reprimanded. A week later he was dismissed for bribing patients with half a gallon of beer disguised as cold tea, to do the pumping for him.

Despite his lapse earlier in the year, Mitchell was well thought of. In December,[10] he was given permission to read with private pupils in his room. He continued to train his apprentices. Percy Lionel Rawlings, son of a solicitor in Market Harborough, was appointed in January 1849.[11] Mitchell was allowed also to accept an outdoor pupil for a premium of £20. The pupils he coached in his room are not named. They were presumably apprentices to local practitioners or medical students of the University. Mitchell's resignation in March 1852 was accepted with regret.

Mitchell's successor as House Surgeon was Edmund Carver (1824–1904). He was born at Melbourn, Cambridgeshire, where his father was schoolmaster. He was apprenticed to William Mann, surgeon, of Royston, from 1841 to 1844. He then became a student at University College Hospital and qualified M.R.C.S. 1848, L.S.A. 1849. He was a House Surgeon to Robert Liston and he also worked under Erickson and Quain. He spent a year in a mining practice in Nantyglo before coming to Addenbrooke's. He was already a man of some experience, such as the duties of the post required. As well as being the only qualified resident, with care of both medical and surgical cases, he was also resident anaesthetist (the introduction of anaesthetics at Addenbrooke's in 1847 is described on p. 139), and was responsible for all post-mortem examinations. Humphry chose him also as his demonstrator in anatomy. He took over Mitchell's apprentice, George Wallis, who had been appointed in 1851, and in 1855 accepted G.F. Holm as apprentice. Carver was also allowed to accept a number of outdoor pupils. In 1854 he became a member of St John's College and was thus able to keep University terms and become eligible to take the M.B. in 1859. Many further residents took advantage of this opportunity of securing a university degree. The Governors formally approved this policy in October 1859.[12]

Carver resigned in June 1859, as he had decided to practise in Cambridge. In 1866, however, he moved to Huntingdon as Surgeon to the County Hospital. George Wallis, formerly an apprentice to Mitchell and then to Carver, was elected Carver's successor as House Surgeon and Apothecary. The only other candidate was Carver's younger brother Eustace.

The Dispensary

The duties of Dispenser were separated from those of the House Surgeon in 1840, but the House Surgeon, who was still referred to as House

Surgeon and Apothecary, continued to have overall responsibility for the work of dispensing.

The Dispenser was to work from 10 a.m. to 3 p.m. on Monday, Wednesday, Thursday, and Saturday, for the salary of £30 per year. William Lyon, the first Dispenser to be appointed, resigned after a few weeks when his request that he might occasionally send his assistant in his place was rejected.[13] The post was advertised, offering 1 guinea a week for attendance daily (except Sundays) for five or six hours from 10 a.m. Smith Hurrell was appointed and carried out his duties to give 'general and great satisfaction' for four years. His successor, Mr Finch, at first attended only three times weekly, but he claimed that this caused great inconvenience to out-patients and asked to be allowed to attend on the same terms as Hurrell. This was agreed to as a temporary measure but was in fact allowed to continue for several years.

Although the Dispenser was employed to take over some of the dispensing, the ultimate responsibility for its accuracy and efficiency remained with the House Surgeon.

On 25 October 1854, the Governors received from the Revd William Cecil, Rector of Longstowe St Michael, a long letter in which he accused the Hospital of negligence and inhumanity. His complaints were specific and were supported by what appeared to be acceptable evidence. (His other complaints are discussed on p. 132.) Of the dispensary he wrote 'In the hurry and precipitation which takes place with the out-patients, Medicines are made up with a carelessness which makes them unfit for use.' The committee of enquiry set up to investigate the allegations did not challenge their truth. The Committee made many recommendations for improving the efficiency of the dispensary. However the quality of the dispensary was from time to time called into question, and Finch was called before the Governors in March 1869, when he promised that he would in future dispense all medicines himself and not allow the surgery boy to do so.[14]

The visiting medical staff

The Hospital staff in 1825 was, with the exception of John Haviland, totally undistinguished. Ingle's resignation in December 1826 provided the opportunity to strengthen the staff by electing Frederic Thackeray, who was proposed by Lord Godolphin, and seconded by John Mortlock, and was elected unanimously.

Thackeray was a popular and influential man.[15] He had entered as a Fellow Commoner at Emmanuel College in 1800, but in 1804 Pennington, as Regius Professor, had refused to allow him to keep an Act for a first degree in medicine, on the grounds that the Elizabethan statutes excluded him because he was in professional practice. The controversy which followed this refusal aroused intense interest in the University, and much sympathy was expressed for Thackeray, but Pennington's interpretation of the statutes was not rescinded until 1815. Later in that year Thackeray took the M.B., in 1817 the M.L., and in 1820 the M.D. In 1817, he had resigned as Surgeon to the Hospital, but as a Governor he had continued to play an active part in the Hospital's affairs. In 1819 he was one of the earliest Fellows of the recently founded Cambridge Philosophical Society, and served as its treasurer from 1825 to 1834. For a number of years from 1835, he was chosen a member of the Caput, the autocratic body any member of which could prevent a Grace from reaching the Senate. The Caput consisted[16] of the Vice Chancellor, a doctor from each of the faculties of Theology, Law and Medicine, and one Regent and one non-Regent Master of Arts.

Thackeray's high standing in the town and in the University enabled him to give influential support to Haviland's endeavours to improve the standards of the Medical School, the quality of the Hospital staff, and the amenities of the Hospital.

In February 1828, Dr Woodhouse resigned. For some reason no immediate steps were taken to appoint a successor, and Haviland and Thackeray agreed to undertake Woodhouse's duties.[17] Nine months later John Barthrop Roberts, M.L. 1828, of Corpus Christi College, was elected unopposed,[18] but he resigned in June 1830, as, so he said, he had decided to practise at Bishops Stortford. He may have done so for a time, but in 1835 he was ordained priest and from 1837 to 1879 he was the incumbent of livings first in Kent and later in Northumberland. In October Henry Hayles Bond was elected to succeed Roberts.[19]

Henry John Hayles Bond (1801–1883) was the son of the Revd William Bond, rector of Wheatacre, Norfolk, former Fellow of Caius College and headmaster of the Perse School, Cambridge, and his wife Martha, daughter of Richard Hayles, surgeon. He was admitted pensioner of Corpus Christi College in 1819. He studied medicine at Cambridge, Edinburgh and Paris, and in London. In 1827, when he was a clinical clerk at St Bartholomew's Hospital, under Peter Mere Latham, he was one of the first in this country to practise auscultation.[20] He was M.B. in 1825 and he took the University licence to practise medicine (M.L.) in 1829 and proceeded M.D. in 1831. He soon acquired a large practice from his home at 56 Trumpington Street, for he was a sound and conscientious physician. He was a retiring man whose shyness made him appear rather abrupt, but he was sincere, considerate and kind-hearted. He succeeded Haviland as Regius Professor of Physic in 1851. His lectures were comprehensive and were regularly delivered. His dislike of ostentation and his refusal to publish more than a syllabus of his lectures, and a few hospital case reports, perhaps account for the lack of recognition he has received for his contributions to the development of the Medical School during his 21 years as Regius Professor. He was the first representative of the University on the General Medical Council from 1858 to 1863. He was not by nature an active reformer, and the initiative had passed into the hands of Paget some years before he actually succeeded Bond.[21]

In 1839 Haviland resigned for reasons of health, and also gave up his practice, but he remained Regius Professor and was active on Hospital committees until his death. He was succeeded as Physician to the Hospital by George Paget.

George Edward Paget (1809–1892) is considered in the next chapter. He shared Haviland's ambitions for the Medical School and the Hospital and he must have played a leading part in the events of 1842, which created a vacancy on the surgical staff for G.M. Humphry.

On 24 August,[22] the medical staff gave notice of their intention to propose that in future appointments to the staff should be for a limited period, at the end of which the Physician or Surgeon should be eligible for re-election. At the General Court on 3 October, before this proposal was discussed, Lestourgeon, Okes and Abbott, submitted their resignations which were formerly accepted. The motion was then proposed by H.J. Adeane, seconded by Christopher Pemberton and carried by a majority of 34 to 14. It was then agreed that the term of future appointments should be 12 years.

Elaborate arrangements were then made for the election of the Surgeons. An attempt was made to forestall manoeuvres which could be applied to the disadvantage of some candidates, by deciding the election, on this occasion only, on a single ballot. Each Governor had three votes, only one of which might be given to any one candidate. Each ballot paper must bear the name of the candidate and the Governor's signature. The

Special Court met on 31 October at 12 o'clock at the Hospital and at once adjourned to the Great Room at the Eagle Inn; the poll was kept open until 5 o'clock when it was closed with the written consent of all the candidates. Two candidates withdrew before the poll. The votes cast for the remaining six were as follows:

C. Lestourgeon	280
J. Hammond	266
G.M. Humphry	221
J.L. Sudbury	103
A.W. Thurnall	85
E. Knowles	20

At the adjourned Special Court on 2 November, Lestourgeon, Hammond and Humphry were declared elected. The convincing majorities secured by the three successful candidates (even Humphry's votes outnumbered the total cast for the three unsuccessful candidates), are evidence of the influence on the Governors of Haviland, Thackeray and Paget. It seems likely that one of the principal objectives of these three reformers was to elect G.M. Humphry to the surgical staff. Humphry was very young and had only just qualified. His potential had been recognised by Paget's brother James, who had recommended him, and he, as well as Bond, Haviland, Thackeray, Paget and Clark, the Professor of Anatomy, had all trained at St Bartholomew's Hospital.

It had been the custom to appoint surgeons from among the general practitioners actively established in the town. Each candidate was supported by such of the Governors as were his patients, and also often by Governors whose votes followed the lead of those who wielded political power and patronage. Lestourgeon was an obvious choice. He was the son and partner of one of the retiring surgeons, and the partner also of John Okes, brother of Richard Okes, Fellow and later provost of King's College. His chances must have been even further improved by his marriage in 1841 to the eldest daughter of Ebenezer Foster of Anstey Hall, Trumpington, a very active and influential Governor. The Okes/Lestourgeon Trinity Street practice numbered among its patients many of the most senior members of the University.

Josiah Hammond, too, was an obvious choice. He had local connections; he had qualified about ten years previously and was well known in practice in Market Hill. He was proposed by the Master of Clare Hall and seconded by the Revd F.A. Brown.

According to traditional values, both Sudbury and Thurnall should have had a better chance than Humphry. Both had been in practice at Cambridge for about ten years. Thurnall's claim was perhaps particularly strong in that he had served as Apothecary's apprentice to the Hospital from 1825 to 1830. His name was proposed by the Master of Peterhouse.

Humphry was proposed by the Master of Trinity College, William Whewell, and seconded by H.J. Adeane, a Babraham landowner who had proposed the motion that appointments to the staff should be for a limited period. Whewell's interest in Humphry may well have been stimulated by Humphry's elder brother, William Gilson Humphry, who was a Fellow of Trinity College, having been senior classic in 1837.

The election brought onto the staff, in Lestourgeon and Hammond, two competent men of at least average ability, and in Humphry one of the most outstanding British surgeons of the nineteenth century, distinguished as anatomist, pathologist, administrator and reformer.

In March 1843, Bond and Thackeray submitted their resignations. Bond pointed out that the letter of the new bye-law did not apply to him, but that as he had taken an active part in introducing it he wished to conform with its spirit. However, Bond and Thackeray both agreed to the request of the Governors that they should withdraw their resignations. In the future, all resignations offered under the 1842 rule were rejected.

Charles Lestourgeon (1808–1891) entered Trinity College in 1824 as a pupil of Dr William Whewell. He was B.A. in 1828 as fifteenth Wrangler. He then studied at St Bartholomew's Hospital and in Paris, was M.R.C.S., L.S.A. in 1831, and M.A. and M.B. in 1833. He joined his father and John Okes in general practice at 34 Trinity Street. In 1843, he became one of the original F.R.C.S., in 1852 he moved to a large house, Howe Close, which he had built himself on the Huntingdon Road, and this was far enough from the centre of the city to lead to a progressive reduction in his professional work. But he was amiable and unambitious and well content to lend his support to the energetic Humphry.

Josiah Hammond (1803–1875) qualified L.S.A. in 1832 from St Bartholomew's Hospital. He was elected one of the original F.R.C.S. in 1843.

George Murray Humphry (1820–1896) is considered in another chapter. For fifty years after his election his life and that of his colleague Paget were to be intimately involved with the development of the Hospital and of the Medical School.

After the excitement of 1842 there were no further changes until 1845 when Dr Thackeray resigned, and the special procedure followed in 1842 was again adopted for the election of his successor. The Special General Court[23] assembled in the Board Room but adjourned to the Operation Room 'for the quiet of the Hospital'. There were three candidates, for whom the Governors voted as follows: W.W. Fisher (130), W.H. Drosier (111), and J.H. Webster (52). Had a second ballot been allowed, Fisher might well have lost to Drosier, who was a Fellow of Caius College, the Master of which proposed him. He was a popular man and a great skater. He soon gave up practice but remained medical lecturer at Caius College for many years. J.H. Webster was the son of the Rector of St Botolph's Church, Cambridge. He had been clinical clerk to Bond at the Hospital and had been in practice in Cambridge for about a year, having qualified M.B. 1843, M.L. 1844.

William Webster Fisher (1793–1874) was certainly the best candidate. He had taken his M.D. in 1825 at Montpellier, where he was friendly with Auguste Comte. He was admitted at Trinity College in 1827, but migrated to Downing College in 1830. He was M.B. in 1834, in which year he was elected Fellow and Bursar of the College. In 1841 he was elected Downing Professor of Medicine, on which occasion *The Times* commented that his politics were anything but conservative and that he enjoyed a European reputation for his professional abilities. From 1842 he gave regular lectures, mainly on materia medica. He resigned as Physician in 1861 but continued to hold his Chair and to carry on a large practice until his death. His successor, as Physician, was Henry James Haviland, third son of John Haviland. He was the only candidate.

Henry Haviland (1825–1900) entered at Pembroke College in 1844 and continued his studies at Edinburgh and at St Bartholomew's Hospital. He was M.B. in 1849 and M.D. in 1854. He resigned in March 1853, as he planned to leave Cambridge (notices in the local press suggest that he probably left Cambridge after his marriage had run into difficulties).

~ 12 ~

Sir George Paget

The rise of the Cambridge Medical School during the nineteenth century to one of the largest and most distinguished in the United Kingdom, was, to a great extent, due to the efforts of George Paget and George Humphry.[1]

Paget (Fig. 15), who was to become the Regius Professor of Physic, was first on the scene and one of his greatest services to the School was when, with his brother James, he introduced Humphry into Cambridge. Humphry was to be Professor of Anatomy and then the first Professor of Surgery.

Paget, who was a Physician at Addenbrooke's for 45 years, should be remembered especially for introducing, in 1842, bedside examinations in clinical medicine, the first in the United Kingdom and a procedure which has since become universal; and also for being instrumental in establishing the Natural Sciences Tripos in the University in 1848, the first examinations being held in 1851.[2] His administrative successes were said[3] to have been 'by a combination of farsightedness, precision, social charm, eloquence and enthusiasm. At the same time he was a teacher and physican of the first rank.'

George Edward Paget was born on 22 December 1809, at Great Yarmouth, Norfolk, at that time a busy port. His father was Samuel Paget, a ship-owner and brewer, and his mother was Sarah Elizabeth Tolver. They had seventeen children and George was the seventh.

His childhood was overshadowed by the national anxiety about Napoleon and his son has written[4] that to the last year of his life he vividly remembered seeing the stage-coach come into Yarmouth with flags flying and the guard shouting the news about the battle of Waterloo.

George attended a day-school in the town and then at 14, following his two older brothers, was sent to Charterhouse; it was at that time the largest of English public schools but taught only the classics. George studied mathematics privately and consequently when the subject was introduced into the school following the remonstrance of one of the fathers, who was an influential banker, he was able to come out top of the

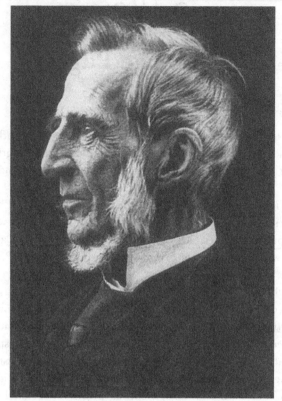

Fig. 15. Sir George Edward Paget (1809–1892). From a
photograph in the Wellcome Institute of the History of Medicine.
By courtesy of 'The Wellcome Trustees'.

initial examination. One of his school fellows was William Makepeace
Thackeray, who later shared rooms in the Inner Temple with Paget's
older brother Arthur Coyte, the prototype of a character in 'Esmond'.[2]

On leaving Charterhouse in 1827 he entered Gonville and Caius
College, Cambridge, again in Arthur's footsteps. He 'worked moderately
and rowed well',[4] but in his third year resolved to do better than predicted
in mathematics and was rewarded by being placed eighth Wrangler. The
following year he was elected a Fellow of his college and according to the
terms of the Fellowship began to study medicine. This was commenced in
Cambridge under the Regius Professorship of Dr Haviland and was
continued in Paris and at St Bartholomew's Hospital.

He returned to Cambridge and took his Bachelor of Medicine degree in
1833, the licence to practise in 1836, and Doctor of Medicine in 1838. He

was Fellow until 1851 and held many College offices, such as catechist (1834), bursar (1835–1838), steward (1839–1841) and registrar (1843). But for his marriage, upon which he had to vacate his Fellowship, he would probably have become Master.[2]

In 1839 he was elected Physician to Addenbrooke's Hospital in place of Dr Haviland who resigned. It may be surmised that he had many friends in Cambridge by this time who would vote for him, and his opponent in the election, Dr W.J. Bayne, Physician at Bury St Edmunds, ruefully withdrew from the encounter after discovering this. Exactly what his friends did is a matter for conjecture but a Hospital subscriber writing to the Editor of the *Cambridge Advertiser and Free Press*, 15 October[5] said: 'I am glad that by the retirement of Dr. Bayne there will be no contest for the office of Physician to Addenbrooke's Hospital, as such contests are usually of an exceedingly unpleasant character. I wished well to Dr. Paget, yet learnt with regret that some over-zeallous and most injudicious friends of that gentleman endavoured to give the election a political turn. I think I know enough of Dr. Paget to say that nothing could be more repugnant to his feelings – I am sure nothing could be more injurious to the best interest of this noble institution.' The correspondent continued by suggesting that there should be four or even five Physicians and Surgeons at the Hospital instead of the three of each permitted at that time.

In 1839 he also became a Fellow of the Royal College of Physicians of London.

Until his election to a medical Fellowship, Paget had not felt any inclination towards medicine,[2] yet he applied himself to it and after his marriage in 1851 to Clara, youngest daughter of the late Revd Thomas Fardell, LL.D. Cantab., Vicar of Sutton in the Isle of Ely, when he was released from many collegiate duties and had to vacate his rooms in college and became the first occupant of 2 St Peter's Terrace in the town, he is said to have pursued his profession as a consulting physician even more vigorously than before.[4]

He had a brother, James, younger by five years, who became a famous surgeon at St Bartholomew's Hospital, and is said rarely to have taken an important step in life without consulting George.[2] The two have been compared to William and John Hunter, who were also physician and surgeon but unlike the Hunters the Paget brothers remained close friends[6] throughout life. In 1842, the year Paget initiated clinical examinations for the final M.B., James and George brought 22-year-old George Murray Humphry from St Bartholomew's to Cambridge where he was elected the youngest hospital surgeon in the country, and able to aid George Paget in his work for the Hospital and the University.

In July 1851, Paget became Linacre lecturer at St John's College and was re-elected until 1872 when, being appointed Regius Professor, he resigned and was succeeded by J.B. Bradbury.[2] In 1855–6 he was President of the Cambridge Philosophical Society and in 1856 he was also elected a member of the first Council of the Senate under the Universities Act.[4] In 1863 he was elected to represent Cambridge University on the General Council of Medical Education and Registration of the United Kingdom and continued to do so until 1869 when he became its President for five years. In 1864 he presided over the British Medical Association when it met for the first time in Cambridge. His speech on this occasion expounded a cause close to his heart, the necessity for more general instruction in natural science:[7] 'If some portion of the natural sciences, and in particular those which treat of the laws of life, should become an established part of the higher general education – of the education, not of medical students only, but of every English gentleman, we may expect that Society will, in course of time, become more conversant with the kind of knowledge required for distinguishing between true science and its counterfeit.' And also, 'if some acquaintance with the natural sciences be so needful for men in general, what should be expected of *us*, the medical profession, who practise daily an art which has its only sound basis in these very sciences'. At this meeting, P.W. Latham, later to be Downing Professor of Medicine, and to throw a hefty spoke in the wheel of the Medical School (see p. 246), was Secretary.

In 1866 Paget delivered the Harveian Oration at the Royal College of Physicians on the text of Harvey's exhortation, 'to search and study out the secrets of nature by way of experiment'. He had a particular interest in William Harvey. Soon after taking his degree he had visited Harvey's tomb in Hempstead, Essex, had four casts made of the bust on his monument and given one each to the College of Physicians, Caius College and St Bartholomew's Hospital, keeping the last for himself.[8] In 1849 he had printed a letter from Harvey to Dr Samuel Ward, Master of Sidney Sussex College, Cambridge (1609–1643), and the following year printed 'A Notice of an unpublished Manuscript of William Harvey'. In his oration he asked: 'Is there nothing more that we may learn from Jenner's discovery?' a question that has earned him a place in history for predicting the subsequent activities of immunology.[2]

In 1872 the Crown appointed him the Regius Professor of Physic, an office he filled with dignity and with more distinction than any of his predecessors save Glisson.[2] His lectures held much of local interest from his personal experience, such as examples of people who had been buried for days in the snow around Cambridge and survived.

In 1873 he was elected a Fellow of the Royal Society.

In 1875, largely through Paget's work, Public Health examinations were held in Cambridge for the first time. It was not a first for Cambridge; that honour belonged to Trinity College, Dublin, in 1871,[9] but the Dublin examinations were restricted to graduates of Trinity, Oxford and Cambridge; the Cambridge examinations were open to all registered medical men. Paget had also been instrumental in the introduction of the examination in Dublin.

In 1884 Paget retired from his position as Physician at Addenbrooke's Hospital and a year later was made a Knight Commander of the Bath. A bust, subscribed for by his friends, was placed in the entrance hall at Addenbrooke's Hospital and now (1988), together with a bust of Sir George Humphry, and a portrait of Sir Thomas Clifford Allbutt, graces the Clinical School Library at the new Hospital. On 29 January 1892, he died suddenly with an attack of epidemic influenza.

His son says:[4]

> To those who knew him, perhaps some of the chief characteristics of Sir George Paget's life were his singular uprightness and his strong sense of honour and justice. He was, besides, exceptionally sympathetic and very generous, and capable of detecting good in those who were generally regarded as worthless. He was, consequently, invariably kind and considerate. He was social by nature, an admirable story-teller, and keenly humorous. His memory was particularly good, even over a very wide range of subjects, and rarely failed him. His business capacities were very marked during the whole of his life, not excepting that period of it when he was most harassed by the duties of his provincial practice, and the necessity of presiding over the meetings of the General Medical Council in London. His papers were always kept carefully arranged, and all his habits were orderly.

~ 13 ~

Sir George Humphry

Sir George Murray Humphry (Fig. 16) was one of the giants of Cambridge medicine in the nineteenth century and did much to raise the Medical School from a position of insignificance to one of world renown. He was Surgeon at Addenbrooke's Hospital for 52 years and, when the Hospital was enlarged and almost rebuilt in 1864 and 1865 at a cost of about £15,000, it was at his instigation and to the designs he drew up with the architect Sir Matthew Digby Wyatt.

George Humphry was the third son in a family of five and was born on 18 July 1820, in Sudbury, Suffolk. His father, William, held the office of distributor of stamps for Suffolk which his father and grandfather had held before him and also qualified as a barrister. He was said to be silent and uncommunicative but a pure and upright character. George's mother, Betsy Anne Gilson was a strong character and had a great influence on her husband. The family had been prominent in the borough for generations and more than one member had been Mayor.[1]

Humphry's family seems to have been well represented in the professions. His oldest brother William Gilson (1815–1880) graduated as senior classic, second Chancellor's Medallist and twenty-seventh Wrangler and was to become a Fellow of Trinity College, Proctor of Cambridge University, Vicar of St Martin-in-the Fields, and author of many works;[2] and his second brother, Joseph, became a barrister in London. Humphry's son, Alfred Paget Humphry, was to be Senior Esquire Bedell of Cambridge University and was also a first class rifle shot, winning the Queen's prize of the National Rifle Association as an undergraduate in 1871. Humphry himself became eminent, with busts of him in Addenbrooke's, in the Medical School and in the Royal College of Surgeons, his portrait in the Fitzwilliam Museum, Cambridge, and engraved; another, painted by his niece, Miss K.M. Humphry in 1892, on the occasion of his enrolement as freeman of his native town, in the public hall at Sudbury.[3]

Although the Humphrys were fairly well off and William went to Shrewsbury School, times became harder, for George was sent to Gram-

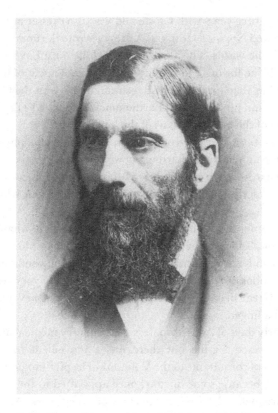

Fig. 16. Sir George Murray Humphry (1820–1896). From an
album of original photographs of officers of the International
Medical Congress, 1881, in the Wellcome Institute of the History
of Medicine. By courtesy of 'The Wellcome Trustees'.

mar school at Sudbury and later Dedham and had to leave at 16 to
become apprenticed to a surgeon at Norwich. His master, John Green
Crosse (1790–1850), was a famous lithotomist and made a Fellow of the
Royal Society in the year that young Humphry joined him. He had a
pathological museum and library alongside his surgery and through his
encouragement his apprentice was to develop a lifelong enthusiasm for
collecting and cataloguing museum specimens.

Later, in his Hunterian Oration (1879) to the Royal College of
Surgeons, Humphry was to say[4] that the medical profession had suffered
in quality, status and practical outcome from being commenced, in many
instances, too early in life. He thought that twenty, which was John
Hunter's age when he started medical work, was the best time to begin.

He stayed three years with Crosse and was also dresser at that time in the Norfolk and Norwich Hospital. A dresser wrote the notes and assisted generally in the wards. This taste of medical life must have awakened a love of medicine for in 1839 he entered St Bartholomew's Hospital as a student and in 1840, in the 1st M.B. examinations, won the Gold Medal for anatomy and physiology. St Bartholomew's, founded 1123, was then, as now, one of the great hospitals of the kingdom.

James Paget, brother of George Paget, the Cambridge physician, was curator of the museum at St Bartholomew's during Humphry's time there and destined to have a great career as a surgeon, being remembered by the eponymous description of diseases of the nipple and of bone which are still in use.[5]

Paget was interested in his students, keeping records of what became of them and publishing these in 1869. He noticed Humphry and it was through the influence of him and his brother that the young man was to get his first appointment, becoming at the age of 22 the youngest hospital surgeon in Great Britain not yet having his M.B. and never yet having amputated a finger![1]

In the early days of Addenbrooke's the honorary medical and surgical staff were elected for life but there was a movement to restrict the appointment of consultants to the Voluntary Hospitals to perhaps five or seven years,[6] because some doctors, once appointed to these prestigious positions, frequently left deputies to carry out their work. An incident of this kind had happened in Cambridge and in 1842 it was proposed that in future surgeons be elected for a term of years.[7] Messrs Lestourgeon, Okes and Abbott resigned and Charles Lestourgeon Junior, Josiah Hammond and George Humphry were elected.

It is possible that this was a carefully planned campaign engineered by Frederic Thackeray, who was ambitious for the Hospital, and John Haviland, who worked energetically for the Medical School, to give the Hospital a staff of higher professional calibre who were eager to teach. Probably both this factor and the wish to end hospital appointments as sinecures contributed as motives for the change.

In the election Lestourgeon obtained 280 votes and his rival Humphry was third with 221 votes. They were to compete again in at least two other elections, with Humphry the winner on these occasions, and also in their practice in Cambridge; both became the owners of large and beautiful houses in the locality.

On 19 November, 1841, Humphry had become a member of the Royal

College of Surgeons and, on 12 May 1842, a Licentiate of the Society of Apothecaries of London, so he was qualified to practise even though he had not yet got his degree. It may be that Sir James Paget, knowing of the possibility of elections at Cambridge urged him to interrupt the studies which he was later to resume at Cambridge.

In the December after the election the Hospital Board gave the medical staff permission to institute a system of clinical lectures. Credit for the advance has been variously given to Dr Frederic Thackeray together with Professor John Haviland, or to Sir George Paget in conjunction with Humphry.[1] Whoever was responsible it gave Humphry the opportunity to teach, and that he proceeded to do.

In 1844, by virtue of his hospital appointment, Humphry was elected one of the original Fellows of the Royal College of Surgeons which under the patronage of King George III had been formed from the Company of Surgeons in 1800. Humphry was a year younger than the statutory age of 25 years, appeared last on the list, and had to wait for formal admission.

The Professor of Anatomy at that time was the Revd William 'Bone' Clark ('Bone' to distinguish him from two other Professors Clarke currently in the University, 'Stone' Clark, Professor of Mineralogy, and 'Tone' Clarke, Professor of Music),[8] and the position covered both human and comparative anatomy. In 1847 Professor Clark invited Humphry to act as his deputy teaching human anatomy, which he did, giving lectures and demonstrations until 1866 when he was elected to his own Chair.

Bodies for dissection were still hard to come by in Humphry's time. In London, prior to the Anatomy Act of 1834, the Company of Surgeons and then the College of Surgeons, had hired a house in Lock Lane where the bodies of criminals could be delivered by the hangman after execution. 'The President in full court dress, it is recorded, awaited the bodies on the first floor. The executioner, coarsely dressed, entered with the body on his back and let it fall with a thud on the table; after which the President made a small incision over the sternum and bowed to the hangman'.[9] Against this recent background Humphry sought his specimens, being aided in his search by one Sims whom he described as 'the most truthful liar I have ever known'.[4]

At St Bartholomew's Humphry had come under the influence of Peter Mere Latham; he often spoke of his lectures later in life and it is believed that the clear emphatic style of the great physician moulded the subsequent lecturing style of his pupil.[1] Humphry is said to have been a magnetic teacher, employing the Socratic method and an interrogative forefinger. His anatomical teaching was known as 'Humphryology' because of the stress on function[4] which his students did not understand to be useful until later. He is also said to have been a keen observer and to have urged this habit on his students in the out-patients' room and wards.

He had a talent for repartee and on one occastion when a student not renowned for ability unexpectedly answered a question correctly and remarked 'You seem surprised, Professor', Humphry retaliated with 'So was Balaam when his ass spoke.' He is reputed to have retorted to a barrister in court, on being asked if he was accustomed to lose many of his cases, that he did not conduct his surgical cases as the cross-examiner did his legal cases, 'otherwise he would lose them all'.[4]

He was slight and of medium height with coal black straight hair and always pictured with a beard. He is said to have had expressive glittering eyes, and a pupil, W.H. Dickinson, wrote: 'There was a fascination in his glance, so piercing and enquiring; like Cassius, he seemed to look quite through the deeds of men'.[1] It was, however, also said that 'he was not an infallible judge of men'.

He did not have a strong constitution and early in life was threatened by pulmonary tuberculosis, so went his rounds by horse on medical advice. Later he used to say that every hair of that horse – bought, it is said, from borrowed funds, he was so poor – was worth a guinea as a means to recovery. He frequently conducted his operations at the house of the patient and, if at night, it might be by the light of a single candle. He would worry before a big operation and have disturbed nights, 'a great operation was a severe trial to him',[10] but he was a good and successful surgeon. After a time he gave up riding and was driven round in a light dog-cart.

In 1847, the same year as he became Professor Clark's deputy, Humphry joined the University as a Fellow Commoner, a modified status of undergraduate, at Downing College, and took the degree of M.B. in 1852 and M.D. in 1859. For his M.D. thesis, presented shortly after a change in the regulations removing the necessity for it to be written in Latin, he utilised his own three experiences of phlebitis, which had occurred in 1843 after pleurisy, in 1847 after typhoid fever, and in 1851 after pleurisy again, as well as other case histories.

As well as teaching anatomy he taught surgery, giving in 1849 a 28 lecture course which was published 1849–1850 in the *Provincial Medical and Surgical Journal*, the forerunner to the *British Medical Journal*, and then in 1851 in book form. For both his surgical lectures and his anatomical demonstrations he was helped by the 2,000 specimens the University bought in 1836 from James Macartney (1770–1843), Professor of Anatomy and Chirurgery at Dublin. Crosse, who had taught Humphry in his youth, had been a favourite pupil and demonstrator of Macartney, and Humphry regarded the specimens with almost filial affection,[1] adding to them with enthusiasm whenever he travelled and constantly cataloguing and working at the specimens. The museum was later called after him. 'Before all things he was a scientific man and a collector'.[3]

In 1849 he married Mary, daughter of Daniel Robert McNab, a surgeon of Epping, Essex. His brother Joseph married her sister. Both girls were considerable heiresses.[1] George and Mary were to have a son and two daughters.

Mary Humphry was a talented artist and substantially helped her husband in his life's work. When his great monograph *A Treatise on the Human Skeleton (including the joints)* was published in 1858, it contained 60 illustrations, all done on stone, by his wife. She also illustrated much of his other work. The 'Treatise', described by Rolleston as 'epoch-making'[1] and making 'the dry bones live'[4] was delved into by many succeeding anatomy teachers, probably won him his F.R.C.S. of the following year, and formed a basis for some of Humphry's own original papers.

In 1849, when Humphry gave his course of surgical lectures, the number of names on the Register of Pupils at Addenbrooke's was averaging six. This it had done since February 1841, when clinical teaching was first introduced as ward rounds, and pupils were obliged to sign the register each month;[11] the number of signatures ranged between one and fifteen, and a number of local practitioners and their apprentices were among those attending.

After Humphry's appointment, however, lectures were given as well as ward rounds and ward visits, and later the lectures and rounds in general medicine and surgery were supplemented by regular lectures on special subjects. By the 1880s the names on the Register of Pupils were averaging over 60, and almost all now were members of the University.

As well as drawing in students for the school, Humphry was concerned about the welfare of his poorer pupils, no doubt remembering his own early days. He established Dr Humphry's Hostel for Medical Students near the Hospital at 56 Trumpington Street, and in 1860 it accommodated five students, in 1861 six, and in 1863 three. It was succeeded by Cavendish College which served the same purpose.[12]

His surgical practice continued. In 1856 he published 'A Report of

Some Cases of Operation: (Division of stricture of the urethra and rectum; amputation at the hip joint; excision of the condyle of the lower jaw; excision of the knee; ovariotomy; encysted urinary calculus; tracheotomy). Treated for the most part in Addenbrooke's Hospital, Cambridge, and in the year 1855.' In this work he describes a number of his cases, not all ending successfully, and tries to draw useful conclusions from them for his colleagues. For example, although his ovariotomy patient succumbed to tetanus and died, he had collected the results of 105 ovariotomies and analysed them, to work out the conditions in which the operation was most likely to be successful and whether in fact it should be done at all. His results with excision of the knee joint so pleased him that later nervous patients were to try to quell his enthusiasm with 'Now Dr. Humphry, I am not going to have my knee took out.'[4]

He reports several of the operations as being conducted under chloroform, the anaesthetic newly discovered and respectable only since Queen Victoria had given it her blessing by accepting it in childbirth in 1853. However, he is said to have sometimes dispensed with anaesthetics altogether and never followed the antiseptic routine, using what he described as the 'open method' of treating wounds, covering them with a piece of gauze. He seems to have been a bold surgeon, removing the whole of the right condyle of the lower jaw from a deformed 22-year-old girl, although 'my colleagues thought it was doubtful to be recommended to the patient'. This boldness may have been due to a quick sympathy for his patients.

In 1864 he was President of the Surgical Section at the Cambridge meeting of the British Medical Association, and showed his clear-sightedness by saying that 'pathology, in all its branches,' was 'the very cornerstone of surgery'. (The Cambridge Chair of Pathology was not established for another 20 years.)

In 1866 Humphry was elected Professor of Human Anatomy. Originally, when the Professorship of Anatomy was founded in 1707, the duties of the Professor had not been specified, and Professor Clark began his term by giving lectures on the anatomy and physiology of the human body, subsequently including also some aspects of comparative anatomy. Then Humphry took over the Department of Human Anatomy and Physiology while lectures in comparative anatomy were given by the Professor or his deputy, Dr Drosier.[13] In 1865 a syndicate appointed to consider the best means of teaching anatomy and zoology recommended a split into two separate disciplines and Dr Clark resigned.

The two applicants for the Professorship of Human Anatomy were Humphry himself and his old rival Charles Lestourgeon, who had annually for 12 years been delivering two courses of lectures on clinical surgery. Later Lestourgeon withdrew his application without stating a reason, although probably it was because of Humphry's superior qualification by virtue of his having taught anatomy and physiology in the University for nearly 20 years as Clark's deputy. Alfred Newton, M.A., was elected Professor of Zoology and Comparative Anatomy.

From that time onwards honours and distinctions were heaped on Humphry and cannot all be detailed here. However, in 1871 he obtained recognition from the Royal College of Surgeons for the teaching of anatomy, surgery and medicine at Cambridge so that these subjects were now on the same plane as at the other great medical schools, and in 1876, through his influence, human anatomy was recognised as a separate branch of science in the Natural Science Tripos.

When Humphry first took over as Professor of Anatomy the emoluments barely covered expenses but by the 1880s, the Medical School now being populous, they were substantial. Humphry, believing with the Special Board for Medicine that a Professor of Surgery was urgently needed in the University, and knowing that funds for such a Chair were not available, offered to give up the Anatomy Chair and take the new position without stipend. In two letters preserved in the University archives he explains why.[14] In the one to the Vice Chancellor he says 'Hitherto I have carried on the work and teaching of Anatomy and the work and teaching of Surgery, the former during great part of the year, the latter chiefly during the summer. Circumstances induced me thus to take up and continue the two subjects, though I was well aware that in attempting both I could not do justice to either.

'The Anatomical class is now so large that the superintendance of it with the teaching and study of the science and practical work of Anatomy require the full time and attention of the Professor; and the efficient performance of the duties of the Professorship is so essential to the success of the Medical School that it is most important for the occupant of the Chair to be able to devote himself wholly and energetically to the work appertaining to it.'

To Paget, he writes: 'Teaching surgery would – indeed always would have been – more congenial and less laborious to me than teaching Anatomy which I have now done in the University for six and thirty years.'

He was the only candidate and was elected to be the first Professor of Surgery on 20 June 1883. The Chair was suspended after his death until 1903 when Howard Marsh was appointed, and then again suspended after his death from 1915 until 1921 when it was discontinued. It was re-established in 1965.

Humphry held the optimistic doctrine that the efficiency of a teacher increases as his salary falls, and that the usefulness of a University is enhanced by every decline in its revenue,[4] and in May 1888, when an assistant, Joseph Griffiths, was appointed for him, he paid Griffiths' salary.

In 1884 he was elected a Professorial Fellow of Kings College, an honour which gave him great pleasure and he delighted in taking weekend visitors to service in the Chapel.[3] In 1891 he was knighted but is said to have preferred being called 'Professor'.[1]

In 1894 he left the staff of Addenbrooke's after 52 years. With his letter of resignation he enclosed a cheque for £500 'to be used for the purpose of improving the accommodation for seeing the surgical out-patients as well as for providing suitable accommodation for the students who may be attending this part of the Hospital practice'. In proposing that the Quarterly Court should accept his resignation. Dr MacAlister spoke of Humphry and 'his enormous influence in making it (Addenbrooke's Hospital) one of the great centres of medical education in this country'.

Two years later, on 24 September 1896, Humphry died at his home, Grove Lodge, with intestinal obstruction, having been confined to bed for six weeks previous resolutely refusing to be operated on for cancer of the caecum. Although strong in spirit he had never been a physically strong man and looked ill; he dressed poorly and though generous was sparing in all that concerned his own comfort; it is remembered of him that once when he sat resting in the outer hall at the Royal College of Surgeons he was noticed by a candidate who took him by the beard and shook him, saying: 'What's the matter with you, my man?'.[3]

In an obituary on Sir George Paget,[15] who died before Humphry, in 1891, a compliment was paid to both of them together:

> For a long period the study of medicine at Cambridge had been neglected. From 1833 to 1858 the average number of persons proceeding to the degree of Bachelor of Medicine was less than four a year. With the exception of Gonville and Caius and St. John's Colleges, no encouragement was given by Fellowships or scholarships to the students of medicine. The degree, itself, although it enabled its holder to practise, was not considered in the

profession as a very high qualification, and there was some danger of the medical faculty becoming extinct. At the present time the Medical School at Cambridge is one of the largest in the United Kingdom, and the possession of a Medical Degree at Cambridge is considered one of the highest professional qualifications. This remarkable change is due to the energy, zeal and perseverance of Sir George Paget and Sir George Humphry, the present Professor of Surgery. Like all great movements, it was a labour of years.

~ 14 ~

Some Hospital extensions

Building

The period following the Bowtell extension of the Hospital (see Chapter 10) was one of consolidation. The Hospital's investments were increased as opportunity offered, to lessen its dependence on annual subscriptions. John Haviland and Frederic Thackeray, joined in 1837 by George Paget, worked successfully to secure recognition of the Hospital as a teaching centre. They were preparing the ground for the rapid development of the Hospital's amenities and prestige, which were to accompany the regeneration of the Medical School in the next four decades.

No important structural changes were contemplated until 1833[1] when it was resolved to construct two fever wards. A Planning Committee was set up under the chairmanship of Lord Godolphin, and at the same time a Repairing Committee with Thomas Hovell as Chairman, for the state of the old buildings was causing concern. The offer of gratuitous services from James Walton, architect of Cambridge, was accepted. The Planning Committee submitted its report the following month.[2] They recommended the erection of a building 49 feet long and 25 feet wide, its south front 'to be in line with the South side of the operation room and the West end of it distant from the operation room about 30 feet'. The building should be on two floors, each with room for an eight-bed ward, a nurses' room, and a water closet. The Governors were concerned about the maintenance costs and after discussion they agreed to a somewhat unusual arrangement. At first only four beds would be opened in each of the new wards, and the total number of patients admitted to the whole Hospital should not be increased and 'as many beds be allowed to remain unoccupied in the old building as there may happen at any time to be patients in the fever wards'.

The tender of Messrs Quinse and Asby, amounting to £1,930 was accepted. Lord Godolphin then became chairman of the Building Committee which met frequently while the work was in progress. 'A drying closet of power sufficient to dry all the linen etc. of the whole Hospital

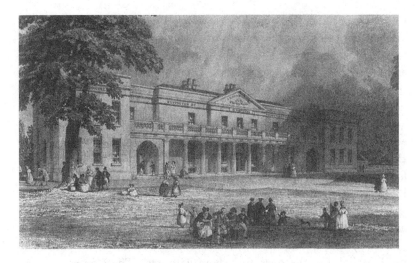

Fig. 17. Addenbrooke's Hospital, 1830. From a drawing by
William Fleetwood Varley.

establishment when filled with patients' was to be installed in the
basement.[3] The new building was completed in 1834.

In 1837 the Governors decided[4] that the number of beds should be
increased by 22 to bring the total to 100. An additional building was
considered but it was decided first to appoint a committee to enquire into
the means of making the best use of available space. The Committee was
fully aware of the advantages of a separate out-patient department, but
could see no way in which this could be accomplished until the Hospital
had obtained possession of some adjacent land which it leased and which
belonged in part to Corpus Christi College and in part to Westfield's
Charity. Prints were ordered to be made of the ground plan of the
Hospital, distinguishing the freehold from the leasehold parts. After very
prolonged negotiation by two successive committees the land was
acquired. The bursar of Corpus Christi struck a hard bargain and an
agreement was not reached until the summer of 1846.

Meanwhile the shortage of accommodation was frequently under
discussion. Lestourgeon had proposed in 1839 'that an extra ward should
be erected for the accommodation of patients suffering from fractures and
other accidents emitting offensive smells'.[5] The medical staff were asked
to prepare a report but no action appears to have been taken about this
particular problem.

The prolonged wrangling between the Governors and the Chancery

Court concerning the purposes to which Bowtell's legacy might be applied, imposed upon the Governors the obligation to use certain wards for specific purposes – the reception of patients applying for vaccination and the relief of personal deformities. There appears to be no evidence in the minutes that the wards erected with the Bowtell bequest were in fact not used from the first as general medical and surgical wards.

A further committee 'to consider the best means of improving the accommodation of the Hospital' was appointed in October 1843. John Haviland was its chairman. In December the Governors[6] approved a plan for two new wards. The total number of patients was not to be increased. By December, 1844, the new building was completed.

In 1848 the Hospital grounds were replanted 'to make a more extensive and airy walking ground for the patients'.

In 1849 a committee considered 'the propriety of lighting the passage of the Hospital and the operating room with gas'. The Committee was informed[7] that St Thomas' and St Bartholomew's Hospitals burned gas in the wards as well as in the passages, but that St George's and Guy's Hospitals used it only in the passages. No ill effects had been experienced. The Committee in its report to the Governors[8] drew attention to a letter from the Surgeons who considered the introduction of gas a matter of great importance, 'in consequence of the very great inconvenience from the use of candlelight in many operations of a very delicate nature, which from time to time require immediate attention at whatever hour they occur'. The Governors accepted the recommendation that gas lighting be introduced in the passages and the operating room. It was estimated that gas would cost very little more than the existing oil lamps.

Dr Paget had for some years been attempting to modernise the Hospital. In 1853[9] the Repairing Committee with three co-opted additional members, regularly referred to as 'the subcommittee to consider the best way of carrying out Dr Paget's proposition', reported to the Governors, and the report was received and adopted. Paget's propositions were hardly revolutionary, 'he wanted to provide separate rooms for the nurses of the four original wards, who still live in bed-sitting rooms on their wards'. He also wanted more water closets and bathrooms, and some single-bedded wards. It was proposed to provide the additional accommodation by knocking down some internal partitions and by erecting small wings, projecting 6 feet beyond the outside wall of the Board Room. Although the Committee thought these projecting wings 'may easily be made ornamental', the Governors had doubts, and rejected the scheme by the Chairman's casting vote.[10]

Apart from these improvements in the amenities Paget and his supporters hoped to erect a new building which would make it possible to separate the medical from the surgical departments.[11] New buildings could be erected only if the Hospital could purchase the freehold of more properties adjoining the Hospital site. A new committee was set up for this purpose towards the end of 1853. The negotiations were fruitless as the owners[12] would not sell, or would do so only on terms which precluded the proposed development. Paget's plan had therefore to be deferred for a time. Meanwhile a committee[13] having first ensured that the quality of the water had been fully tested, entered into an agreement with the Cambridge Water Works Company and the mains installations were made during the course of 1857.

Matron and nurses

Charlotte Whybrow was, as we have seen, an outstanding Matron, perhaps the best of the housekeeping matrons, who were not to be replaced by nursing superintendents for another 40 years. Such references as the Minutes make to the Matron's activities almost invariably concern some aspect of housekeeping or hospital management. In April 1830, Colonel Rushbrook, Chairman of the West Suffolk Hospital, asked if their matron 'might be allowed to witness the mode of conducting the system of management in the housekeeping department of the Hospital'. The Board gave their approval.

Mrs Whybrow resigned in 1834 and was succeeded by Charlotte Spelling. She was the only candidate. We know little about her except that she was under 50 and 'was free from the burden of children'. Her personality was perhaps more abrasive than that of Mrs Whybrow, for complaints about the conduct of the apprentices, porters and others, became frequent after she was appointed. From 1840 onwards, the Matron was allowed exclusive use of her sitting room except on Monday and Saturday mornings when Dr Paget used it for his out-patient clinic.[14]

There is evidence of increasing control by the Board over the activities of its officers. In 1847 the Matron was asked to keep the expenses of the household separate from those of the patients.[15] The following month she was ordered to keep a detailed register of all servants (including under this heading the nurses), and lay the register before each Weekly Board.

The Minutes provide much information about the Matron's duties when she neglected them, and seldom mention them when she did not. The increasing complexity of her job was evidently beyond Mrs Spelling's capacity. A committee set up on 12 July 1848, found complaints of mismanagement and of inattention to the Rules to be justified. Mrs Spelling resigned in April 1849.

The next Matron, Jane Bishop, elected by ballot after three candidates had been rejected when certificates of baptism showed them to be over 45, had a stormy career. On 2 April 1850, she dismissed the cook and the kitchen maid for stealing cheese, and on this occasion the Weekly Board approved her action. In January 1851,[16] complaints about the food were investigated by a committee which in its report blamed the Matron for inadequate supervision of the catering and for intimidating her staff. Miss Bishop's very long letter of protest throws light on the day to day working of the Hospital and on the personality of the Matron.

She claimed that the Committee's report 'must have been framed from misrepresentation or error of judgement'. She insisted that the quality of the meat had been excellent – 'I see it myself when it comes in'. She accused the nurse of Maynard Ward of adding milk gruel and water to the broth intended for that ward 'as a revenge for my not allowing her favorite patient to sit in the kitchen after he had spoken very rudely to myself and the servants'.

If she had erred in her deportment towards the nurses, she said, 'it has been in being too indulgent to them. They have never paid proper respect to me.' There followed pages of rambling self-justification.

The letter was copied into the minute book, but was 'expunged' on the orders of the Board[17] which had expressed itself 'fully convinced of the efficiency of management displayed by Miss Bishop'.[18]

Miss Bishop's letter, which fortunately remains legible, suggests that relations between her and Mitchell, the Apothecary, were openly hostile. A committee was appointed in March[19] 'to define the duties of the Apothecary and Matron'. The Committee's resolutions all tactfully reinforce the Apothecary's authority; for example, it was 'resolved that all letters addressed to the Hospital except those addressed specifically to any particular person be handed to the House Apothecary to open', and 'resolved that the Matron engage as extra nurses such persons only as may be recommended or approved by the House Apothecary'.

That some of the ten nurses were undisciplined is suggested by the notice, ordered in 1856[20] to 'be printed in good sized type and kept hung up in all the wards'. The notice, headed 'Caution', warned the nurses that they would be dismissed if they were caught giving to patients or taking out of the Hospital the provisions issued to them; or accepting money from patients on any pretence whatsoever.

In 1856 the wages of the nurses were increased to £15 in the general wards, and to £16 in the fever wards, increasing in each case by £1 after five years' service and a further £1 after ten years.

There were to be no fundamental changes until 1865 in the type of woman employed as nurses, or in the organisation of nursing in the Hospital.

The Addenbrooke's of Paget and Humphry

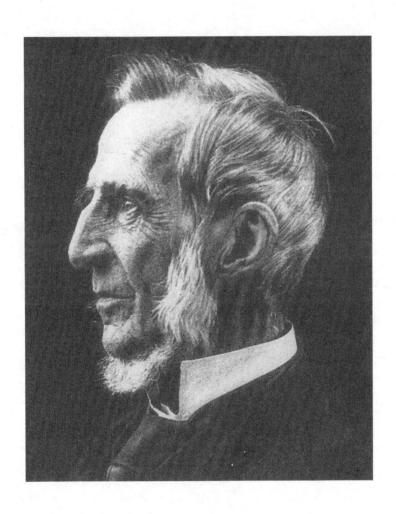

~ 15 ~

The catchment area

The new Poor Law

As we have seen, the parishes functioned as administrative units for the care of sick paupers, under the Poor Law Act of Queen Elizabeth I. The parish overseers had frequently to be reminded by the Hospital Secretary of their financial responsibilites. In 1834 the Poor Law Amendment Act grouped parishes into unions, each under the control of a Board of Guardians, for the administration of poor relief. Each union built a workhouse to which paupers could be admitted under a rigid classification which separated husbands from wives and children from parents. The workhouses were not primarily hospitals but found themselves increasingly obliged to provide accommodation and care for those chronically sick paupers who were excluded by the Rules for admission to hospital; many were indeed paupers because they were sick. As parishes surrendered their responsibility for the sick poor to the unions, the latter became subscribers to the Hospital, and the Clerks to the Boards of Guardians took over from the parish officers the often voluminous correspondence with the Hospital Secretary.

The area covered by each union was divided into a number of districts to each of which a medical officer was appointed. The workhouse itself had a medical officer who sometimes combined these duties with those of a district, often that in which the workhouse was situated. Since many Boards of Guardians gave their medical appointments to the local practitioner who would accept the lowest salary, the Poor Law Medical Service did not everywhere secure the services of the best doctors, particularly in the larger towns. In Cambridge and in other predominantly rural areas however, the union medical officers were commonly successful and popular general practitioners, well able to resist pressure from the local notabilities who were the Guardians.

The Cambridge Union consisted of the fourteen parishes of the Borough. The workhouse was erected in Mill Road in 1838 with accommodation for 250 persons.

Table 3. *Subscribing parishes, 1825–1860*

	Cambridge	Cambridgeshire	Huntingdonshire	Essex	Hertfordshire	Suffolk
1825	13	54	9		1	3

(In 1826 26 of all subscribing parishes were in arrears, nine of them for three years)

	Cambridge	Cambridgeshire	Huntingdonshire	Essex	Hertfordshire	Suffolk
1830	14	59	7		1	1

(all Cambridge parishes)

1834	14	52	6		1	1

(New Poor Law)

1835	14	51	5		1	1
1836	13	47	4		1	1
1837	12	49	4		1	1

(Linton and Newmarket Unions subscribe for first time)

1838	12	36	3		1	1

(North Witchford and Whittlesea Unions also subscribing)

1839	8	29	1		1	

(5 unions subscribing)

1840	8	32	1		2	

(6 unions subscribing)

1845	4	26	1		1	
1850	3	9	1		1	

(8 unions subscribing)

1855	3	34	1			

(12 unions subscribing)

1860	2	6				

(12 unions subscribing)

The Chesterton Union covered 38 parishes in an area of 120 square miles surrounding Cambridge. The workhouse, which accommodated 300 persons, was in Chesterton village.

The Linton Union comprised 22 parishes and 74 square miles. The workhouse could accommodate 230 paupers. The area was divided into Linton, Balsham and Duxford districts.

Newmarket lay partly in Cambridgeshire (parish of All Saints), and partly in Suffolk (parish of St Mary). Both parishes had subscribed to the Hospital and so did the Union of which they formed a small part. The Union covered 29 parishes in an area of 150 square miles including Burwell, Fordham, Soham and the Swaffhams. The large workhouse, erected in 1836 in Exning, accommodated 380 persons.

The first unions to become in 1837 subscribers to the Hospital, were Linton (11 guineas) and Newmarket (6 guineas).

By 1838 the number of subscribing parishes in Cambridgeshire

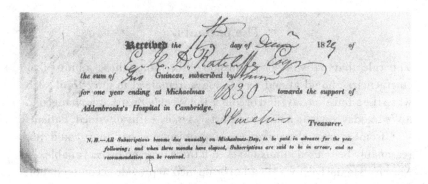

Fig. 18. Receipt for a two guinea subscription for the year ended
Michaelmas, 1830.

(excluding Cambridge), had dropped to 36 (see Table 3), and the unions
at Whittlesea and Witchford had taken the place of some of those parishes
which had ceased to subscribe.

By 1847 two further unions had joined the subscribers, bringing the
total to five, as a number of unions did not renew their subscriptions with
complete regularity. The new subscribers were Caxton and Royston.

It is interesting that the two local unions, Cambridge and Chesterton,
first became subscribers in 1851 and 1849 respectively although the
number of subscribing parishes in the Borough had fallen to three by 1846.
It is possible that subscribers' letters were more readily available in the
Borough and the surrounding villages, because of the higher density of
private subscribers, than in more distant rural areas.

The Ely and Wisbech Unions began to subscribe in 1849.

By 1855 there were twelve subscribing unions. In 1856 their combined
subscriptions amounted to £175, a significant contribution to the total
income from subscriptions of £1,281. The Hospital's association with the
new Poor Law organisation was complete for Cambridgeshire and the Isle
of Ely, and adjoining areas of neighbouring counties, for example the St
Ives and Saffron Walden Unions. More distant unions, such as those of
Bishop's Stortford and Buntingford and King's Lynn, were less regular
subscribers. The majority of parishes ceased to subscribe once the unions
of which they formed part were doing so (there were 74 subscribing
parishes in 1833, but only three in 1873). There were none by 1888 except
Great and Little Eversden which were perpetual subscribers by virtue of a
legacy of £50 to each in 1775.

The patients

The rule that patients for admission, other than those admitted as emergencies, should attend on Mondays, remained in force until 1836 when the admission day, and of course the Weekly Board, was changed to a Wednesday, on which day transport was more easily obtained. Patients sent from a great distance were a problem in that they could not reasonably be refused admission even if there were no beds available. In March 1843 the fever ward had to be opened to provide accommodation for seven such patients. The fever wards had frequently been used in this way,[1] and it was ordered that steps should be taken to avoid such admissions in future. This was not a realistic policy and in 1851 it was agreed[2] that if patients with fever were admitted any other patients then in the fever ward should be transferred to the main hospital. In fact the fever wards continued to be used for other patients when the pressure on beds was heavy.

The medical criteria for admission had remained unchanged since 1766. In 1844 the Governors, on the advice of a committee which had considered the matter, agreed that 'no prostitute labouring under the venereal disease be admitted as an in-patient without an especial permission granted by the Weekly Board, and by the Recommendation of the medical gentlemen under whose care she may be placed'.

The financial criteria for admission had also remained unchanged. Until about 1850 it was usually the lay Governors who complained that patients admitted were not 'proper objects of the Charity'. After that date such complaints came more often from the doctors (e.g. Bond in 1859)[3], for competition in medical practice had become more severe. The medical journals frequently published letters deploring 'the abuse of hospitals'.

The conditions in the wards and among out-patients are not described or even mentioned when they were considered normal. The occasional complaints are informative, particularly when they were detailed. In 1854 a long letter[4] from the Rector of Longstowe St Michael described in convincing detail the experiences at the Hospital of some of his parishioners.

A young woman was admitted with typhus. The Hospital gave her mother her infected clothing to wash at home. The mother and father and seven siblings all contracted typhus. The Rector felt that the mother should have been informed that the washing could be done at the Hospital.

The out-patients attending on Saturdays complained of disorder and inhumanity. They were brought from their villages to the Hospital in carriers' carts and had to wait several hours before they could get their medicine and return home. There was 'a general scuffle and struggle' to get access to the Dispenser.

A committee of enquiry admitted the truth of these and other allegations. Arrangements were made to issue numbered tickets to patients on arrival; they were seen by the doctor and received their medicines in order according to their numbers. 'Many of the patients are very grateful for the order and quiet which has by this means ensued.' The Dispensary was improved too, but the lack of a separate out-patient department placed strict limits on the possibilities for improvement.

The railways

Most of the population in the area served by the Hospital lived in small towns or villages, and we have seen that transport, even between the main centres was scanty and was often available only on one or two days a week. The development of a network of railway lines throughout the Eastern counties had important implications for the Hospital. In the early days serious accidents to 'navvies' constructing the lines led to claims on the railway companies for the cost of their treatment. Later as the network effectively covered a wider and wider area, transport to and from the Hospital became easier and patients from a considerable distance could attend the Hospital and return home the same day (Fig. 19).

A line from Bishop's Stortford to Clayhythe was projected as early as 1821,[5] but did not materialise. The Northern and Eastern Railway in 1836 planned a line from London to Cambridge, but by 1842 had reached no further than Bishop's Stortford and it was extended to Newport by 1845, in which year the Eastern Counties Railway opened a line from Newport to Cambridge, Ely and Brandon. Between 1846 and 1851 lines were constructed linking Cambridge to Peterborough, Wisbech, Huntingdon, King's Lynn, and Bury St Edmunds, Newmarket, and Royston, and branch lines served all but the smallest villages. In 1862 the Cambridge to Bedford line was opened.[6]

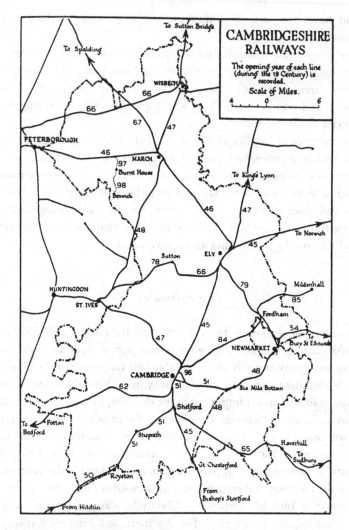

Fig. 19. Cambridgeshire railways in the nineteenth century.
Figure reproduced from *The Cambridge Region*, edited by H.C.
Darby, Cambridge at the University Press, 1938.[6]

The development of the railway system also increased the drift of the rural population into the towns. The population of Cambridgeshire increased by about 25% between 1841 and 1911 but the population of Cambridge more than doubled.[7]

In December 1844 the Governors were first officially informed of the number of railway accident cases which had been admitted during the previous three months.[8] The following May the Secretary was ordered to send to the Northern and Eastern Railway Company a report which stated that, since October 1844, 56 'Railway Patients' had been admitted, 34 as in-patients and 22 as out-patients and that, of these 56, 29 had been accident cases without letters of recommendation.[9] The Company's solicitor acknowledged receipt of the letter.

In June the Quarterly Court agreed to restrict the admission of accidents without recommendation to those taking place in Cambridgeshire and the Isle of Ely. This would of course have had the effect of excluding the accident cases from the Northern and Eastern Railway lines under construction in Essex and Hertfordshire, and also all those from the Great Eastern Railway, from the county boundary to Newport. Accident cases from the latter company's lines, within the county, could not of course be excluded, so the Secretary was ordered to write to the Directors informing them that on Wednesday next a Dahlia Show, partly in aid of Hospital funds, would be held in Cambridge, and suggesting that the Company might run an excursion train to increase the attendance at the show, as the numerous accidents during the construction of their line had put the Hospital to very great expense. The Company did not provide a train, but later sent a donation of 20 guineas.

The number of accidents remained high, as they did in railway construction throughout the country, for the work was inherently hazardous and the gangs of men were unskilled and undisciplined.[10] In 1847 the Secretary was asked to prepare a detailed return of such accidents admitted since 1844, and a return of all sums paid by the railway companies or contractors during this period.

The Secretary ascertained that the number of persons employed by the Eastern Counties Railway admitted as in-patients up to May 1847 was 69, and that their average length of stay was 37 days. Over the same period 36 employees had been treated as out-patients.

Dr Paget, Dr Webster and Mr H.H. Harris were then appointed a committee to apply to the directors of the railway companies concerned.[11] This so-called Railway Committee met on 15 July and agreed a statement to be sent to George Hudson, M.P., Chairman of the Eastern Counties Railway Company. They quoted the statistics given above and estimated that each in-patient had cost the Hospital at least £5. 'The great majority of them required a very generous diet, including (in many cases) large quantities of wine or brandy. They required also the attendance of night nurses who had to be hired as extra hands.' The total cost to the Hospital of these in-patients had therefore been at least £345. The cost of the out-patients was estimated at 3s.10d. each. Moreover, further similar cases had been admitted since the figures were compiled. The Committee trusted that 'it is only necessary to make the above simple statement of facts in order to obtain that support . . . which its Governors have desired us to solicit at your hands'.

On 28 July a letter was received from the Company to the effect that they intended to subscribe five guineas a year.

The Railway Committee met again on 15 September and agreed a similar letter to the Chairman of the Newmarket and Chesterford Railway Company, 19 of whose employees had been treated.

The Eastern Counties Railway increased its subscription to 10 gui-neas,[12] but the cost of the 'Railway Patients' continued to be a source of grievance and protest.

The Census of 1851

The 1851 Census returns list the name, age, occupation and place of birth of every person who spent the night of 30 March of that year in the Hospital. Miss Bishop, the Matron, is listed as head of family, followed by the House Surgeon and his apprentice, six maids, thirteen nurses, the porter and the errand boy, and 84 patients.

Of the 46 male patients, 29 were agricultural labourers, one was a retired farmer. Six of the agricultural labourers were aged 16 or less, the youngest being 12. There was one patient in each of the following occupations: saddler; chemist errand boy; coal porter; carrier; boat builder; railway labourer; plumber; waterman; college waiter; green grocer; groom; pedlar of lucifer matches (aged 16). There were also four scholars aged 7 to 16. Eighteen of the female patients were general servants, eleven of them aged 20 or under. Seven were housewives, and one was a grocer's wife; there were also two laundresses, one lace-maker and one shoebinder. Four of five girls aged 13 or under are listed as scholars, one has no occupation.

The age distribution of the patients is interesting. There is not one child under 7 for the policy of the Hospital was to exclude children, except for lithotomy or serious accidental injury. There were only three patients over 60, a housewife aged 63 and a retired farmer and a farm labourer, both aged 74. Those old people who could not support themselves and whose relations could not afford to help them found their way into the workhouses and, if sick, into the workhouse infirmaries. The farm labourer is listed specifically as a pauper, and was no doubt admitted with a letter from his subscribing parish.

The birth places of the patients also are of considerable interest, and it is probable that in the majority of cases the patients still lived in or near their birth places. Fifty-three of the patients had been born in Cambridgeshire or the Isle of Ely, four in Cambridge itself; nine in villages in Essex, near the county boundary; eight in Huntingdonshire; four in Norfolk, including one housewife, the greengrocer, and the college waiter, and two in Hertfordshire including the young pedlar. Only four had been born outside the Eastern counties. The joiner and plumber was born in Liverpool, one housewife in Buckinghamshire and one laundress in Ireland. A girl aged 13 had been born in Van Diemen's Land.

In 1840 the transportation of convicts to New South Wales, Australia, had ceased, but they were still sending considerable numbers to Van Diemen's Land until 1853 in which year that colony was renamed Tasmania. One can only speculate concerning this child's travels. Were her parents among the free settlers who at about that time were dissatisfied with their form of government? Many moved to Australia but some returned home.

~ 16 ~

Early surgery and anaesthetics

Surgery

Little information has survived concerning the surgery undertaken in the Hospital in pre-anaesthetic days, other than amputation of limbs for compound fractures. The number of other operations is likely to have been small. Kidney stones were particularly common in East Anglia, and would cause such agonising pain that patients were prepared to submit to lithotomy. In 1818[1] John Okes presented a cabinet containing stones extracted from patients with short notes on each case. The Surgeons were asked to add to the collection which should be open to inspection by the Governors and their friends, and by any medical or scientific man. The collection was presented to the University in 1866.

The usual operation for removal of stone was by the lateral approach. In 1848 Humphry successfully removed a stone the size of a hen's egg from the bladder of a boy aged 14, by the 'high' operation which involved an extra-peritoneal approach to the bladder through an abdominal incision.

In 1832 Romilly's diary[2] refers to the Talicotian operation to be performed by Okes the following day. He means the operation of rhinoplasty, reconstruction of a mutilated nose by a graft from the arm, revived in 1597 by Tagliaccozzi of Bologna, Italy.

Although the number of operations increased considerably after the introduction of anaesthesia, the risk of infection was usually too great to justify opening the body cavities. An exception was the operation of ovariotomy – the removal of a diseased ovary. This operation was first successfully carried out in Danville, U.S.A., by Ephraim McDowell in 1809. Humphry attempted the operation in or about 1855, but the patient died of tetanus.

The lectures on surgery delivered by G.M. Humphry were reprinted in a collected edition in 1851. They give a very clear account of the scope of surgical practice at that time. Chronic inflammatory disorders were treated by blistering or by other methods of counter irritation. Abscesses were incised and drained. Chronic ulcers of the legs 'form a considerable proportion of the cases admitted into our hospitals'.[3] Scrofula (tuberculous glands) was common, naevi cysts and superficial tumours were excised.

Table 4 gives notes on some operations Humphry carried out in about 1855.

The introduction of anaesthesia

The first successful public administration of ether for a surgical operation was in Boston, U.S.A. on 16 October 1846. Within weeks it was being given at the North London Hospital (now University College Hospital) for a major operation by Robert Liston. The press gave the occasion the publicity it deserved and, before the end of January 1847, surgeons in many parts of Britain had used, or attempted to use, ether anaesthesia. The success or failure of these initial personal experiences may have deeply influenced each surgeon's attitude to the further use of ether, and since the information available concerning the method of administering ether and the possible contra-indications to its use, was necessarily scanty, a large element of chance entered into every such operation.

The Minute Books do not mention the first anaesthetic at Addenbrooke's Hospital, perhaps because it was successful. However, a local weekly newspaper, the *Cambridge Chronicle*, published with other local news a series of short notes on the exciting events at the Hospital.[4] The first operation at Addenbrooke's Hospital under ether anaesthesia was the amputation of a finger by G.M. Humphry on Saturday 2 January 1847. The ether was administered with an apparatus devised by William Swan Daniel, the House Apprentice. It is not clear whether Daniel, or Mitchell, the House Surgeon, actually gave the anaesthetic.

By the middle of March[5] over 50 operations had been successfully performed under ether, without ill effects. The surgeons were aware of the need for caution in selecting suitable cases, but the number of operations performed during this period was so much above the average, that it has to be assumed that large numbers of patients who had been refusing operations before the introduction of anaesthesia, now came forward.

In March[6] the first death occurred of a patient who had received ether; he was a young man who had been run over by a train and whose leg had been amputated by Mr Hammond. The inquest exonerated ether as a possible factor in his death. The *Chronicle* devoted a weekly paragraph to

Table 4. *Some treatments mentioned by Professor Humphry in his book,[7] 'A Report of some Cases of Operation Treated for the Most Part in Addenbrooke's Hospital, Cambridge, and in the year 1855'*

Case	Operation	Comment
Three cases of urethral stricture causing poor flow or retention of urine.	'Symes operation', at least one case done under chloroform.	Involved cutting through the perineum down onto a staff passed through the ureter and later substituting a catheter around which the wound healed. Sounds similar to the modern Wheelhouse's operation.[8] In one case clots in the bladder, presumably proceeding from the vessels of the bulb, were 'stopped at last under the influence of gallic acid and opium'. (Gallic acid was a preparation of galls which was used in haemorrhages, increased mucous and other discharges, and was powerfully astringent.)[9]
Three cases of stricture of the rectum.	Treated by incision; two of the three cases done under chloroform.	Nowadays treatment is by a variety of methods. In the text clysters of cold water are mentioned as having been given to one patient. Also it is recommended that, prior to operations of this nature, 'having secured, if possible, the complete evacuation of the bowels by means of aperients and clysters, to prevent their action for some days afterwards by the administration of opium'.
Chronic rheumatic arthritis of condyle of lower jaw, producing displacement and deformity in girl of 21.	Excised whole condyle with attached end of pterygoid muscle.	In January 1854, for a year before the operation, the patient attended Out-patients. 'After several blisters, iodine was perseveringly applied, without any decent benefit. Indeed it was scarcely to be expected that much benefit would result either from external applications or medicines. (Blisters were used as counter-irritants and iodine was used to promote the removal of non-malignant swellings.)
Three cases of knee joint trouble: a woman aged 20 with a diseased joint; a sailor of 47 who had broken his patella; and a boy aged 12 with former disease of the knee that had left the joint bent to a right angle.	All three treated by removing a slice off condyles of femur and upper end of fibia and splinting the two bones in a straight line so that they fused.	A patella injury with separated fragments such as described in the sailor could be wired together or removed nowadays with reconstruction of the exterior apparatus. Some diseased joints can be replaced.[8] Before it was decided to operate on the boy's knee it was straightened under chloroform and bound up in a 'gum chalk bandage', but progress was unsatisfactory so the excision operation was decided upon.
Ovarian cysts	Ovariotomy on 18 July. Development of tetanus on 27 July. Died on 30 July.	On 17th and 18th bowels relieved with a dose of castor oil. On 19th 'two grains of opium were given – one last night and one this morning', for pain. Rx: Calomelanos gr.i; opii gr.ss M. Sumatur 34 tis horis. On the 20th: 'Sumat opii gr. iss. Applicand. acetum cantharadis abdomini. Ung. hyd. femori infricend.'

application vesicant. Unguentum Hydragyri (mercury ointment) was used as a topical stimulant to indurated and topically inflamed parts and sometimes for introducing the metal into the system.)[10] On the 21st more opium was given. 'Gave a little brandy and water and then injected one pint of water, by the tube of stomach pump, into the colon.' Acetum cantharidis reapplied. On the 27th, when tetanus developed, the patient was given a pill containing croton oil. (Croton oil a powerful hydragogue purgative.)[9]

Two cases of encysted urinary calculus.	One patient was given lithotrity three times and lithotomy five times. He died. The other patient had lithotrity and lithotomy twice.	The lithotrite was a device for crushing the stone whereas lithotomy removes it by operation. Between lithotomies both patients took small quantities of dilute nitric acid daily, presumably in an attempt to remove the remaining stones. In the case of the second patient this took the form of about 15 minims of dilute nitric acid three times a day for at least a month. After the final lithotomy the first patient suffered pain above the pubes and there was a small quantity of blood fluid in the sheet. He was given a warm fomentation. Later the abdominal muscles were rigid and the abdomen tender (peritonitis). He was given 12 leeches and a fomentation; calomel gr.i, opii gr.½, 3 tiis horis. Both patients had at least one operation under chloroform, one patient being on the table for 50 minutes. Both lithotomies were done on the second patient at his home.
Difficulty in breathing, and speaking, and cough, in man of 35.	Tracheotomy	'Being unwilling to resort to operative proceedings at once, as the symptoms were not very urgent, and thinking it right to watch the case a little while, and endeavour quickly to establish a mercurial influence, I directed mercurial ointment to be rubbed well into both thighs; and a pill containing three grains of calomel with a quarter of a grain of opium, to be taken every three hours. He got through that night pretty well.' (Mercury with chalk was thought to have, amongst other effects, that of increasing the various secretions. It also acted as a cholagogue and purgative, affected the mucous membranes of the intestinal canal powerfully, caused the absorption and prevented the formation of morbid fluids, and was of great use in syphillis.)[10]
Tetanus in woman of 50	Tracheotomy under chloroform. Patient died.	Soon after the operation the spasms returned, 'the progressive loss of strength continued; and the crepitations in the trachea, bronchi and smaller air-tubes, with shortness of breath, indicated that disease was going on in the lungs. To meet these symptoms acetum canth. and blisters were applied, 'to no purpose'.

accidents and another to inquests. From these two sources it is possible to determine the outcome of the more serious accidents. From the end of March 1847, the administration of ether had become such a routine procedure that ether is mentioned only if the surgeons considered that the patient's condition made its use inadvisable.[4]

Although general anaesthesia had so rapidly been adopted as a routine procedure, many years were to pass before, even in big cities, the administration of anaesthetics was accepted as an independent speciality requiring special skill and experience. The House Surgeon was expected to anaesthetise all hospital patients. In private practice the patient's general practitioner commonly accepted this responsibility.

~ 17 ~

Reports on the Hospital

Information concerning the diseases from which patients suffered, and the treatment they received, is generally as scanty and indirect for the greater part of the nineteenth century as it is for the eighteenth, as few case records survive. However, in 1863, the Hospital was visited by two men who placed their observations on record. The first was Timothy Holmes (1825–1907), surgeon to St George's Hospital, who was reporting to the Medical Officer of the Privy Council.[1] The second was Benjamin Ward Richardson (1828–1896) who practised as a physician in London and visited many hospitals throughout the country to collect material for a series of articles on 'The Medical History of England'.[2]

Holmes was critical of the Hospital's facilities, but in spite of these objections 'the practice of the Hospital is not unsuccessful. Surgical operations are known to do very well here.' 'Hospital infections generally are rare; erysipelas is seldom seen and appears never to prove fatal. It does, however, sometimes prevail in the town and is at such times more common in the Hospital. Phagedena is still more rare, but a fatal case had occurred shortly before our visit.'

Holmes thought that these good results were to be attributed to weekly admission by the letter system (i.e. the system of admission by subscriber's letter) which 'tends to restrict the scope of the charity and to lessen the gravity of the cases. Out of 1,911 patients admitted in three years, only 231 were taken in without letters' (i.e. admitted as emergencies), 'Therefore the cases of urgent danger are few and of these fewer still are cases of acute and profuse suppuration. There is little traumatic atmosphere in the wards and this is further diminished by the practice, which we hold to be a very salutary one in such hospitals, of mixing the surgical and medical cases in the same wards.' (Paget and Humphry were eager to separate medical and surgical cases.) 'A great many chronic cases and nervous disorders are admitted; epilepsy is often admitted and kept a long time.'

The mortality rate over three years was 5.5% of patients admitted, which compared very favourably with most hospitals, and Holmes was at pains to explain it, 'Again the Hospital appears to be never at all full. Out of 102 beds which it contains only an average of 78 were occupied in 1862. At the time of our visit there were only 62, but this was in the middle of summer and at a time when there happened to be no fever in the town. Lastly the patients are almost all agricultural labourers of good constitution and quiet regular habits, who do not require and are not used to the alcoholic stimulants which appear necessary in large cities and who are for the most part operated on for chronic strumous diseases (i.e. tuberculosis) of the joints, the most favourable class of cases for recovery.' Richardson's assessment[2] of the nutritional status of the agricultural workers is probably more accurate. He wrote that bread and butter and tea were their staple article of diet, and that they were housed in low thatched huts. He found the dwellings of the poor in the town to be less miserable than those in most towns.

Holmes referred to the 'propriety and advantage of having separate fever wards'. He noted that it was the practice at Addenbrooke's Hospital to exclude from the fever wards 'the most deadly contagious diseases, small-pox and scarlet fever'. He concludes that most cases 'may be placed in the ordinary wards without excessive danger, so long as these wards are properly constructed and the beds sufficiently far apart'. The 67 patients in the Hospital at the time of Holmes' visit consisted of 31 medical patients, of whom five or six had acute diseases, and 36 surgical patients (seven accidents, including one simple and one compound fracture and one burn; eight acute surgical, including one lithotomy and one excision of a knee joint, and 21 chronic surgical including 19 open wounds). Humphry at that time sutured wounds and then left them dry and uncovered with no local application for a few days; they did well.[2]

There is no information available concerning out-patients at this period, but venereal diseases are said to have been very prevalent; 'very few young men escape one or the other'.[2] At least 200 prostitutes were known to the authorities.

As in most hospitals, anaesthetic practice had changed. The first enthusiasm for ether resulted in a number of deaths. It had been replaced by chloroform which long remained in favour although it was eventually to prove more dangerous than ether. In 1863 anaesthetics were still given by the House Surgeon, who gave chloroform by the method of Skinner of Liverpool.[2] Thomas Skinner, an obstetric physician in Liverpool, had published an account of this method in 1862; it consisted in dropping chloroform from a special bottle onto a wool and cotton fabric stretched

Table 5. *Operations carried out at Addenbrooke's Hospital 1860–1862*

Amputations	Thigh	Primary	3	2 deaths (1 from tetanus)
		For disease	11	
		After excision of knee	3	3 deaths (1 from pyaemia)
	Leg	Primary	1	1 death
		For disease	6	1 death
	Arm	Primary	3	
		Primary at shoulder	1	1 death
		For disease of shoulder joint	1	
	Forearm	For disease	8	
Excision of joints		Knee	8	3 deaths (after amputation)
		Elbow	1	
		Shoulder	2	1 death
		Wrist	1	
		Ankle	2	1 death, 1 amputation
Strangulated hernia			5	1 death
Lithotomy		Adults	3	
		Children	7	

over a wire frame. This wire mask would fold up so that it could be carried in the pocket, hat or case. Skinner carried his mask in his hat.[3]

Holmes[1] analysed the operations performed in the Hospital during the three year period 1860–1862; there were 66 in all (see Table 5), an average of fewer than two each month.

The mortality rate after amputation was about 27%, which was almost double the average of 14.99% reported in 1863 for 117 hospitals in England and Wales.[4] The mortality after lithotomy was on the other hand vastly better than the national average of 12.5%. The overall mortality rate of 5.5% of patients admitted may be compared with 7.607% for the hospitals of England and Wales, and 9.19% for the 18 Metropolitan hospitals in 1863.

~ 18 ~

A major reconstruction

By 1860, not only was the Hospital accommodation overcrowded, it was also old-fashioned in design, and inconvenient. A New Building Committee was appointed[1] primarily to consider the possibility of building an Out-patient Department. The Committee was confronted once again with the problem of acquiring the freehold of additional land, notably the plot on the north side of the Hospital belonging to Westfield's Charity, and that on the south side belonging to Corpus Christi College.

The Committee met deputations from Corpus Christi College and from the Trustees of Westfield's Charity. The negotiations may have been aided by the fact that the three Trustees were all Governors of the Hospital, as was Emery, the Bursar of Corpus Christi College who was also Chairman of the Hospital's Improvement Committee. Eventually the College sold the land for £637, including compensation for the surrender of the lease. The Charity Commissioners refused their consent to the proposed sale of the other plot, except on such terms as would secure the Westfield Trustees an income from Consols equal to the £21.10s. they now received in rent. The purchase was finally authorised in June 1862.

The re-appointed Committee accepted on 22 September a report by Bond and Paget on the requirements for the Hospital. These were:

(a) In Out-patients' – a large waiting hall and a large dispensary and three separate rooms for the Surgeons.

(b) In the wards – more cubic space per bed. The Committee recommended 1,600 cubic feet. Martha's, the worst of the four old wards in the central building, had only 808 cubic feet per bed. Water closets should be improved and there should be a bathroom for each ward or contiguous pair of wards. Some two- or three-bed wards were needed for patients who were noisy, had stinking wounds, or suffered from strongly infectious diseases.

(c) The kitchens should be enlarged, 'the health of the servants would be more assured'.

(d) Other desirable improvements were speaking tubes and lifts 'serving to economise labour'.

(e) A porter's lodge was needed.

The Committee recommended that an architect be engaged and that his instructions should include 'certain matters of detail' of importance. Some of these details are of interest. The drains should not be under the Hospital. The walls of the new or enlarged wards should be of white polished Parian cement. There should be ample windows on more than one side of each ward. The plan should include two day-rooms for convalescent patients. The operation room should be in the upper storey of the Hospital and conveniently situated with regards to the wards.

The report was adopted[2] and the Committee was authorised to invite four architects to submit plans. It was to be a competition, with no payment for the unsuccessful competitors. From nine names proposed by various members of the Committee, four were selected by ballot.[3] Three of the four accepted the invitation and an additional architect was approached to take the place of one who declined. The plans were ordered to be hung up in the Board Room in February, and on 5 March Digby Wyatt's plan was selected, but he was asked if he could accept some modifications which the Committee thought would improve it.

At the next General Quarterly Court[4] a proposal that the plan be formally accepted was defeated by an amended proposal by H.H. Harris, seconded by Humphry, which was carried. The plan was referred back to Committee 'to consider whether it is practicable to build a new hospital upon the present or on any other site'. The Governors felt that the minimum cost of the proposed alteration to the old hospital – £7,000 – was too high and they were not satisfied that they would achieve the desired objectives.

Wyatt, replying to the Committee's enquiries, said that 'a very good plain Hospital' for 100 patients might be built on the present site for £12,000 and the old materials, or for 110 patients for £12,500. He found it more difficult to comment on the suggested changes in his original plan because, though he considered some of the objections reasonable, others 'were opposed to what the best authorities have agreed upon as to the arrangement of efficient hospitals'.

He asked that the objections should be sent to him in a clearer form. They had so far reached him only as 'Newspaper abstracts of what has been said under the heat of public discussion'. 'I freely admit the Dean of

Ely's charge of "ugliness" which I should be delighted to do my best to remedy at an extra cost of from one to several thousand pounds, according to the style adopted and the materials I might be permitted to make use of.'

Wyatt's plan seems to have been 'a scheme of extension and incorporation of the existing structure. This, apparently, presented a large central block for the main facilities, with north and south wings on a line of the pre-existent wards.'[5] The Secretary wrote to Wyatt explaining that, apart from the objections to the central front mass, the main defects were that two small wards were accessible only through the operating room, and that there was too much ward space on the ground floor.

On 26 June the Committee received a letter and a memorandum from Wyatt. He felt that in his revised plans he had met all the objections, which he had discussed with the medical staff. However, on 6 July the Committee learned that the Surgeons still considered. that the operating room and surgical wards should be separate from the medical wards in an additional upper storey. The Surgeons were asked to put their proposals in writing and in greater detail.

Digby Wyatt attended a meeting of the Committee on 12 August. They agreed a report from the next Quarterly Court. They thought that Wyatt's amended plan removed most of the objections made to his original plan. The appearance of the exterior would be 'more of an old English style'. The estimated cost was £9,000. The alternative plan suggested by the Surgeons, notably Humphry, would involve lengthening the front of the Hospital and adding another storey in the existing style. The estimated cost was £7,000.

An entirely new building in the style proposed by Wyatt would cost £13,000.

When the three plans were placed before the Governors[6] each found some supporters, but Humphry's plan was approved by 32 votes to 9. The Committee was re-appointed to put the plan into effect, and informed Wyatt of the Governors' decision. 'The idea is to retain the present front of the Hospital with its colonnade etc., but with such modifications as will be necessitated by the alterations and as they may seem to you best fitted to prevent heaviness in the wings and to give a good appearance to the building'.

By 2 December Wyatt had evidently submitted his revised plans, for the Committee selected 'Elevation No. 2'. A sub-committee was set up 'with a view to the diminishing of the expense'. They proposed thirteen modifications in the plans and wrote to ask Wyatt how much money these would save. The long-suffering Wyatt sent an amended plan incorporating the requested modifications which would, he said, reduce the cost from £9,700 to £9,080. He pointed out that 'rigid economy' and 'careful contrivance' would be essential to keep the cost down to this level. The proposed hospital would be 'a good substantial building, wholesome, cheerful and airy, but one in which evidence of pinching cannot be concealed'. 'I only desire to remind the Committee that it is almost impossible to unite excellence and cheapness.' In its report to the Governors the Committee merely recommended that the Hospital be erected. Wyatt's reservations were not mentioned.

Builders in Cambridge and in London were invited to submit tenders, but progress was delayed by the indisposition of Wyatt.[7] On 2 May 1864, six tenders were received, four of them over £14,000. The tender of Thoday and Clayton at £10,975 was accepted.[8] On the following day the contractors who were represented at a meeting of the Committee, agreed to complete the central building and the south wing in seven months, and be allowed up to ten months to complete the rest of the work. In June[9] the Corporate Seal was affixed to the contract, but not before a proposal by the Mayor that an entirely new hospital be built had been put to the vote and lost by seven to fifteen.

The steady progress of the work was reported step by step in the Minutes of the Committee. By 2 August the Committee was able to authorise the first payment of £2,500 to the contractor, and by 28 October the second payment of £2,000. No details are given of the arrangements made for the care of the patients during the reconstruction, but the disorganisation must have been considerable. The number of beds occupied on various dates between 27 July and 21 December, ranged from 22 to 28, and of out-patients per week from 16 to 36. By 8 February the payment to the contractors of the third instalment of £2,000 was authorised. It was agreed that the inscription ' "Addenbrooke's Hospital" should be cut in the stonework on either side of the centre'. The payment of a further instalment of £2,500 was authorised on 18 May, but the Governors were far from satisfied with the progress of the work and, in June 1865,[10] they reminded the contractors of the penalty clauses in their contract. This reminder must have been effective for the Committee, at its meeting on 16 August, discussed bedsteads, mattresses, and the best ways of celebrating the re-opening of the Hospital. On 29 September it was reported that 110 iron bedsteads had been ordered from Swan Hurrell at 17s.6d. each.

On 17 October the Committee ordered that the five male wards be named Bowtell, Maynard, Griffith, Turton and Abbott, and that the four female wards be named Victoria, Elizabeth, Mary and Anne. Soon afterwards[11] Elizabeth Ward was renamed Hatton Ward, after Miss E.A. Hatton who had in 1846 established the building fund with a gift of £1,200. The admission of patients to the new wards on the upper storey, at the discretion of Paget and Lestourgeon, was sanctioned on 17 October. The number of occupied beds increased from 29 on 1 November to 41 on 20 December, and by the end of the year the whole of the top floor and one ward on first floor were in use.[12]

Meanwhile the Committee had asked Wyatt to look at the fever wards and the laundry and other buildings in the old hospital not covered by the scheme in progress, to see whether they could be improved.

Wyatt listed the principal defects:[12] the laundry was too small and neither it nor the rooms occupied by the residential medical staff and pupils were satisfactorily separated from the fever wards. These and some other defects could be remedied at a cost of £385. The Committee received the Governors' approval to carry out improvements at a cost not exceeding £400.[13]

On 14 May the Hospital was opened to the public. 'Upwards of 2,000 persons visited the Hospital . . . the buildings having been decorated with flowers and plants lent from the Horticultural Fete – the visitors were most orderly and expressed themselves much pleased with all they saw.'[14] The Building Committee, meeting on 27 September for the last time, also expressed its satisfaction with what had been achieved. The total expenditure had been £15,565.9s.11d.; £14,573.6s.9d. on the building, £952.3s.2d. on bedsteads, bedding and furniture, and £40 on the garden.

In their final report they congratulated the Governors on 'the possession of a building for novelty and beauty of elevation and convenience of internal arrangements equal to any provincial hospital in the Kingdom'.

Sir Matthew Digby Wyatt (1820–1887), was an architect of some distinction. His first important work was Paddington Station. According to Pevsner[15] he was undeniably a remarkable man, but undeniably a bad architect. Pevsner writes

> Nowhere else in Wyatt's oeuvre does this embarrassing loss of concentration come out more distressingly than in Addenbrooke's Hospital. It is sufficient to look at these symmetrical wings with their buttresses holding up an arcade with closely set columns, and the two broader arcades with a third above displaying a kind of weak Gothic lintels, which connect the wings with a weakly recessed Tudor centre, and one cannot fail to feel that deliberation must have dictated to the architect this covering of his whole

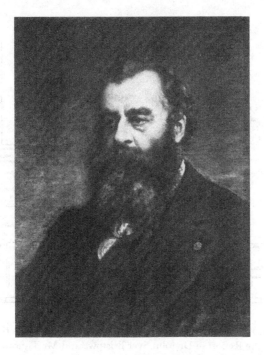

Fig. 20. Matthew Digby Wyatt, from the portrait in the R.I.B.A.
by Ossani (c.1870).

surface, with whatever motives, but that the quality and juxtaposition of
these motives show him to have been a highly insensitive architect.

Wyatt's contemporaries thought highly of his work. The author of a
long editorial in *The Lancet*[16] praised the Hospital as, for its size, a model
hospital. He praised its artistic merits: 'the front of the building presents a
noble façade, great variety and picturesqueness being obtained by the
judicious use of stone, terra-cotta and encaustic tiles, and coloured bricks;
the general effect being heightened by recessed exercising colonnades and
a continuous arcade of coloured brickwork springing from terra-cotta
columns with foliated caps and moulded bases'.

The artistic judgement of the leader writer is of less interest than his
account of the amenities of the Hospital after the completion of the
rebuilding, for it may be compared with an account of conditions in 1863,
just before this was commenced, written by Mr Timothy Holmes, the
London surgeon[17] mentioned in the previous chapter. His report included
a plan of the hospital (Fig. 21). The original (1766) building contained

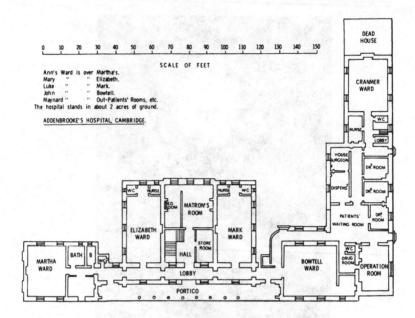

Fig. 21. Plan of Addenbrooke's before the 1860s reconstruction,
from the Report of Dr John Syer Bristowe and Mr Timothy
Holmes.[1] The ground and first floors only were used as wards at
this time.

four wards: Elizabeth and Mark on the ground floor, with Anne and Luke
above them. The Bowtell extensions had added the wings, providing
Martha and Bowtell Wards on the ground floor and Anne and John
Wards upstairs. The fever wards were added on two floors of a separate
building, which was then connected to the main building by a block
containing the Out-patient Department on the ground floor with Maynard Ward above it. Holmes was very critical of the accommodation. He
commented that the lack of any regular plan prevented any adequate
through-ventilation. The accommodation for in-patients was insufficient,
the beds being too crowded. The sanitary arrangements were defective,
with water closets in the corners of most wards. The small size of the wards
made nursing and supervision costly and imperfect.

The Lancet visited the Hospital in 1866 and was very impressed by the
accommodation. The water closets were in projected pavilions at the
extreme angles of the wards. The cubic feet of air allowed to each bed
varied from 1,500 to nearly 2,000 in different wards. The day-rooms,
which were prettily decorated, communicated with an exercising arcade

~ 152 ~

above the colonnade. The day-rooms and the principal wards had a dark green skirting, a cheerful red dado, and warm green walls with stencilled ornaments in various colours. 'The whole effect is that of great comfort and homeliness, entirely doing away with the workhouselike look which is so apt on entering ordinary hospital wards to impress the patient with a sense of dreariness and isolation.' 'On the whole, the new Addenbrooke's Hospital must be seen to be appreciated. It is a great ornament to the town . . .'

~ 19 ~

The sick, 1860 to 1900

Throughout the 1860s the alleged 'abuse of the Charity' by patients well able to pay, continued to be discussed. Some cases were brought to the notice of the Governors by the medical staff or by general practitioners. For example, one case of 'abuse' accepted as such by the Governors[1] was reported by Mr R.O. Arnold of Waterbeach. He complained that the child of a farmer and merchant, 'in every way well off' had been admitted to hospital with a simple fracture of the leg. 'What with the abuse of the Hospital, the Clubs and the Unions, there is very little private practice for any medical man in this part of the country'.

Another problem was the cost of railway travel. In 1866 the Vicar of Wisbech informed the Governors that the return ticket to Cambridge cost 8s.1od. on Wednesday (out-patients' day) but only 4s.5d. on Saturdays.[2] The Great Eastern Railway refused to allow a reduced fare on Wednesdays for patients of the Hospital. The Governors agreed[3] that patients coming more than 8 miles by rail, or from places where carriers did not come on Wednesdays, might attend on Saturdays.

Infectious diseases

Infectious disease was a constant problem. On several occasions special accommodation had been constructed for infectious cases, but shortage of beds had each time resulted in the use of the designated accommodation for general medical and surgical cases. In the early 1870s a hospital as short of money as Addenbrooke's was particularly reluctant to spend it on isolation wards since it was known that legislation was planned giving local authorities the general power to erect special hospitals; such legislation was in fact included in the great Public Health Act of 1875.[4]

However, early in 1871[5] the number of cases of smallpox, typhoid and scarlet fever in the wards began to alarm the Governors and the nursing staff. The admission of further cases of smallpox was forbidden[6] and a report on the outbreak was called for.[7] Four patients with smallpox had been admitted between 10 December and 7 February. Six patients and the Assistant Porter had contracted smallpox in the hospital. Another patient developed smallpox in April.[8] The Minutes do not suggest that admission of smallpox cases to general wards was considered hazardous.

In 1883 Albert and Hatton Wards were closed for two months because of an outbreak of erysipelas. The medical staff decided that they could be re-opened 'if the beds are thoroughly disinfected'.[9] But erysipelas continued to present serious problems. In 1886 a committee was 'empowered to take steps at once for dealing with the erysipelas cases in the Hospital'.[10] These cases were to be isolated in the 'so-called fever wards' and attended only by the House Surgeon (H.S.). The bedrooms adjacent to the fever wards were to be occupied only by nurses working in these fever wards.

The difficulty of controlling infection in wards heavily crowded with furniture and draperies (see Fig. 22) would have been great enough had the cause and mode of transmission of streptococcal infection been clearly known. In the absence of such knowledge the problem was virtually insurmountable. Mr Wherry blamed one case on the centrally opening windows of the water closets.[11] A complaint from a patient adds a picturesque detail to our knowledge of the state of the wards. The complaint concerned birds in Victoria Ward. An investigation by two Governors established 'that the patients unanimously approved of the birds': two canaries, a blackbird and a jackdaw.[12]

The confused attitude towards venereal disease was strikingly illustrated in 1885 when Dr Perowne, Master of Corpus Christi College, wrote in his capacity as Chairman of the Managing Committee of the Cambridge Female Refuge, to ask why the Hospital had refused a patient from the Refuge on the grounds 'that there was no ward for the reception of cases of this kind'.[13] Dr Perowne was referred to Rule 79 which excluded patients with venereal disease. He reminded the Board, quite correctly, that a ward had recently been provided specifically for such patients. The Secretary assured him that the rearrangement of the wards was in preparation, but it seems that, as on numerous previous occasions in the past, beds provided for isolation had been quickly brought into general use.

On 17 November 1886[14] there were ten cases of typhoid in the Hospital and two more were expected that day. One of the probationers looking after them died and another was severely ill.[15] In 1887 an Infectious Diseases Hospital was opened in Mill Road. A patient with scarlet fever was transferred there in October of that year. The Hospital agreed to pay a general practitioner 5s. per visit to attend her.

In January 1888,[16] the House Surgeon reported five cases of erysipelas.

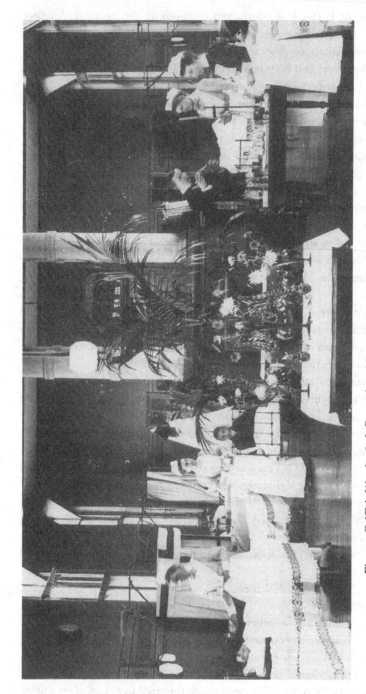

Fig. 22. Griffith Ward, 1896. Reproduced by permission of the Cambridgeshire Collection.

The Weekly Board asked the medical staff whether it would be practicable not to admit patients known to be suffering from smallpox, typhoid, scarlet fever, diphtheria or erysipelas. The medical staff accepted this regulation if the two diseases last named were excluded but nevertheless failed to comply with it. They were criticised by the Medical Officer of Health (M.O.H.) for this refusal to accept Borough cases of typhoid (which were eligible for admission to the isolation hospital) whilst continuing to admit those from elsewhere.[17] The M.O.H. refused to accept a patient with measles from the children's ward.[18] He was strictly within his rights for measles was not covered by the Infectious Diseases Act.

The high incidence of infections led the medical staff to ask on many occasions in 1887 and 1888 for an inspection of the drains, the defective state of which they suspected as causing the infection. The Board was not convinced, and only minor inspections were made.[19] Infections, and the overcrowding which contributed to them, continued to be a serious problem, partly because concepts of infection remained ill-defined. Latham complained[20] that cases of gangrene, erysipelas and whooping cough 'were put into the fever wards which prevented their being put to their proper use'. It was agreed that erysipelas cases should be admitted to the Hope Ward and not to the fever wards. Hope Ward was intended for women with venereal disease. One consequence of the admission of erysipelas cases to this ward was the decision in March 1890 not to admit women with venereal disease until suitable separate accommodation was available!

New cases of erysipelas continued to be reported. The Governors asked the medical officers to send cases to 'The Sanatorium' (i.e. the Infectious Diseases Hospital, Brookfields), but the M.O.H. would accept only Borough patients. A County hospital for infectious diseases was an obvious need.[21] The medical staff, and Professor Latham in particular, continued to press for an investigation of the insanitary state of the wards. Latham blamed sore throats and diphtheria on 'emanations from the sewers'. At last, in April 1892, the Governors agreed to set up a committee[22] with the consequences described on p. 224.

The curious relationship between Brookfields and Addenbrooke's remained a source of vigorous dispute between Whitehead, the Town Clerk, and the Hospital Secretary. The Town Clerk expected the Hospital to pay £1.1s. weekly to his office for any patient, not a resident of the Borough, transferred from the Hospital to Brookfields. Whitehead, a

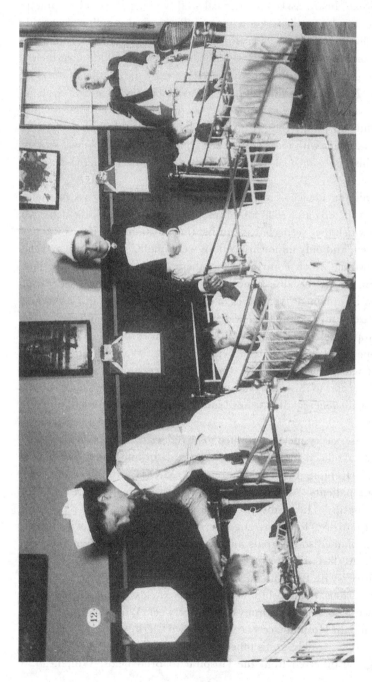

Fig. 23. Children's ward, July 1894. Central figure is believed to be the Matron, Miss Mary Cureton. Reproduced by permission of the Cambridgeshire Collection.

Select Governor of the Hospital, was present when the Weekly Board[23] decided to write to the Sanatorium Committee of the Cambridge Town Council, asking whether they would receive in the Sanatorium cases of infectious disease which had been sent to the Hospital from the County and elsewhere, and on what terms. Whitehead replied to this letter in his capacity as Town Clerk.[24] The Sanatorium Committee had agreed to recommend the Council to accept cases of typhoid, scarlet fever, diptheria or smallpox. They proposed to charge £2.2s. per week and, in addition to the actual cost of the ambulance (4s.), another £2.2s. per week for a day or night nurse 'when directly necessitated by the admission of such patients', 'Addenbrooke's Hospital is to supply medical attention, medicines and medical extras.' These very ungenerous terms were accepted when the Solicitor to the Hospitals' Association advised the Governors that their argument that 'a person resident outside the district but who had found his way into the Hospital, thereby became an inhabitant of the district',[25] was not valid.

The coprolite miners

When any special source of emergency admissions came to the notice of the Governors they sought some means of reducing the frequency of the accidents and recovering the cost of treating them; emergencies were not required to bring subscribers' letters. The railway companies had been approached when accidents to men engaged on construction work were frequent, and road traffic accidents were later to form another category of patients expensive to the Hospital. In 1875 the numerous accidents to coprolite workmen led the Governors[26] to write to the Secretary of State to bring to his notice this situation in the hope that steps might be taken to prevent these accidents. The Secretary of State replied that as coprolite pits were 'not within the Coal Mine Regulation Act' he had no jurisdiction over them. He had, however, sent an Inspector of Mines who informed him that the accidents were the result of carelessness.

Coprolites are phosphatic nodules which were found in deposits in certain geological formations in Cambridgeshire.[27] They were first discovered in 1851 and shown to be a valuable source of fertiliser. From the late 1850s the coprolite industry expanded rapidly to reach its peak in 1885, after which it declined.

George Wherry, who was House Surgeon from 1874 to 1878 remembered these accidents, and recalled that they continued until coprolite mining ceased. They were mostly severe crush injuries, such as fractured pelvis.[28]

Out-patients

The Governors, looking for possible economies, expressed their concern about the increase in the number of out-patients. The House Physician was asked to prepare a report.[29] He found that total attendances for 1 January to 10 March had been 2,779 in 1881, 3,008 in 1882, and 3,330 in 1883. He considered that the Out-patient Department was abused by patients who could afford to pay, but also 'by persons who ought to come under the care of the Parish, people whose diseases are largely due to want and destitution, and they receive almost no benefit from hospital treatment in Out-patients'. Finally, there were patients, mainly women, who 'although far from being malingerers had scarcely any complaint except an insatiable desire for medicines'.

The Committee on Out-patients considered this report.[30] Their only proposal was that patients who had attended for two months should not be allowed to renew their recommendations (i.e. obtain another subscriber's letter) unless the Physician or Surgeon had certified in writing that this was desirable.

The first seriously planned attempt to restrict the so-called abuse of the Out-patient Department was devised by a committee set up in December 1890[31] to confer with the Committee of the National Provident Association. They met a month later when Mr Huddlestone explained the working of the Association.[32] The Committee resolved that a notice be printed on the recommendation papers used by subscribers in referring patients. 'Proper recipients of the benefits of charity are 1) persons whose condition in consequence of bodily suffering requires immediate and special treatment. 2) Those, who having had medical advice at their own cost and who, in consequence of narrow circumstances are unable to continue to have such advice. 3) And in general – persons whose earnings if single, do not exceed 16/- per week or if married 21/- per week, with an allowance of 2/- per week for each child.' Persons earning more than this should be encouraged to join a Medical Provident Institution or Sick Benefit Club.

The very poor were, of course, entitled to medical care by the Unions whose medical officers could arrange for them to be referred to the

Hospital at the expense of the Union. The Committee recommended also 'that it is advisable to supply a person . . . to enquire into the condition of all persons applying from the Parliamentary Borough of Cambridge as Out-patients'. The Committee met again on 6 March[33] and approved the amendments to the recommendation paper but, for item 3 above, they substituted 'persons who are unable to pay for medical assistance themselves'. The regulations covering out-patients were then revised but without significant changes. The only infections excluded were smallpox, scarlet fever and erysipelas.

However, a necessary change in the regulations for in-patients was introduced in 1893 when Tubbs, the House Surgeon, complained that the number of visitors to each patient was unlimited, and often exceeded ten, most of them trying to sit on the bed. The wards became crowded and 'the atmosphere foul and oppressive'. There were also a number of people wandering aimlessly around visiting no-one in particular.[34] The number of visitors was reduced to two at a time and the visiting hours were reduced. To enforce these regulations two numbered tickets were issued for each occupied bed.[35]

Medical records

The earliest surviving case records concerned medical in-patients; they are bound in now tattered volumes and some information from them is given in the next chapter. Previous references to medical records mention only the 'bed tickets', which, according to the rules of the Hospital, gave the name of the member of the staff in charge of the patient, and particulars of diet and treatment. In 1895 it was resolved[36] that the Surgeon in Charge of the Gynaecological Department be requested to keep a register and case book of gynaecological out-patients, that the Assistant Surgeon should be requested to keep similar records of surgical out-patients, and the House Surgeon be requested to keep a register of operations and anaesthetics.

Out-patient amenities

A first attempt to improve the amenities of the Out-patient Department was made in 1889 when backs were fitted to ten of the nineteen forms in the Waiting Room.[37] A further step forward was taken in 1896[38] when the

Cambridge Branch of the British Women's Temperance Association was granted permission for their 'small hand coffee cart' to stand in the corridor of the Out-patient Department 'in charge of a very respectable young man'. The waiting time was often exceedingly long as all patients were required to attend at the same time and as there were frequently further queues for the Dispensary.

Recommendation papers

The Governors had ordered in 1891 that all particulars appearing on the recommendation papers should be recorded in a book.[39] The report of the committee analysing this information was received on 31 May 1899. The Committee considered that fewer recommendation papers should be given to subscribers. At present about 10,000 were issued, but only 6,000 came back. They thought that this 'superabundance' of forms led Governors to give them to those who were not deserving people. There were also many irregularities; Governors sometimes gave signed blank forms to others; out-of-date forms were used.

They thought that the submission of a weekly list of patients' names, addresses and occupations, with the name of the referring subscriber, should be presented to the Weekly Board. To the report the Committee attached a list of the occupations of all patients referred between 1 October 1898 and 16 May 1899. Over 20% of the forms had omitted the occupation of the patient. Also attached was a list of names of some sixty persons, the status of which they felt should be investigated. Many of those listed were publicans or farmers or held managerial positions and therefore seemed likely to be ineligible on financial grounds.

The Committee reported again in July and August.[40] It was agreed that the Hospital must try to avoid admitting improper recipients of the advantages of the Institution but 'every precaution must be taken not to lessen the efficiency or popularity of the Hospital'. A change in the form was agreed but the Board recognised the 'extreme difficulty or perhaps the utter impossibility' of determining fairly who could afford to pay and who could not.

～20～

Some of Addenbrooke's earliest medical records

Medical

The earliest (extant) set of medical records for Addenbrooke's Hospital date from 1876 and are for Dr Latham's patients. A slightly later set labelled 'Dr. MacAlister Oct 1884 – Oct 1888' were examined and analysed. They contain part of an index for 152 patients and case notes, mostly complete, for 141 admissions, all male medical. The book is battered and crumbling and of the type known as a guard book, pages stuck onto a spine of one-inch wide strips after they have been written.

Taking a series of patients at random the diagnoses are: 'Chronic Bright's, Bronchitis; Phthisis; Bronchitis, Emphysema, Dilated right heart; Lateral sclerosis; Locomotor ataxy (sic); Hepatitis; Groph. Goitre; Pleural Effusion; Phthisis & tuberc. peritonitis; Cancer of liver; Double mitral disease; ?tuberculosis.'

Tuberculosis seems to have been the most prevalent complaint overall. Seventeen patients were diagnosed as suffering from it and there were at least another eleven likely cases giving a total of 28 (20%). In addition, from the patients' family histories it appears that at least 36 patients (26%) had one or more relatives who had suffered, or were suffering, from tuberculosis.

Amongst the other cases, heart disease was diagnosed 22 times (16%); nervous cases and tumours sixteen times each (11% each); bronchitis eight times; no illness (sometimes 'nihilitis') six times; syphilis five; rheumatism, pneumonia and Bright's disease four times each; alcoholism three times; typhoid, poisoning and rheumatic fever twice each.[1]

The treatment given to the patients was often not mentioned in the notes and at the end of one case it says 'For Medicines See Dispensary Sheet'. Only two of these have been found for this period, folded loose in the notes. Sometimes, however, the medicines are reported. Many are illegible but some interpretations are given in Table 6.

Table 6. *Some medicines given to Dr MacAlister's medical patients, 1884–1888*

Case	Medicine	Comment – derived from contemporary textbooks
Cardiac disease	Ether	A powerful, diffusible stimulant, expectorant, antispasmodic and narcotic, and is of great use in dyspnoea and gastralgia. Used to expel flatus from the stomach and to allay pain and cramp in that organ. In nausea given as a cordial.[2]
Cardiac disease	Digitalis	Digitalis Folia (from the Foxglove). Sedative and diuretic, useful in acute dropsy when disturbance arises from over-action of the heart.[2]
Cardiac disease	Chloroform water	Internally chloroform is a sedative, narcotic and anti-spasmodic, given on sugar for sea-sickness. May be given as an antiperiodic. Externally a stimulant in senile gangrene and sloughing ulcers. The vapour is often applied to the eye, and also to the rectum or vagina.
Cardiac disease	Infus Sennae	Infusum Sennae (from Cassia). A general and efficient laxative.
Tertiary Syphilis	Potassium Bromide	Introduced for chronic enlargements of the liver. Employed in enlargement of the spleen, and in bronchocele and scrofula. It exerts a powerful influence on the generative organs, lowering their functions to a marked degree. Useful in mania and nymphomania, epilepsy, spasmodic asthma etc.[2]
Tertiary Syphilis	Dec Sarsae Co	Decoctum Sarsa Compositum (Decoction of Sarsae compound, from the dried root of Jamaica Sarsaparilla). It is an alternative and tonic; of special service in secondary syphilis, in chronic rheumatism, in cachetic diseases, chronic abcesses attended with profuse discharge, and many maladies connected with a depraved state of the system.[2]
Mitral Obstruction	Enema of oil	
Phthisis	Antipyrine – used to control temperature	Phenazone. Antipyretic and analgesic nervine sedative. Given to reduce temperature in all forms of febrile disease.[3]
Phthisis	Pil Belladonna c Quinine	Pilulae (pills) of Belladonna with Quinine. Belladonna (Deadly Nightshade) is a powerful narcotic with diaphoretic and diuretic properties. Quinine (from Cinchona bark) was used in ague and other chronic diseases and cases of direct debility.[2]

Condition	Treatment	Notes
?Hypertrophied Heart	Encf. Bellad to precordial area	Possibly Emplastrum (plaster) Belladonna which should be spread with a moderately warm iron.[2]
Angina Pectoris	Sodium nitrite	Vaso-dilator and antispasmodic used with the object of warding off the attack in angina pectoris and asthma, as well as relieving the symptoms during an attack.[3]
Tubercular pleurisy and Peritonitis (Patient died)	Turpentine Enema	Oil of Turpentine is antiseptic, haemostatic, diuretic, anthelminthic. Antispasmodic in hysterical affections and in hiccough, it is said to dissolve gallstones. Used as an inhalation in chronic bronchitis. As an enema for obstinate constipation, for flatulency and typanitic distension of the bowels, and in threadworm. Externally rubiefacient and counter-irritant; employed as a liniment in chronic inflammations and rheumatism.[3]
Glioma of brain	Physostigmine on eyes	Physostigmine Sulphate. Used to contract the pupil in ciliary paralysis due e.g. to diphtheria; to reduce intra-ocular tension in glaucoma etc; to prevent or reduce prolapse of the iris after corneal wounds etc.[3]
Sciatica, disease of ankle	Scotts dressing to ankle	Ankle was swollen and tender. Scotts ointment of mercury.[2]
Splenic Leucocythaemia	Quinine	From Cinchona bark. Used in ague and also in many chronic diseases in which intermissions do not occur, and in cases of direct debility.[2]
Dyspepsia, Hypochondriasis	Liq: arsenic Hydroch	Liquor Arsenici Hydrochloricus (from Arsenious acid). A nerve tonic given in Eczema, in chronic cutaneous diseases, and in chronic rheumatism of the joints. It is an anti-periodic in agues and neuralgic affections.[2]
Dyspepsia	Ac Carbol	Carbolic Acid. Given to check sickness, to arrest diarrhoea, to remove intestinal worms etc. It produces profuse perspiration, lowers the pulse and is thus useful in fever, scarlatina, measles and smallpox. Externally, used alone is a powerful caustic; as a lotion for foul or syphilitic ulcers, carbuncles, scabies and lepra; excellent for eczema etc.[2]
Tracheotomy for Laryngitis	Collodion painted round red swollen wound	Chiefly used for coating diseased or wounded parts with a protecting film.[2]

As well as being given medicines the patients were also occasionally subjected to minor surgical procedures. One patient with laryngitis was 'Put under chloroform and tracheotomy done with the greatest skill and celerity by Mr Rivers Pollock (H.S.)', and when two days later 'wound and surrounding read (sic) and swollen', the area was painted with collodion. This patient recovered.

Another, with epithelioma of the gullet, had a catheter passed into his stomach; and two had oesophageal bougies passed, one for oesophageal carcinoma, and the other with 'dyspepsia and pulsating abdominal aorta'.

Others had swellings opened or aspirated; several had their chests tapped; Professor Humphry himself aspirated a hydatid cyst of the liver; and one had acupuncture of the lumbar region for pleurisy. Three had blisters or plasters applied and another was 'to be blistered behind ears' – he had tubercular meningitis and was apparently discharged on the day he was described as having 'constant gurgling in throat and scattered rales through lungs. Constantly working arms as though on a treadmill or else picking at bedclothes.'

Not much was said about the patients' diet. One patient with 'Fatty Brights' who eventually died in hospital 'Has not been sick but takes very little, only milk. Was cupped, right side, last night, gave relief to pain.' Two days later 'Takes milk well and eggs, but was sick after mutton broth.' This patient was also given brandy.

Another patient with Bright's disease was given eggs and milk pudding and took Turkish Baths.

The two patients whose dispensary sheets were folded into the notes were both prescribed brandy as part of their regular diet and one also had a pint of beer prescribed. Alcohol, particularly brandy, was often given medicinally 'to rouse the system in some cases of extreme debility'.[4] There were diets described on the sheet as 'Admission' and 'Full' and although exactly what these were has not survived, a copy of the diets* approved in

* The daily nutrient value of the full diet has been worked out[5] as follows.
Men: energy 2070 kilocalories; protein 112 g; calcium 1030 mg; iron 15 mg.
Women: energy 2000 kilocalories; protein 103 g; calcium 1030 mg; iron 14 mg.
The medical patients received extra food, and their daily intake was:
Men: energy 3020 kilocalories; protein 167 g; calcium 2530 mg; iron 18 mg.
Women: energy 2956 kilocalories; protein 157.6 g; calcium 2530 mg; iron 17 mg.
The medical patients in particular appear to have received a diet in excess of modern recommendations (see Chapter 10), although the vitamin content cannot be determined owing to insufficient detail regarding the fruit and vegetables consumed.

Adopted 27 November 1905

DIETS

Full Diet: Bread 12oz
Beef or Mutton* Men 4oz. Women 3oz.
Pudding 8oz
Milk ¾ pt
Broth ¾ pt
Potatoes 6oz. Other vegetables when convenient

Fish Diet: The same as full diet but 8oz fish instead of 4oz meat.

Admission Diet: Bread 12oz
Pudding 8oz (rice, sago or tapioca)
Broth or soup 1 pint
Milk 2 pints

Milk Diet: Milk 3 pints

Diet of those on Colonnade: Full diet with the addition either of:†
2 pints of milk, or
2 eggs, or
1 egg and bacon, and sometimes also porridge.

Children's Diet: (Between the ages of two and ten) A child of 7 years to have half an adult's diet and the apportionment to be arranged in the wards according to the age and needs of each child.

---

* If it is convenient rabbit can be substituted for beef or mutton, one rabbit to four diets.
Extras Fowl (one fowl to four diets)
Meat juice

† Surgical cases. Full diet plus milk 1 pint, bacon.
Medical cases. *Men*: Full diet plus milk 2 pints; bacon and one egg, or eggs two.
Medical cases. *Women*: Full diet plus milk 2 pints, bacon.

Alteration recommended by the honorary staff, December 1906, and approved by the General Committee of January 1907.

1905 and 1907 has been found in the Minute Book (see above). The outcome of the treatment received by the patients was not good at this time. Twenty-five of the 141 died (18%) and four became worse. There were three re-admissions but two of these were for unknown patients, their original case notes possibly in another book.

Three patients were self-discharged and one, in whom nothing was found wrong, was discharged to 'Bowtell'. The rest were discharged either without comment or with remarks such as 'much improved', 'improved', 'well', 'in status quo'; one was 'fair' and one case of rheumatic fever was a 'cure'.

The patients were mostly men employed in jobs likely to be lowly paid such as labourer (56 out of 126 employed were labourers, i.e. 44%), bricklayer, painter, trumpeter, engineer, sawyer, messenger, and there were only four men for whom no occupation was stated, including one 15-year-old imbecile.

Children were included in the case notes and nine boys were at school; there was no 'occupation' recorded for two but presumably they were at school too.

The ages of the patients ranged from 8 to 71 years, 21 were below 18 years (15%) and 17 were above 60 years (12%). The average age was 38.78 years. For four no age was given and one of these was a boy.

They came mostly from Cambridge itself and surrounding towns and villages, but occasionally hailed from more distant places, such as Forest Hill, Bishops Stortford, Sevenoaks and even Germany.

The case histories were quite full and included past medical histories. Ten had a probable or definite history of syphilis (7%), and six had had gonorrhea (4%), one patient having had it four times. Only two were recorded as having had tuberculosis. Many patients had their drinking habits recorded, including 47 who took a daily quantity of beer averaging 2.97 pints. Some also took spirits or drank during harvest or when working only. Five had been drinkers but were now either temperate or abstainers.

There were 141 sets of notes but for two a discharge date could not be determined. Of the remaining 139 the average duration of stay in hospital was 28.94 days. However, the discharge date on the notes was not always exact as sometimes it appeared to be a day or so prior to a date on the temperature chart; in these cases it was the latter that was noted.

Other points of interest were that urine was analysed routinely, and reports included acidity, albumen, sugar, cells, casts, phosphates and specific gravity. There were occasional reports of the microscopic examination of fluids – blood, urine, sputum and tumour serum – and these included three mentions of searches for tubercle bacilli, two of these in sputum and the third presumably so.

Temperature charts were kept frequently but not in every case. Pulse and respiration rates were quite often recorded, and 11 patients had pulses of 60 or below (a low pulse rate may be related to a high degree of fitness).

One patient with tuberculosis had a laryngoscopic examination, and another with paralysis of the extensors of the right hand was given Faradism. In four cardiovascular cases oblongs of smoked paper marked

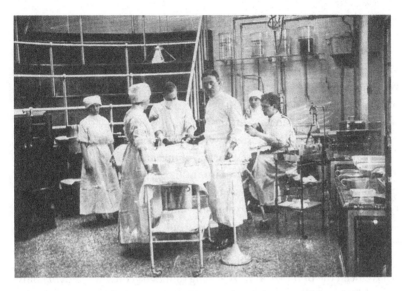

Fig. 24.Operating theatre as it was in the early 1900s although the
group is thought to be of slightly later date.

with a trace had been stuck into the notes and these are thought to be
sphygmographic tracings of the pulse, one set was labelled 'left radial' and
'right radial', and another 'mit regurg'. Electrical currents in the heart
were not demonstrated until 1887.

Surgical

The earliest surgical records are for 1896. A well-preserved volume for the
year 1900 was examined. The notes were arranged in alphabetical order
and extended over two volumes. The first 141 admissions were studied;
these filled more than a third of the first volume and extended to surnames
beginning CH-. Three general surgeons shared the cases, Griffiths,
Deighton and Wherry, and a fourth, Mr Higgins, operated once.

The first eleven cases in the book were diagnosed as: 'old spinal caries;
Rt. Fract Femur; L. Varicocoele; Gon. Opthalmica; Ulcer – Erysipelas;
Burn (2 degrees) – Buttocks & shoulders; Abscess of cheek; Gangrene of
Rt. Foot (Diabetic); comminuted fractured Rt. Tib & Fib – middle $\frac{1}{3}$;
ulcerated corn; Glandular abscess of neck. Lupus of (L) thigh.'

Traumatic injury was the most common presenting complaint, ten patients having fractures, and there being thirteen other injuries, making a total of 23 cases (16%) in all.

Tuberculosis was the second most common presenting complaint; it was explicit in twelve cases (including two re-admissions) and there were five others who sounded tubercular – presenting with glands in the neck for example. This made a total of 17 (12%). Only eight patients had tuberculosis in their family histories (6%), however.

Of the other complaints there were eleven connected with eyes, nine each of abscesses and ulcers, seven each of tumours and hernias, five each of spinal complaints, cellulitis and urethral complaints, four cleft palates, three fistulae-in-ano or perineal fistulae, and two each of varicocoeles, hydrocoeles, burns, cysts, erysipelas, malformed feet and intestinal obstructions. Surprisingly there was only one appendicitis and that was a relapse.

In Addenbrooke's around the beginning of this century, there appears to have been the practice, at least among some surgeons, of removing only part of the appendix when doing an appendicectomy. This was obviously not a general practice because it has been commented on[6] by the distinguished pathologist Sir Philip Panton (born 1877) who was Assistant House Surgeon and Senior House Surgeon at Addenbrooke's in 1904–1905.

He was a medical student at Cambridge and says he went down in 1900. He qualified M.R.C.S., L.R.C.P. in 1903 and was House Physician and Assistant Pathologist at St Thomas' Hospital, going on to Addenbrooke's from there. He says: 'The change from house physician at St. Thomas's to house surgeon at Addenbrooke's was rather like transferring from a Cunard Liner to a tramp steamer.'

Later he continued: 'The really appalling aspect of the hospital practice lay with the surgery. The senior surgeon could not do a simple appendicectomy, but contented himself with the removal of the top of that organ. Shortly after my arrival, I had to inform him that a patient whose appendix he was supposed to have removed a month previously had been admitted with acute appendicitis. There were other surgical incidents too disastrous to record, and finally I admitted all patients requiring surgical intervention to one of the junior surgeons, retaining the simpler cases for myself.'

In the appendicitis case found in the notes it says that $1\frac{3}{4}''$ of the appendix was removed and a faecal concretion found inside. Half an inch was left and sewn up and a portion of the meso-appendix was ligatured.

The surgeon was Mr Wherry and the physician Professor Bradbury. The notes were very detailed and included frequent blood counts, the only obvious use of pathological services in those notes examined apart from the frequent, probably routine, reports of tests on urine for specific gravity, acidity, albumen, sugar and sometimes blood and phosphates. These appendicitis notes also include pulse and respiration records which were not found in the other notes.

The surgical notes are brief, averaging perhaps a single page, and family histories and medical histories are nearly always sketchy or not given. However, the notes are neat and orderly, and most had a temperature chart attached or a note to say that it was uneventful.

Sometimes the treatment given the patient was not recorded in the notes and sometimes it was medical, but sometimes operative details were given. In these cases usually the practice was basically similar to, although obviously often not so advanced as, current practice. The main differences were due to the absence of modern antibiotics, for example the treatment of tubercular joints involved in one case excision of the head of the femur, in another scraping and opening of abscesses in the hips and draining, in a third case a splint of the knee. Nowadays chemotherapy would be employed before any operative procedure. Similarly lupus vulgaris was scraped here where nowadays chemotherapy would be used.

Scoliosis was treated with a plaster jacket in both a child and an adult. Nowadays for a child a brace might be used or a cast plus operative procedure; other options include operative correction such as hooks to vertebrae connected to a rod with a ratchet for gradual correction.

Radiotherapy was not used at all and the notes suggest that resection for malignancy was restricted to the pathological area only, rather than including an amount of sound surrounding tissues as is the case today.

The surgeons did not seem so inclined to look for the causes of symptoms and signs as we do today (and the medicines of the day seem largely symptomatic): for example, they resected swollen glands in the neck, which could be symptoms of infection elsewhere, and apparently were content to leave, without looking further, faecal matter discharging to the outside in a case of intestinal obstruction in which the colon had been entered. However, a case of epithelioma of the lip was noted as 'smoker but never held his pipe this side', which does suggest a search for cause and effect.

X-ray was only mentioned twice – it was discovered by Röntgen in 1895. In the first instance a tubercular diseased hip had been operated on and the head of the femur removed; during operation the femur was accidentally fractured and it was X-rayed about 13 days later. In the second case the embedded tip of a needle was located in a lady's hand by skiagraph before it was removed. X-rays may have been used more frequently than appears, however, since in another case a break is described as if it has been viewed, 'fracture is oblique – & there is slight splintering of the bone', although there is no mention of use of a machine.

Splints were frequently used, both for fractures and for other injuries or malformations. Dr Griffiths is recorded as having used some 'Griffiths' splints, perhaps his own design.

Leeches, which in the 1980s, enjoyed a resurgence for micro-surgery, were mentioned twice. They were applied once to the right temporal region in connection with an inflamed right eye which had three months previously been operated on for glaucoma, and 'Hirudo' was also used in a case of hyphaema. Both apparently improved.

The anaesthetics used for the operations were often mentioned but not the name of the administering doctor. A variety of anaesthetics and combinations of anaesthetics were used, based no doubt on the personal preference of the surgeon and the received wisdom of the day. A list of those anaesthetics recorded in the first 70 cases in the notes is given in Table 7.

Martindale's *Extra Pharmacopoeia*[7] gives some details on the various anaesthetics that would be available to the medical practitioners of the age.

A.C.E. was a combination of alcohol, 1 volume, chloroform, 2 volumes, and ether, 3 volumes. These proportions were held to be such that they would evaporate uniformly from the mixture. It was said to be safer than chloroform and quicker than ether and as effective as pure chloroform when deep and prolonged anaesthesia was to be produced.

Chloroform was at one time the most generally used of anaesthetics but it fell into disfavour and by the end of the nineteenth century had been somewhat supplanted by ether. Chloroform lowered the blood pressure and weakened the heart's action but deaths were more often due to its checking the power of respiration than to arrest of the heart's action. Effects during and subsequent to inhalation were less disagreeable to the patient than ether, however, although the death rate was higher.

Death rate of chloroform: 1 in 2,300 cases
Death rate of A.C.E.:   1 in 5,000 cases
Death rate of ether: 1 in 13,500 cases
Death rate of nitrous oxide: almost nil

Table 7. *Anaesthetics used in the first 70 cases of the first volume of surgical case notes, 1900, at Addenbrooke's Hospital*

Surgeon	Case
Anaesthetic: chloroform	
Griffiths	Setting fractured femur.
	Refracturing and resetting same patient as above.
	Surgery on feet then setting.
	Opening hip joint.
Deighton	Removing growth plus piece of lower jaw.
	Removing nasal polypus fibroid with forceps.
Anaesthetic: ether	
Griffiths	Excising ulcerated corn.
	Re-opening tuberculous knee, scraping and plugging.
	Operation to free right testicle and close external abdominal ring.
	Opening fistula-in-ano and packing with gauze.
Wherry	Setting comminuted fracture of tibia and fibula in splint.
	Excising and cauterising urethral carbuncle.
	Sewing up crushed fingers.
Anaesthetic: A.C.E. (alcohol, chloroform, ether)	
Deighton	Sewing up tears in shin of infant aged 1 year 8 months.
Anaesthetic: gas (nitrous oxide)	
Griffiths	Incisions to dorsum of foot and inserting drainage tubes.
	Incisions to leg to reduce cellulitis tension.
	Opening sinus after operation for tubercular patella.
Deighton	Opening abscess in cheek.
Anaesthetic: chloroform and A.C.E.	
Griffiths	Removal of tuberculous glands from neck. Patient aged 26.
Deighton	Removal of naevus from ankle. Patient aged 8.
Wherry	Removal of glands from neck, open sinus in neck, and scrape lupus of thigh. Patient aged 11.
Anaesthetic: G & E (gas and ether)	
Griffiths	Amputating foot in mid leg.
	Opening abscess in neck.
	Operation for inguinal hernia.
Deighton	Removing varicocoele.
	Removal of haemorrhoids.
	Abdominal hysterectomy.
Wherry	Incision in hand to remove $\frac{1}{4}''$ of embedded needle.
	Removal of hydrocoele.
Anaesthetic: G & E & chloroform	
Deighton	Dissecting out bursal cyst of neck.
Anaesthetic: cocaine	
Deighton	Incision and evacuation of Nybomian cyst.
Wherry	'Cocaine needling' in operation for double cataract.
	Readmission of above patient, 'extrusion of lens' operation.

Ether was said to produce less depression on the heart than either ethidene dichloride or chloroform but its use was unpleasant to both the patient and the operator. Also it had a suffocating action on the patient which could prove fatal in a lung or bronchial affection, and was very inflammable which was a handicap at first when operations were being carried out by candlelight.

The administration of nitrous oxide preceding ether was recommended in a *British Medical Journal* article, and appears to have been used in some cases at Addenbrooke's Hospital.

Nitrous oxide[3] was sometimes used together with ether for minor operations in dentistry and surgery. Here, however, the combination has been used for some quite major operations, including an abdominal hysterectomy.

Cocaine, from Coca leaves, was used for its local anaesthetic action on mucous membranes. Martindale[7] says: 'Evil results having followed the application of cocaine as an anaesthetic in several dental and eye operations, the bad effects have been attributed to fungoid growths . . . salicylic acid has been found to be the most effective preservative, and its addition is ordered in the official hypodermic injection'. It was used at Addenbrooke's for three eye operations.

Sir Philip Panton[6] had something to say on the subject of asepsis in Addenbrooke's during his time there.

> The amateur Management Committee, with whom I came to have so many disputes did their best with a hopeless staff and utterly inadequate funds; but my first shock was the discovery that there was not a single sterile dressing in the hospital, owing to the unattainable cost of dressing tins. Dressings were taken out of the ancient steriliser by unwashed hands, placed in open receivers and deposited round the wards. A local grocer came to my rescue and, at a cost of less than five pounds, provided an assortment of tea, coffee and biscuit tins and stamped them with the ward names. These makeshift, but quite effective, dressing tins were still in service some years later.
>
> The conception that a piece of lint once sterilised remained sterilised for ever was typical of the general attitude towards infection. All infected wounds were conceived to be of the same nature, and the nurses went from one patient to another using time and again the same set of dirty instruments. Such patients as escaped alive must have been immunised to every known pus-producing organism. On one occasion a nurse whom I had diagnosed in the morning as suffering from diphtheria was discovered later that night transferred to the children's ward.

With these, and other, comments in mind the outcomes of the surgical cases at Addenbrooke's in the early 1900s are of particular interest (see Table 8), and similarly the temperature charts, as guides to the infections sustained by the patients after surgery.

Only three of the 141 admissions died in hospital (2%) and a fourth was recorded as dying within one month of discharge. Of these deaths one case was a van driver who had been pitched off a Great Eastern Railway van after a collision and only lived ten minutes after admission to hospital. A second had a strangulated hernia, was pale and collapsed when admitted and died about three hours after his operation. The third had malignant disease of the peritoneum and died about a month after admission; and the last, who died after discharge, had a sarcoma of the axillary glands. All these deaths seem readily understandable and unless a goodly number of patients died after discharge then the record must be considered good even by modern standards. There were five re-admissions during the year (4%).

Of the remainder of the patients one was sent to a convalescent home, one transferred to a medical ward, and one 'discharged to come up to side room'; fifteen were said to be cured, two healed and one was a 'recovery'; sixteen were relieved; three were discharged at their own request and two at their parents' requests; there was one unknown and the rest were merely discharged. Disregarding the patient with no discharge date the average stay for the 140 patients was 26.9 days.

Regarding infection, four patients operated on for tuberculous joints experienced severe problems, there was difficulty with a patient with a strangulated hernia and undescended testis, with another with an axillary tumour, and with a third who had a urethral carbuncle removed. A boy of ten who had a fractured femur had a temperature of 99–100 °F for 50 days.

Patients often had a temperature peak for a day or so immediately after their operation and sometimes came in with a high temperature but for the most part they were either uninfected during treatment or any infection quickly vanished. This seems a good record for an age without the powerful modern antibiotics although it was, of course, true that the patients in general were young.

All ages from babies to the elderly were included among the patients and the average age was only 29.97 years. Both men's and women's notes were included in this first volume of surgical records and among those examined there were 85 males and 56 females; 17 men and women were over 60 (12%), and 46 (33%) were under 18 years.

There must have been virtually full employment in the community

Table 8. *Some preparations used in surgical cases, 1900*

Case	Medicine	Comment – derived from contemporary textbooks
Operation for Varicocele	Boracic fom[ts] after the operation	Borax is a salt with antiseptic and antiparasitic properties.[3] A fomentation was the application of a flannel, or spongiopiline, wet with warm water or some medicinal concoction, to a part of the body. Dry fomentation consisted of the application of warmth without moisture, e.g. a hot brick wrapped in flannel.[8]
Gon. opthalmica	Hg d. Perchlor	Probably mercuric chloride. Antiseptic disinfectant, escharotic alternative. Given in syphilitic affections and in syphilitic and other skin diseases.[3]
Ulcers & Erysipelas	Ferri Perchlor[m]	Ferri Perchloridum. The strong solution of ferric chloride is a powerful local styptic and astringent.[3]
Burns	Zinc ointment	An astringent application in eczema and slight excoriations and ulcerations.[3]
Tubercular disease of tarsus, bone scraped then later incised again because infected.	'dressed cyanide'	Gauze prepared with mercury zinco-cyanide which had been found by Lord Lister to have antiseptic properties.[3]
Later leg incised for cellulitis.	'dressed sodae chlor'	Sodae Chlorinate Liquor (solution of chlorinated soda). Antiseptic and disinfectant.[3]
Later patient's body shows bed sore and signs of pressure.	Packed with wool and boracic powder	See Borax.
Readmission of above case with erysipelas of stump and abscess in neck.	Opened abscess and 'plugged Iodoform emulsion'	Iodoform is an antiseptic, deodorant, alternative and local anaesthetic. In emulsion with Glyerin and water is for local use.[3]

Patient kicked in abdomen – injuries include scrotum.	Lot. Plumbi	Lotio Plumbi Acetatis. Lead acetate in small doses is sedative and astringent, lessening morbid mucous discharges and haemorrhages in the gastro-intestinal and genito-urinary tracts, and even diminishing natural secretions.[3]
Fractured tibia	Sod. Salicyl.	Sodium Salicylate. Given as specific in acute rheumatism; and as a powerful antipyretic in pneumonia, typhoid and all pyrexial affections. A soluble form of Salicylic Acid.[3]
Patient dying from injuries caused by accident.	Strychnine	Similar properties to Nux Vomica; useful in the treatment of reflex or functional paralysis and of peripheral neuritis and paralysis due to alcohol, tobacco or diptheria. A bitter tonic.[3]
After sewing up cleft palate	Morph. hypoderm	Injectio Morphinae Hypodermica (hypodermic injection of morphine). Morphine is the principal alkaloid obtained from Opium. The salts of morphine possess the anodyne, soporific and other actions of opium.[3]
Fractured femur	Chloral	Chloral Hydrate. An excellent hypnotic.
Malignant disease of peritoneum	Nepenthe	Nepenthes opiatum (opium pills) from the term 'Nepenthes', removing all sorrow.[8]
Fractured tibia	After a month 'silicate case applied'	Presumably some sort of supporting structure.[3]
Intestinal obstruction	Liq. Extract. Casc Sagrad	Extractum Cascara Sagradae Liquidum (Liquid extract of Cascara Sagrada). Cascara Sagrada is a tonic laxative that acts principally on the large intestine. Indicated in obstinate and habitual constipation.[3]
Artifical anus constructed	Aq	Aqua Destillata (distilled water).[3] This would be clean.

from which these patients were drawn. There were only eight male admissions over the age of 16 for whom employment was not specified: four of these were over 60, three were only 17 and only relate to two patients as one was admitted twice, and the last was 38 years. There were 62 men over the age of 16, therefore although 13% had no given occupation most of these probably either did not want one or had not started work yet.

There were 43 women over the age of 16. Of these only two single women did not have occupations specified, one aged 17 and another of 22; another two women aged 18 of uncertain marital status were also without jobs together with eight married women under 60, two of 68 years and one of 75 years. Therefore although 15 women (35%) were without jobs the majority again were probably not seeking them.

A large number of the female patients were stated to be single and this percentage was calculated. There were 39 female patients over 20 years and of these 20 (including two re-admissions) were single, i.e. 51%. Only two of the married women were under 30. Fourteen of the female patients between 20 and 30 were single, but apart from four cases of tuberculosis their complaints were all different, for example, burns, abscess of cheek, double cataract, etc.

As previously, the occupations of the patients were all low paid – coachman, parlour maid, tobacconist – and again a large proportion were labourers. There were 37 labourers out of 57 employed males, i.e. 54%. An even larger proportion of the females were in domestic service, 19 out of 24 employed females, i.e. 79%. Two of the patients enjoyed a certain amount of role reversal in their occupations, there was one 70-year-old single female 'helper in the fields', and one 29-year-old male housekeeper.

～ 2 1 ～

The first House Physician

The resident medical staff

George Wallis was Apothecary and House Surgeon from 1859 to 1867. After serving as Apothecary's apprentice from 1852 to 1854 he had qualified M.R.C.S. 1857 and L.S.A. 1858 from St Bartholomew's Hospital. Although he was House Surgeon for eight years he did not take the opportunity of becoming a member of the University. Ill health may have forced him to restrict his activities; he was given 25 guineas in March 1864 towards the 'expenses he has sustained by reason of his late severe illness'. He had obviously impressed his chiefs very favourably for he was elected Surgeon in 1879, although he never obtained the F.R.C.S.

His successor as House Surgeon was George Lucas.[1] In 1868 he was allowed to take Stephen Ashton as an apprentice.[2] Ashton, a doctor's son, who already had some experience as an apprentice, appears to have been a satisfactory pupil, but his successor, Morice, apprenticed in 1871, was not, and his behaviour forced the medical staff to discuss whether it was reasonable to continue the existing system of employing only one qualified resident with a young unqualified pupil. Their recommendation that in future there should be a House Physician and a House Surgeon and no resident pupils was approved.[3] Each man would receive £65 per annum.[4]

Detailed rules, applicable to both the House Physician and the House Surgeon, were drawn up, together with 'Special Directions' relating to each of them.[5] The rules stated that they were with the assistance of the Dispenser to dispense the medicines prescribed by the Physicians and Surgeons respectively, but they were to prescribe no medicines except in emergency. They were to furnish the Matron every day with a list of the diets required for their patients. They were to 'make reports to the Weekly Board of all patients received into the Hospital in the foregoing week and deliver lists at every Board of such patients as have been in the Hospital two months'. 'When either of them is aware that any order has been or is likely to be infringed he mention the same to the Weekly Board.'

The striking feature of these rules is the degree of authority they gave to the Governors, largely and often exclusively laymen, who attended the Weekly Board. The House Physician and House Surgeon were obliged also to maintain, for submission to the Board, detailed registers of all in- and out-patients, 'the parish to which the patients belong, their age and disease, by whom recommended, when admitted, when discharged, and in what state'. They had to keep a separate register of the out-patients who required admission, but were excluded for lack of beds. Finally they had to keep lists 'of such patients as have been discharged by the Governors for improper conduct, stating therein the respective causes of their discharge and that such lists be suspended in the Waiting Room'.

The 'Special Directions' are interesting. The House Physician was still responsible for the duties that were formerly undertaken by the Apothecary, and the Dispenser helped to dispense and did no more. The relevant directions read: 'That he allow no drugs or medicines to be deposited among the stores 'til he have first inspected them. That he keep a daily account of such things as are brought into the Hospital for the use of the dispensary, and that he examine and certify all bills quarterly, and also that he take an account on Michaelmas Day of the Stock of Drugs in the Hospital for the use of the Auditors.' The numerous other 'Special Directions' for the House Physician make him responsible for the supervision of the clinical clerks, the discipline of the medical wards (he is to report any misconduct on the part of clerks, pupils or nurses) and for performing post-mortem examinations when required.

The House Surgeon too had to perform post-mortem examinations, and he was responsible for discipline in the surgical wards. He was to administer chloroform, and he was responsible for keeping a list of the surgical instruments and ensuring that they were in good order.

In October 1871, Arthur Brailey was appointed the first House Physician. He was the first of many of great ability who were attracted by Paget and Latham. A scholar of Downing College, he obtained first class honours in the Natural Sciences Tripos in 1867. He was a popular coach in the natural sciences and in 1869 was college lecturer. He worked at Guy's Hospital and qualified M.B. in 1871. In 1872 he was elected a Fellow of Downing College. In 1880 he was appointed ophthalmic surgeon to Guy's Hospital. He died in 1915.

In February, 1872, George Lucas gave one month's notice and settled in general practice in Uckfield, Sussex.* He and Brailey had been

---

* Several generations of the Lucas family practised in Cambridgeshire and Huntingdonshire. George Lucas' son, George Humphrey Lucas (1874–1960), was in practice at Wisbech from 1903 until his death.

appointed under the old system: a majority of the votes of the Governors attending the meeting, often called specially for the purpose. Under the new system the appointment of the House Physician and House Surgeon was entrusted exclusively to the medical staff, subject of course to the approval of the Governors. The Quarterly Court of 25 March 1870, agreed that the 'new Scheme' should now come into effect, but that Brailey be invited to continue in office until the next Court. The medical staff met on 29 June and recommended Brailey for re-appointment as House Physician and W.P. Addis[†] for appointment as House Surgeon. Whether a genuine mistake was made, or whether the Governors resented the slight erosion of their authority, the next Court, having elected Addis as House Surgeon, proceeded to elect Theodore Maxwell[‡] as House Physician by a majority of 23 votes to 2 and also resolved that rules for the nomination and election of House Physicians and House Surgeons should be drawn up.

The September Court[6] referred back to the Board the Board's proposal that it consider 'by what means the additional expenditure or some part thereof caused by the appointment of two medical officers can be met'. Evidently some Governors resented not only the new method of election of house officers, but also the creation of the new post. The atmosphere in the Hospital must have been far from friendly. In November Maxwell resigned, and shortly afterwards was reported by Latham for being absent without providing a substitute. Maxwell replied that he had been absent on account of abscesses of the hands following a post-mortem examination, and with the approval of Dr Paget; he greatly resented Dr Latham's complaint. He was given permission to leave at once[7] and Addis's resignation was received and accepted.

The new method of election, which did not so heavily favour local candidates known to the Governors, resulted in a larger number of applicants. However, in the event a local man, H.F. Banham,[§] was appointed House Physician. R.W. Edginton was elected House Surgeon.

[†] W.P. Addis had qualified M.R.C.S. from University College Hospital in 1872. He was later a general practitioner in Buckinghamshire.

[‡] Theodore Maxwell (1847–1914) entered King's College in 1866, was M.B. 1872, and F.R.C.S. 1873. He practised at Woolwich.

[§] Henry French Banham (1846–1932), Sidney Sussex College 1865. Migrated to St John's 1866. B.A. 1869. St Thomas' Hospital, L.S.A. 1872. He was Lecturer in Medicine at Sheffield 1876–1885 and Physician to the Royal Berkshire Hospital, Reading, 1885–1890. He was ordained in 1892 and from 1901 to 1932 was Vicar of Assington, Suffolk.

[‖] Robert William Edginton, educated at Queen's College, Birmingham, qualified M.R.C.S. in 1871. He later practised at Edgbaston, Birmingham.

There were five candidates for the post of House Surgeon when Edginton resigned in January 1874. The Board[8] accepted George Wherry on the recommendation of the medical staff. At the next Quarterly Court[9] an attempt was made to censure the Board for recommending any individual, but the motion was withdrawn. On a show of hands there were 43 for Wherry and 33 for his only rival. A poll was held and Wherry gained 118 votes and his rival 77.

The procedure for the election of the resident medical officers was clearly not fully acceptable to the Governors. In March 1874, a modified procedure was approved.[10] The Select Governors and the medical staff would constitute a committee to examine the testimonials of candidates and make recommendations to the Governors. They were authorised to call up selected candidates for interview and to pay reasonable travelling expenses. Banham's resignation in September, 1875, led to the first appointment under the new regulations. The Committee recommended the appointment of William Ewart,* who had been acting as Banham's locum. The Court confirmed the appointment without discussion.[11] Ewart resigned after almost a year to take an appointment in London. There were seven applicants for the post. J.K. Fowler† was elected.

Wherry and Fowler were criticised[12] for not carrying out their duties in the Dispensary. As a result of their protest the rules were changed and they were made responsible for dispensing only in the absence of the Dispenser.

When Wherry resigned in 1877 there were fifteen applicants for the post of House Surgeon. Edward Ground, M.R.C.S. from King's College Hospital, was elected. He held the appointment for the three years necessary for a University degree and resigned in 1880 on his election as Surgeon to the West Kent Hospital at Maidstone.

When in due course Fowler resigned there were sixteen applicants for the post of House Physician. The opportunity of obtaining a University

---

* William Ewart (1848–1929). As a senior medical student at St George's Hospital he had served with the French army in the Franco-Prussian war. He was M.R.C.S. 1871. He entered Caius College in 1873 and gained first class honours in the Natural Sciences Tripos. He was subsequently Physician to St George's Hospital and Physician and Pathologist to the Brompton Hospital.

† James Kingston Fowler (1852–1934) had qualified M.R.C.S. in 1874 and L.R.C.P. 1876 from King's College Hospital. During the three years he spent as House Physician he obtained the M.B. as a member of Caius College and proceeded M.D. 1884. He became Physician to the Middlesex Hospital and the Brompton Hospital. He was appointed K.C.M.G. in 1930.

degree certainly attracted many candidates, some of high calibre. W.A. Shann* was elected.

Many of the house officers stayed for three years but those who were already Cambridge graduates tended to stay for a shorter period. There were numerous applicants, sometimes more than 20; the majority held the conjoint qualifications, or Scottish diplomas. Some later achieved some distinction. A.M. Shield (1856–1922) became Surgeon to St George's Hospital, W.R. Pollock (1859–1909) was to become obstetric physician to the Westminster Hospital and Queen Charlotte's Hospital. Ashton Street (1864–1946) became Professor of Anatomy in Bombay. F.W. Burton (1863–1937), later Burton-Fanning, became Physician to the Norfolk and Norwich Hospital and an authority on pulmonary tuberculosis. A.F. Stabb (1867–1944), House Physician from 1891 to 1894 was University Lecturer in midwifery from 1897–1903 and subsequently Physician and Lecturer in midwifery at St George's Hospital.

The general pattern of the duties of the resident staff appears to have changed very little between 1860 and 1890. Wherry recalled[13] that as House Surgeon he was also anaesthetist and dental surgeon (his dental patients included Humphry himself), and had to carry out all post-mortem examinations including those for the coroner, as there was no public mortuary in the town. For the coroner's cases he received no extra payment until, by threatening to write to the Home Secretary, he induced Mr Gotobed, the Coroner, to pay a fee of one guinea.

In 1889 minor changes in the rules were introduced.[14] The House Surgeon was not to admit medical cases under the Surgeons nor surgical cases under the Physicians, and he was to make and keep an inventory of all surgical and medical instruments and apparatus.

The visiting medical staff

The resignation of Henry Haviland left a vacancy for a Physician. The 1842 single ballot procedure was planned, but in the event the only candidate, P.W. Latham, was elected unopposed on 4 May 1863.

Peter Wallwork Latham (1832–1923) was indeed a very strong candi-

---

* William Arthur Shann (1857–1940) had qualified M.R.C.S. at St George's Hospital. He passed the M.B. soon after leaving Addenbrooke's Hospital, then joined his father in practice at York. He later moved to Lowestoft.

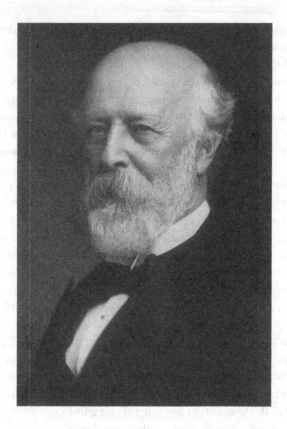

Fig. 25. Peter Wallwork Latham, Honorary Physician to
Addenbrooke's, 1863–1899.

date of undoubted academic distinction. He was born in Wigan, where his
father was in general practice. He worked as his father's apprentice, and
at Glasgow University, before entering Caius College in 1854. He gained
high mathematical honours in 1858 (nineteenth Wrangler) and in the
following year first class honours in the Natural Sciences Tripos in which
he secured the top mark in all five subjects. He then studied at St
Bartholomew's Hospital and in Germany, and was elected a Fellow of
Downing College in 1860, the year before he qualified M.B. In 1862 he
was appointed Assistant Physician to the Westminster Hospital, but
resigned on his election to Addenbrooke's Hospital.

His many publications were concerned largely with the application of
organic chemistry to medicine. He acquired a very large practice and was
popular with his patients and with general practitioners. When he retired

from practice in 1912[15] his friends in the town and the University presented him with a silver tray at a ceremony in Trinity Hall at which Deighton spoke of his kindness, boundless energy and geniality. At a second ceremony in Caius College the local medical men made a presentation; Allbutt presided.

He was the first provincial Fellow to serve on the Council of the Royal College of Physicians of which he had been elected Fellow in 1866, and was Croonian Lecturer in 1886 and Harveian Orator in 1888.[16] These College Honours are an indication of his high standing nationally as a physician. His standing in Cambridge was equally high. He was elected Downing Professor of Medicine in 1874, and for many years he worked with Paget and Humphry to build up the Medical School. He was, however, a man of combative temperament, who often held strongly individual opinions. He never forgave the University when Allbutt was appointed to succeed Paget as Regius Professor of Physic in 1892, considering with some justification that he himself was the obvious candidate. He opposed Allbutt by every means in his power and succeeded in keeping him off the staff of the Hospital until 1900. He resigned the Downing professorship in 1894 and his Hospital appointment in 1899, but he continued to live in Cambridge until 1912, when he moved to London. He died in Clifton in 1923.

In 1863 Paget offered his resignation under the twelve-year rule, but he was asked to continue as Physician, as were all other members of the staff who offered to resign under this rule which was gradually allowed to become obsolete. Paget had married in 1851 and there were ten children of the marriage, three of whom died young, but his family responsibilities did not reduce his capacity for work. He had a very large practice and he was active in University and Hospital affairs. His medical publications were relatively few.[17] They demonstrate his interest in neurological disorders, particularly epilepsy, and in psychiatry.

In 1872 Dr Bond resigned. For two years previously, with the approval of the Governors[18], J.B. Bradbury had been acting as deputy if any of the Physicians was unable to attend the Hospital, and was therefore a strong candidate to succeed Bond. Proposed by Mortlock and seconded by Paget, he was unanimously elected.[19]

John Buckley Bradbury (1841–1930), was born at Saddleworth, Yorkshire, apprenticed to a general practitioner and then attended King's College, London, before entering Caius College in 1862. He migrated to Downing College the following year, on winning a scholarship there.

After obtaining first class honours in the Natural Sciences Tripos, he spent two years at King's College Hospital and returned to Cambridge in 1866 as Assistant Lecturer in medicine and natural sciences to Downing College. He was M.B. and M.R.C.P. in 1867 and F.R.C.P. in 1874. In 1894 he succeeded Latham as Downing Professor. Bradbury was interested in pharmacology and in 1895 he gave the Bradshaw lectures at the College of Physicians on 'Some New Vasodilators', but he devoted most of the time to his extensive practice and was still seeing patients until his final illness. In 1872[20] he submitted his resignation as Physician, on the grounds that he intended to work as a general practitioner. He withdrew his resignation the following week, having decided to continue to practise as a physician. In fact, his practice throughout his long career was that of a physician in general practice and he was at times criticised for his willingness to accept patients not referred by their own doctors.

In October 1870, Hammond resigned as Surgeon.[21] In his letter he referred to the 'harmony of feeling' and friendship of his two surgical colleagues. Later that month E.J. Carver was elected Surgeon by 22 votes to 4; the only other candidate was F.R. Hall.[22] Edmund Carver had been House Surgeon from 1852 to 1859 and from 1866 had been Surgeon to Huntingdon County Hospital until his health failed. He recovered after a voyage round the world and was Surgeon to Addenbrooke's Hospital from 1870 to 1898. He died in 1904.

In 1875[23] Latham 'applied to be retired from the care of Out-patients'. It was the practice in many hospitals for honorary staff to hold the rank of Assistant Physician or Surgeon when first elected, and to have the care of out-patients only. On becoming full Physician or Surgeon they had charge of beds and in some hospitals gave up their out-patient work. Latham's application was referred to the next Weekly Board for discussion. Paget, who was unable to be present, wrote a letter to the Board. For years, 'with continually increasing inconvenience', he had seen all out-patients himself. This was now impossible. For a year or two Bradbury had accepted responsibility for Paget's out-patients, but he had recently been unable to do so and Paget's patients had been seen chiefly by Banham, the House Physician. Paget felt that as Banham had had considerable experience there no reason to believe the patients were neglected.

The Board approved Latham's application as Dr Bradbury had agreed that, with the assistance of Banham, he would see the out-patients given up by Latham. However, many Governors obviously found this state of affairs unsatisfactory, for in June the Board resolved[24] 'That the attention of the Quarterly Court be called to the state of the Medical and Surgical staff as shown by the minutes of this Board'. The Quarterly Court referred the matter back to the Board asking them to submit a report after discussion with the medical staff. The Physicians then modified their proposal[25] – 'that the Physicians be authorised to transfer to the charge of the House Physician those among their Out-patients whose cases properly admit of being so transferred; it being understood that the Physician's attention will be called again to any of these cases if, in their progress, his opinion should be needed'. The Court referred this report back to the Board, which on 22 December recommended that the Physicians' proposal be sanctioned. The December Court was doubtful and reluctant to agree. By this stage feelings were running high. Latham gave notice that at the next Quarterly Court he would move that an Assistant Physician be appointed to take charge of out-patients. Bradbury then gave notice that, if such a proposal were made, he intended to move, as an amendment, that those Physicians who declined properly to attend to their out-patients be requested to resign their appointments. This unseemly controversy had now continued for two months and it was receiving regular publicity in the local press. The Board[26] therefore set up a committee (the Revd H. Hall, the Revd Dr Pelling, the Revd Dr Campion, the Revd J. Martin and Mr Gotobed), to confer with the medical officers 'with the view of arranging a table of attendance'.

The Committee met the next day and agreed to recommend[27] a change in the rules to specify precisely the times of attendance on in-patients of the Senior, Second and Junior Physicians. The Physicians would attend in turn every Wednesday to examine new out-patients, with authority to transfer to the care of the House Physician 'those among their out-patients whose cases properly admit of being so transfered'. The Junior Physician would examine new out-patients attending on Saturdays and such patients would remain under his care. The report was adopted.[28]

In 1879 Lestourgeon resigned.[29] The Board[30] recommended the number of Surgeons be increased from three to four. The Court agreed[31] and set up a committee to consider the number and duties of the Physicians. The increase in the number of Surgeons seems to have been made to allow the election of both of two local candidates, rather than because the pressure of general surgical work required the additional appointment. Moreover, the number of ophthalmic cases attending the Hospital had led the Governors in 1877[32] to set up a committee to consider the possibility of appointing an ophthalmic surgeon. This Committee had accepted the arrangement proposed by the Surgeons, to place the ophthalmic cases under the care of one or other of their number.[33] In November 1879, George Wallis and George Wherry were elected Surgeons.[34]

George Wallis had been the Apothecary's apprentice from 1851 to 1854. He had then worked at St Bartholomew's Hospital, and had qualified M.R.C.S. in 1857, and L.S.A. in 1858. He had returned to Cambridge as House Surgeon and Apothecary 1859–1867, and had practised in Cambridge from 1870.

George Edward Wherry (1852–1925), of Cornish descent, was the son of a corn merchant at Bourne, Lincolnshire, and was educated at the Grammar School there, and at St Thomas' Hospital where he qualified M.R.C.S. in 1873. In 1874 he came to Addenbrooke's Hospital as House Surgeon. He must have impressed the Governors very favourably for it was the Chairman of the Weekly Board who nominated him as 'a fit and proper person to be elected . . . to the post of Surgeon'. As House Surgeon he had shown great interest in ophthalmic cases and although he was elected as a general surgeon and no mention of ophthalmology was made in the Minutes at that time, he immediately opened an ophthalmic out-patients' clinic. The number of ophthalmic out-patients increased rapidly. By 1884 the accommodation was already inadequate,[35] and the need for additional accommodation for ophthalmic out-patients was often discussed. In 1889 Wherry stated[36] that he had seen 46 ophthalmic patients on 4 March.

Wherry was a protégé of Humphry and was appointed University Lecturer in surgery when that post was established in 1883, and held the post until it was suppressed in 1911. He continued until his retirement from the Hospital in 1915 to practise both as a general and as an ophthalmic surgeon. Throughout the First World War he served as Surgeon to the Eastern General Hospital in the rank of Lieutenant-Colonel. His scientific publications were few but he was an active member of the Cambridge Medical Society to which he presented over 60 communications. They illustrate the very wide range of the work of a general surgeon of the period; twenty-two were concerned with ortho-paedics, twenty with ophthalmology, nine with abdominal surgery (including three on appendicitis, the earliest in 1895), eight with gynae-cology, three with urology and two with ear, nose and throat surgery. He also published papers on comparative anatomy. He was kindly, shy and self-effacing. He was an enthusiastic mountaineer and served on the committee of the Alpine Club. His interests were varied. He published two books of Alpine reminiscences and a small volume on 'Cambridge and Charles Lamb'. He died in 1925, on holiday in Switzerland.

The Committee on the Number and Duties of Physicians made a preliminary report in December 1879, recommending no changes. Dr Bradbury dissented. In June 1884,[37] Paget resigned as Physician as he found it necessary to reduce his work. Latham proposed that in future there should be two Physicians and two Assistant Physicians. A committee appointed to consider the matter recommended that there should be three Physicians and one Assistant Physician. They also recommended that every year from 1 October to 30 June, the two senior of these Physicians should be responsible for in-patients. The junior of the three would be in charge of four women's and four men's beds and all the beds in the children's ward. The care of out-patients should be the responsibility of the Junior Physician and the Assistant Physician and if any out-patients were admitted such patients should have a prior claim to the beds reserved for the Junior Physician. The posts of Physician and Assistant Physician were advertised in the usual way, but the names of the applicants were not recorded in the Minute Book. Donald MacAlister was elected Physician and Laurence Humphry Assistant Physician.

Donald MacAlister (1854–1933)[38] was born in Perth, Scotland, and was educated at Perth and at High schools in Liverpool. He entered St John's College in 1873 and in 1877 was Senior Wrangler, that is to say he won the first place in the mathematical honours list. He was elected a Fellow of his college. He then spent two years at St Bartholomew's Hospital and in 1880 qualified M.B. and L.S.A. During his years as a clinical student he published a number of articles, mainly comprehensive reviews on aspects of physics. In 1880 he worked under Ludwig in Leipzig, and in 1882 he was appointed co-editor of the 'Practitioner' with Lauder Brunton and also a member of the editorial committee of the British Medical Journal. He was a prominent and influential figure in the medical world from an early stage of his career. At the Royal College of Physicians he was Goulstonian Lecturer in 1887, and Croonian Lecturer in 1883. The following year he was elected the Cambridge representative on the General Medical Council.

From 1881, when he became Tutor and Medical Lecturer at St John's College, until 1904, he was very active in University administration. He was Secretary to the Medical Board and was a member of the General

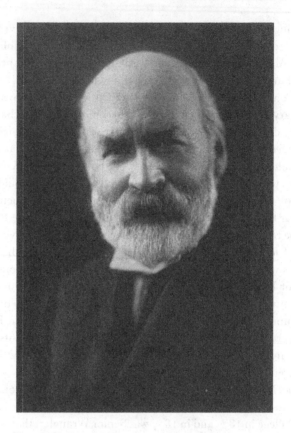

Fig. 26. Sir Donald MacAlister, Honorary Physician to
Addenbrooke's, 1884–1902.

Board and of the Council of the Senate. He was a key personality during
the years of heightened tension between the University and the Hospital
in the 1890s. Despite his administrative commitments he was actively
concerned with his hospital duties and also saw many private patients at
home and in his college rooms. According to his wife, it was generally
expected that he would succeed Paget as Regius Professor.[38] From 1907 to
1929 he was Principal of Glasgow University. He was knighted in 1908.

Laurence Humphry (1856–1920), the recently appointed Assistant
Physician was born at Richmond, Surrey, the son of G.M. Humphry's
barrister brother, Joseph. Educated at Haileybury, Trinity College and
St Bartholomew's Hospital, he qualified in 1880, and after holding junior
appointments at his own hospital and at the City of London Hospital for
Diseases of the Chest, he settled in practice at Cambridge on the advice of
his uncle. He was a competent, conscientious physician, but self-effacing

and unambitious. He taught pathology and was, from 1901 to 1911, Lecturer in Medicine.

When in 1884 the Governors had decided the division of duties between the Physicians, they had made no special provision for the months of July, August and September. Difficulties soon arose. In July 1887, Dr Joseph Griffiths, who had recently joined the department of pathology, was accepted as MacAlister's deputy, while the latter was visiting the United States. The following summer MacAlister asked if, during the absence of Latham and Bradbury, he might ask Dr William Hunter to help him. Hunter was John Lucas Walker Student in the department of pathology. He subsequently became a distinguished Physician at the Charing Cross Hospital. The Board agreed, but pointed out that, as Hunter was not on the staff of the Hospital, the approval of the medical staff must be obtained. This was given and the staff reported that in future years they would divide among themselves the medical work during the summer months. Meanwhile Joseph Griffiths, who in 1887 had deputised for a Physician, was accepted as deputy for the Surgeons, G.M. Humphry and Carver.[39]

It was now the turn of the Surgeons to re-organise their staffing arrangements, on lines similar to those followed by the Physicians. In September 1891, Humphry, Wallis and Wherry submitted their resignations under the twelve-year rule. Wallis did not seek re-election. The Governors agreed, after a poll, that there should in future be three Surgeons and one Assistant Surgeon.[40] Humphry and Wherry were re-elected Surgeons.[41] At the same Court, F. Deighton, E.H. Douty and J. Griffiths were the candidates for the junior post. The voting was so close (Griffiths 21, Deighton 18 and Douty 16)– that a poll was demanded. At the poll which took place on 24 November, Deighton obtained 164 votes, Douty 150, and Griffiths 129; Deighton was declared elected. However, all three candidates were to be closely concerned with the development of the Hospital during the next two decades.

On 28 March 1892, the Governors paid tribute to Sir George Paget who had died on 29 January of influenza. Amongst his massive contributions to the development of the Hospital and the Medical School, his interest in psychiatry had found practical expression when the psychiatric clinic was inaugurated. His services to medicine were recognised by Trinity College, Dublin, and the Universities of Oxford, Durham and Edinburgh, who conferred honorary doctorates on him. There is a window to his memory in the chapel at Caius College.

~ 22 ~

The influence of Florence Nightingale

In many hospitals in the late 1800s trained and educated nurses were imposed by the Governors on a reluctant medical staff. At Addenbrooke's Hospital the medical staff took the initiative in nursing reform. Humphry suggested in June 1865 'the employment of a better class of nurses', and the Medical Officers were authorised 'to make arrangements for providing such nurses to the Hospital'.[1]

An advertisement was placed in the Cambridge, Norfolk and Suffolk papers, 'Nurses are required for Addenbrooke's Hospital: not to be over 40 years of age . . . Previous experience in nursing not required.' It is not clear whether there was any connection between that advertisement and Paget's announcement in October[2] that they had 'engaged four nurses of a superior kind who have been trained at St Thomas' Hospital under the regulations of the Nightingale Fund, and five under nurses who seem capable of becoming fit for the situation of upper nurses, when they shall have had some experience and instruction in Addenbrooke's Hospital'. The 'superior nurses' should be paid a salary of £25; the wages of the 'under nurses' should be from £16 to £18.

The new nurses, whose names are not recorded in the Minutes, but who included Elizabeth Smith, Elizabeth Cox, Elizabeth Wetton, and Esther Mandell, started work at the end of October. From the beginning the Governors and the medical staff had to struggle to keep the peace between the new nurses and the Matron. In January 1866,[3] the Matron complained 'that Sister Albert had not behaved with proper deference to her as Matron'. Sister Albert and three other Sisters were called before the Board and reminded that suggestions and complaints must be addressed in the first instance to the Matron. (The term 'Sister' for the head nurse of a ward came to the Hospital with the Nightingale nurses and left with them.) The Matron was ordered to keep a diary in which were recorded her daily visits to the wards, her comments and suggestions, and to submit the diary to the Board every week.

The Matron treated the new nurses as she had the old and it would not be reasonable to assume that she sought deliberately to humiliate them, though she undoubtedly resented their pretensions and the fact that many of the Governors appeared to take their side in any dispute. Soon after the complaint against Sister Albert the Board was informed[4] that one of the nurses had been employed in scrubbing a ward. There was a certain lack of understanding in the Matron's comment: she 'promised to give more particular attention to the matter if necessary'. Despite the difficulties the Board continued its efforts to improve the nursing.[5] They agreed to the engagement of two night nurses to live in the Hospital and to be paid the same wages as other nurses. Until then 'night nursing' had been carried out by the casual engagement of a 'watcher' when required for a restless or difficult patient. The same Board agreed to engage on a week's trial 'a man named Fletcher, for looking after the patients'.

The struggle with the Matron continued throughout the year, with charges and countercharges. Most of these were petty, but some of them throw light on the basic problem: the social status which the new nurses considered to be their due, and the reluctance of the Matron to acknowledge it. At the end of January three of the nurses attended the Board to complain that the cook shared their table at dinner, and that dinners were 'irregular and unsatisfactory'. The matter was referred to the Matron, who appears to have taken no action. On 1 August the Matron was directed to allow the Sisters to dine in the dining hall and to have it cleared for that purpose.[6] A fortnight later this order was repeated,[7] 'the Hall to be used for that purpose by next Wednesday' (i.e. two days later).

At the end of the year[8] the Board agreed a report for submission to the Quarterly Court: 'This Weekly Board has been chiefly occupied in adjusting differences between the Matron and the Nursing Sisters arising probably from the introduction of a new and improved system of nursing, and beg to report that they consider the domestic arrangements are far from satisfactory. The Board hopes that this notice to the Quarterly Court will have its proper effect.'

This report was not laid before the Court on 31 December, presumably because there had been no time to include it in the advertised agenda, but it was not discussed at the April or the July Court. However, the July Court[9] received a letter from the Matron: 'I beg respectfully to state that lately the power has been taken out of my hands, which has caused insubordination throughout the House. I ask therefore to be reinstated that I may be enabled to manage your valuable institution as in the

previous 17 years with advantage to the Charity and credit to myself.'
There were many Governors whose sympathies lay with the Matron.
Whatever their real motives for opposing the new nursing they could
safely attack it on the undeniable grounds that it was much more
expensive than the old system: and this they did.

The Court of 1 July adjourned to 15 July when it received a report from
the medical officers. This report proposed reducing the number of Sisters
from five to three, retaining one for each floor. The salary of Sister Bowtell
should be reduced from £23, as this ward was smaller than the others, and
the nurse of that ward should wash the floor. There should be only one
night nurse. These economies would save £145 a year. The Board was
asked also to consider 'whether some economy could not be effected by the
nurses and servants dining together'. The report was received and
adopted. The same adjourned Court received the resignations of the
Sisters of Bowtell, Hatton, Griffith and Victoria Wards, and a letter from
them which was read to the Court. The letter was a spirited reply to a
letter in the *Cambridge Chronicle* by Mr Nicholl, in which he had claimed
that the Sisters were more ornamental than useful. He described in some
detail the duties of a Sister. They would, they wrote, tolerate insults and
injustice and lack of encouragement, but would not put up with ridicule.
The Governors resolved that the medical officers be required to explain to
the 'Superior Nurses' that their services were appreciated by the Governors, and to arrange for three of them to stay on.

The Matron's letter was then read. Revd J. Martin proposed, and Dr
Latham seconded, a resolution holding Miss Bishop responsible for the
'difficulties of the Hospital management' and calling for the appointment
of another Matron. The proposal was, however, withdrawn, and the
problem was referred back to the Finance Committee. This Committee[10]
recommended unanimously that 'the Matron be given notice to leave her
situation'. The Board[11] considered the Finance Committee's recommendations and in the course of their discussion referred to the departure of
the Sisters, but they did not discuss the Matron.

In December[12] the Finance Committee reported 'that the Matron does
not appear to be able to cope with the difficulties of her situation'. The
Court, meeting later the same day, adjourned to 10 February on which
day the Finance Committee would be required to give the facts on which
this statement was founded. This Committee,[13] in its report, stated that it
had wished to avoid making specific charges, but that, since further
information was demanded, they would provide it. The Matron was

unable to control the servants, she failed to observe the rules laid down for her direction, she repeatedly broke other rules, and she caused unnecessary expenditure by unauthorised purchases.

The next Court[14] received this report and a letter of protest from the Matron, and discussed both at considerable length. It resolved that Miss Bishop be requested to resign and a committee was appointed to consider what gratuity or allowance should be granted to her. The Matron submitted her resignation and protested that the proposed gratuity of £200 was poor recompense for nineteen years of service.

The unfortunate Miss Bishop was again in trouble with the Governors in July, as her explanation of her reasons for cutting pages from account books was considered unsatisfactory. The Committee's earlier assessment that the job was beyond her capacity seems to have been fully justified.

A large committee was then appointed to supervise the arrangements for the appointment of a new Matron. Advertisements, which were placed in *The Times*, *The Daily Telegraph*, *The Lancet*, and the *British Medical Journal* as well as in the local papers, invited applications from candidates aged between 28 and 40 and stated that the Governors discouraged canvassing. There were 14 candidates: the usual procedures were followed, and Mrs Agnes Robertson was appointed.[15]

The Governors were very conscious of the need to improve the nursing arrangements. Professor Babington[16] felt that the appointment of a new Matron provided the opportunity of doing so, and he sent, for the consideration of the Court, a memorandum prepared by the Lady Visitors of Victoria Ward.[17] Victoria Ward was the 23-bed female surgical and accident ward, and connected to it was the three-bed Mary Ward. Since the reduction of nursing staff in the interests of economy about a year earlier there had been only one nurse for these two wards. She worked from 5.30 a.m. to 10.30 p.m. She was under the superintendance of the Sister who was also responsible for the male ward at the other end of the Hospital.

The organisation of the nursing was, at this stage, curiously neglected by the medical staff. When they were asked to prepare a report on the duties of Upper and Under Nurses[18] they suggested that the arrangements should be left to the discretion and direction of the Matron.[19] The well-attended Weekly Board on 11 November requested its chairman, the Revd J. Martin 'to speak to the nurses and to direct them to see that the patients have a bath on admission when necessary'.

After the failure of the 'Superior Nurses' to come to terms with Miss

Bishop, the Hospital had reverted to the old system of advertising for nurses in the local papers, or selecting them from the domestic staff. Problems of discipline were frequent, though less so than a century earlier. The medical staff was aware that an improved standard of nursing at a cost which the Hospital could afford could be achieved only by establishing a training school. The wives of many Governors were, in the capacity of Lady Visitors, becoming increasingly interested in the Hospital's nursing problems. An association of ladies, most of them the wives of senior members of the University, who were active also as Governors, resolved to establish at Cambridge a home and training school for nurses (see Appendix I).

The first official notification of this important development was given by Humphry to a Weekly Board in December 1872,[20] when on behalf of the thirteen lady signatories of the document he read their request for the approval and cooperation of medical officers and.governors. They asked for permission to send two or more probationers into the wards for instruction; whilst in the wards they would be subject to Hospital discipline. For the first three to six months of their training period no remuneration would be expected from the Hospital for their services. The Board appointed Revd J. Martin, Dr Paget and Mr Lestourgeon a committee to confer with Miss Pelling and the other ladies. By the end of the year[21] the admission of probationers to the wards had been approved. Some probationers certainly worked in the wards in 1873, as one was voted a gratuity for her help in the fever ward, but no regular training programme was established. Agnes Robertson resigned as Matron in August[22] and was succeeded by Mrs Lavinia Stanley.

In April 1874,[23] the Board decided to accept no more probationers until rules for their conduct had been drawn up by the medical staff. The Staff referred the matter to a committee on which they were represented by Bradbury and Carver. The rules, slightly amended by the Board, were approved at the end of the month.[24] Many of the rules were designed to subject the probationers to normal Hospital discipline, but some were of considerable interest. Probationers were 'to wear no dress indicating a Sisterhood or a connection with a Sisterhood'. The Protestant Sisterhood of St John had developed nursing at King's College Hospital in London. The Addenbrooke's probationers were to belong to no such organisation, but they were obliged 'to attend public worship on Sundays twice, if their duty permits, and always once except for some grave excuse'. The Matron was to report to the Weekly Board 'such Head Nurses as seek in any way to contravene these regulations, and the purpose of these, viz. the teaching the probationers how to nurse properly'. Every Head Nurse was to be paid 2s.6d. (raised by the next Board to 3s.6d.) for each week during which she had a probationer in her ward. On 29 April 1874, the Board accepted as a probationer, Mary Whittlesey, aged 24, from the Ladies Institution for Training Nurses. Her hours of attendance at the Hospital were to be:

Monday to Saturday	7.00 a.m.–1.15 p.m. and	3.45 p.m.–8.00 p.m.
Sundays alternately	7.00 a.m.–1.15 p.m. and	7.00 a.m.–10.00 a.m.
	and also	5.30 p.m.–8.00 p.m.

The probationers lived in 'The Home for Nurses' at 1 Bene't Close. The Lady Superintendent of the Home was Miss S.M. Henslow. She regularly recommended girls who had to be approved individually by the Weekly Board and she withdrew, after a month's trial, any considered 'not likely to make a desirable nurse'.[25]

In June 1874, the Matron resigned, giving no reason and apparently on cordial terms with the Governors. There were 23 applicants for the appointment and the Governors conscientiously followed the usual procedure in making their selection, and invited four of the candidates for interview. Mrs M.E. Sale of London was elected.[26]

Mrs Sale had been in office a little over two years when a committee appointed to investigate recent excessive expenditure resolved 'that the services of a Matron better skilled in housekeeping than the present Matron are needed'. The Matron accepted the suggestion that she might like to anticipate their report by resigning.

Since the departure of Miss Bishop in 1868 the Hospital had had three Matrons in eight years. This lack of stability and continuity obviously caused the Governors great concern. They appointed a Select Committee 'to make enquiries in relation to the appointment of a Matron'.[27] The Minutes are not explicit, but it appears that the general subject of 'Matronship' was discussed. Miss Henslow and Miss Pelling, who as ladies could not sit on the Committee, were consulted. The Committee's report[28] considered that the Matron should be capable of supervising both the nursing and the housekeeping but that because of 'the possible need of further organisation in the management of the Hospital, they are of opinion that any arrangement now made with a Matron should be temporary'. Miss Henslow, Superintendent of the Nurses' Home (now in Fitzwilliam Street), was prepared to act as Matron for six months, provided that she could retain the office of Superintendent of the Home.

The Committee recommended Miss Henslow's appointment for six months 'in the present emergency'. One member of the Committee, Mr J.H. Turner, refused to sign the report.

The Court on 9 April was well attended.[29] After the report had been read, Mr Turner's reasons for not signing it were also read. Turner's 'general reasons' for not signing were the Committee's failure to consider the claims of candidates other than Miss Henslow and their insistence on appointing her to an office not yet in existence – 'virtually lady-superintendent'. He also had some objections to Miss Henslow herself – her refusal to apply for the appointment, which she would accept if invited, and her admitted dislike of keeping accounts. According to Turner 'the nursing of the Hospital is said to be in a bad state'. He gave evidence to support his contention that 'Our nursing may be at fault but not our nurses.' He gave some reasons for his belief that 'if Miss Henslow be elected our best nurses will leave'.

Miss Henslow was proposed by Revd H. Hall and seconded by Dr Bradbury. Mrs Olwen Roe, previously strongly recommended to the Select Committee,[30] was proposed by Mr Turner. Mr Cockerell proposed, and Mr Cooper seconded, as an amendment that the vacancy in the office of Matron be filled in the usual manner. The amendment was carried by 22 votes to 18. Of the 23 candidates, four were interviewed. Mrs Olwen Roe was the first to be eliminated, but only by the casting vote of the Chairman. Eventually Miss Alice Fisher (Fig. 27) was elected.[31]

The fortunate choice of Alice Fisher brought to the Hospital at a critical stage in its history a remarkable woman with a strong but warm personality and high intelligence. Not only was the nursing of the Hospital in a bad state; the financial situation was desperate. Miss Fisher did much to remedy both.

Alice Fisher,[32] was the elder daughter of the Revd George Fisher, F.R.S., astronomer, mathematician and headmaster. In 1873 she published a novel, *Too Bright to Last*, and in 1875 another in three volumes, *His Queen*. In 1874 she was accepted at the Nightingale Training School at St Thomas' Hospital, where she spent one year as a Lady Probationer. Miss Nightingale noted about her: 'talkative, exaggerates, an authoress, but keeps the rules'. On leaving the Training School Miss Fisher went to the Edinburgh Royal Infirmary where Miss Pringle had recently been elected Superintendent of Nursing. Miss Pringle wrote of her to Florence Nightingale: 'it is a great privilege to have her. She is so sunny-tempered and unexacting'. In June 1876, she was appointed Matron of the

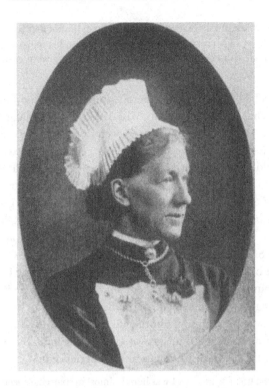

Fig. 27. Alice Fisher (1839–1888). Figure reproduced by kind
permission of the Editor of *Nursing Times/Nursing Mirror*.

Newcastle Fever Hospital and during the eleven months she spent there
she collaborated with Rachel Williams in writing 'Hints for Hospital
Nurses' (This was a small practical manual of 170 pages).

Like so many of Miss Nightingale's young ladies, Alice Fisher continued to correspond with her and these very frank letters add life and
colour to the bare record of the Minute Books. Not long after her
appointment to Addenbrooke's Hospital she wrote[32]

> My chief recommendation, I understand, in the eyes of the Governors who
> appointed me was that I had a good knowledge of housekeeping and knew
> something of book-keeping; that I had been trained in a Hospital was quite
> of minor importance, and the widow of a man who kept an inn in the town
> was very nearly placed here instead of me.
>
> The finances of the Hospital were in a very bad state, and indeed I found
> everything in confusion. There were no trained nurses, the night nursing
> was done by old women of indifferent character who did not live in the
> house, and the ward-maids who were the only assistants to the nurses were

dirty and ignorant girls of seventeen who slept in the kitchen attached to the wards. The head-nurses and ward nurses dined together and during dinner, which by all accounts lasted a long time, the wards were entirely unattended to.

The recollections[33] of George Wherry, appointed House Surgeon in 1874, suggest that in these criticisms Miss Fisher did not exaggerate. He once found a night nurse asleep in an easy chair with her legs across the legs of the restless man of whom she was in charge. Had he tried to get out of bed he would have awakened her. Wherry reminds us that at that time nurses wore no uniform and could dress as they wished. He recollected doing a round of Albert Ward with a nurse dressed in bright green silk.

Miss Fisher tackled her problems with energy and with tact. Soon after her arrival she transferred the care and issue of wines and spirits to the Dispensary.[34] She continued to accept probationers from the Cambridge Nurses' Home but took them also from other organisations and from other parts of the country, for example Fakenham,[35] and Newcastle.[36] She was allowed to engage an additional permanent nurse[37] to be available wherever she was needed, and another to serve as Night Superintendent.[38] The Minutes suggest that she was given a free hand but a letter to Miss Nightingale tells of the difficulties she experienced.[32]

> During the first few months I was here I almost despaired, especially as the committee were of opinion that the nursing arrangements were quite perfect. However, I thought I had better begin with the expenditure and if I effected a reform there they might perhaps be induced to listen favourably to anything else I had to suggest, and the first quarter, to my great joy, there was a saving of £300 as compared with the corresponding quarter of last year. This emboldened me to take some steps about the nursing. I replaced all the tipsy old night nurses with young women, partially trained only, but respectable and as good as I could get for £16.
> Then a further saving of £300 for the next quarter gave me confidence to take another step and substitute probationers for ward servants. These probationers are sent to be trained for private nursing by different nursing homes – we pay them nothing and are thus able to afford scrubbers who do all the scrubbing and stove cleaning but nothing else.

The Governors, at a Quarterly Court on 1 October, did not accept the Board's authorisation to the Matron 'to make such arrangements as she considered expedient'.[39] They ordered the Board to consider the rules governing the admission and duties of probationers and to report back to the next Court. The Select Governors and the medical officers appointed a Committee (Revd H. Hall, Mr Knowles, Mr Gotobed and Professor

Humphry), which produced a plan for the accommodation of the extra nurses and the probationers.

Another committee[40] considered the financial implications of the probationers. Their recommendations were based on discussions with the Matron.

The staff was to consist of

7 nurses at £30 each	£210
3 charwomen (on an average), boarding but not lodging, at 1s.0d. a day	say £55
a Superintendent Night Nurse at	£35
(and 5 ward servants).	

These would be the only paid attendants. In addition there
would be 5 probationers of the 1st class, who would pay 12s.0d.
a week if boarding in the hospital,
10 probationers of the 2nd class. These last would pay nothing as
they would take the place of ward servants and night nurses
and do the cleaning of the wards except scrubbing and grate
cleaning.

At the request of the Board,[41] Revd H. Hall and Mr Knowles, in consultation with the Matron, drew up a 'tabulated statement of the regulations for probationers'.[42]

Timetable

6.00 a.m.	Probationers rise
6.30 a.m.	Prayers and Breakfast
7.00 a.m.	On duty in the wards, probationers having previously made their own beds and left their rooms in order.

Apart from 30 minutes break for luncheon, 30 minutes for dinner (at 1.30 or 2.00 p.m.) and one hour for tea (at 5.00 p.m.), the probationers were on the wards all day until Prayers and Supper at 8.30 p.m.

10.00 p.m.	Probationers go to the dormitories.
10.30 p.m.	All lights to be put out, after which perfect silence is to be observed.

There were no regular days off but every probationer had, each day, a short period off duty, either from 11.15 a.m. to 12.15 p.m. or from 3.00 p.m. to 4.30 p.m. Nurse probationers attended classes from 12.15 to 12.45 p.m. every day except Friday, and special probationers on Monday, Wednesday and Friday, from 4.30 to 5.00 p.m. The general rules for probationers were strict but in no way unusual. There was still no uniform, but 'when in the Hospital whether on duty or not the dress must be studiously simple and no jewellery is to be worn'.

The number of applications from prospective probationers increased steadily. Some were still accepted from Miss Henslow, now referred to as the Matron of the Nurses' Home, but relations with her seem, at best, to have been formal. She was asked to submit her applications to the Secretary.[43]

Miss Fisher wrote to Florence Nightingale in July 1878:[32]

> We have not outlived prejudice yet and only the most severe economy keeps me right in the eyes of a large number of the Governors. It was long before I could get proper accommodation for even a part of my probationers; ten are now well provided for, but they will not fit up a room properly for the rest till I manage to get the money for it, they tell me. So there is to be a bazaar in the hospital in October, when I hope to get £300 to pay for all the probationers' rooms and to furnish a children's ward. I do not like bazaars but we have no other means of raising money.

So successful was the training scheme that the scale of fees was raised in February 1880.[44]

First Class or Special Probationers	£13.13s.0d. per quarter
but if they remain for one year	£7.10s.0d. per quarter
Second Class or Nurse Probationers	£7.10s.0d. per quarter
but if they remain for one year	Free of charge

All probationers are charged an entrance fee of £1.1s.0d.

Nurses were certainly hired out for private work, which brought the Hospital into competition with Miss Henslow's Home. There are occasional entries in the Minutes such as[45] 'The Matron paid £6.9s.6d. she had received for services of Nurses.'

In March 1880, Miss Fisher apparently considered leaving, for she asked the Finance Committee and the Weekly Board for testimonials. These were provided and were unrestrained in their praise of her ability, tact and judgement. However, Miss Fisher decided to stay, and the School of Nursing prospered (see Chapter 39). In November 1881, it was agreed that £5 per quarter should be paid to those members of the medical staff who gave lectures to the probationers.

Miss Fisher resigned in March 1882, on her appointment as Matron to the Radcliffe Infirmary, Oxford. She left Oxford in October of the same year and, from then until October 1884, she was Matron of the Birmingham General Hospital. From October 1884, until shortly before her death in June 1888, she was Matron of Blockley Hospital, Philadelphia, where William Osler was a Physician. He is believed to have been the author of an appreciation for *Medical News*: she had demonstrated 'the fact that the profession of nursing affords an ample as well as a most suitable field to women of the highest culture and intelligence'.[32]

Miss Fisher's work at Addenbrooke's Hospital had provided an effective and apparently durable structure for the organisation of the nursing. Most of the staff she had appointed stayed on to work for her successor; Miss Barnacle, the efficient Night Superintendent and Deputy Matron who had also kept the accounts, was one of the few to resign almost immediately.

Alice F. Brown, of the National Hospital for the Deformed, Great Portland Street, was appointed to succeed Miss Fisher.[46] It would have taken a woman of exceptional charm and ability to take over her organisation, which depended for its success, to a greater degree than most Governors appear to have realised, on Miss Fisher's personal qualities. Miss Brown had little opportunity to demonstrate her capabilities. She was taken ill in September, 1884. Mary Young acted as her Deputy during her prolonged leave. In December 1885, Miss Brown underwent major surgery, but although she made a good recovery from the operation she was not physically or emotionally fit for her duties. Frances Hole, who took over as Deputy Matron in July 1886,[47] effectively ran the Hospital. In April 1887, the Matron was asked to tender her resignation as 'conducive to the general interests of the Hospital'. She resigned a week later – 'the business and worries connected with this Hospital are more than my strength can stand'.

The causes of the Matron's worries deserve our attention. The problem of accommodation for the probationers had not been adequately resolved. Early in 1884, before Miss Brown's election, the building of a nurses' home was at last considered (see p. 227) and the solution to this long-standing problem was at last in sight.

In August[48] the Board drew up and ordered to be printed the rules for nurses engaged in private nursing. The 'ordering fee' for the services of a nurse was one guinea weekly, double in cases of infection, and £1.11s.6d. 'if a nurse be required to do duty both day and night'. Hours on duty were 9.00 a.m. to 9.00 p.m. for day nurses, and 9.00 p.m. to 9.00 a.m. for night nurses. Each day nurse should receive three, and each night nurse two, meals whilst on duty. 'It is requested that they be not required to take their meals in the kitchen.' The Hospital uniform was to be worn by all nurses when on duty.

In February 1886[49] a Committee recommended improvement in the nurses' diet and later in the month one of the probationers wrote on behalf of 25 other probationers and herself to thank the Board for 'additional provisions and fires in the cubicles'.

All these changes can only have simplified the Matron's task, until Miss Hole, the Deputy Matron, received a letter from Jessie Murray, a Staff Nurse at King's College Hospital, and this letter was read to the Board.[50] Jessie Murray was one of four staff nurses at King's College Hospital who had moved there from Addenbrooke's Hospital some four months previously. They had heard, she wrote, of discontent which seemed to prevail amongst the new set of nurses. She wrote to criticise the new nurses for she and her three colleagues had felt that their life at Addenbrooke's 'was one of the happiest we had ever lived'. She wrote 'as a protest against the discontent at present prevailing amongst you and as a tribute to Miss Brown's invariable kindness to her nurses'.

The discontent continued. In August one probationer resigned 'owing to the treatment and "training" I have received during the last six months'. A Committee was set up in August to consider 'possible changes in the admission, training and general treatment of probationers'. The first proposal of the Committee was that a scrubber be engaged to relieve probationers from the duty of scrubbing and carrying coals. However, the revised rules for probationers, sent to the printer in October,[51] showed little relaxation of the rigid regime established six years before. For example, probationers, who after all were paying for their training, could still be sent out to earn money for the Hospital as private nurses.

Another source of tension within the nursing staff, is suggested by the action of the Board[52] in censoring the Matron for showing class distinction by failing to invite the staff nurses of Victoria and Bowtell Wards to a supper party she had given soon after Christmas, and to which she had invited all of the other staff nurses.

From 1886 the Board had gradually come to realise that the demands made upon the Matron were beyond the capacity of any woman other than a Miss Fisher. In May 1887, the Board[53] set up a committee to consider the duties of the Matron, before the Governors appointed Miss Brown's successor.

~ 23 ~

Administrative reform

It will be seen from Appendix III that, despite a healthy sum in investments, the Hospital had, since the beginning of the nineteenth century, frequently been left with a debit balance on the annual account. It entered the 1860s in chronic financial difficulties but with the Governors opposing those suggestions of the Improvement Committee which seemed most likely to increase the Hospital's income: a proposal that the Hospital should lend the Corporation of Cambridge £16,000 at 4%, for example, and another that the collection of churches or chapels should be increased by giving the clergy the right to refer patients.

The only substantial legacy received during the 1860s was the sum of £3,423 from the Revd J. Griffith of Ely in 1862, and this was paid into the Building Fund Account.

In September 1864, the Governors set up a committee to distribute circulars appealing for more subscriptions. The appeal was moderately successful but did little to solve the Hospital's problems. On 26 June 1867, a Financial Committee, appointed in the previous March to examine a report on the income and expenditure of the Hospital, presented its report. They estimated that the income for the present year, at £3,347, would fall over £500 below expenditure; either wards must be closed or income increased and economies made. As another committee was concerned with improving the funds, the Finance Committee made only two suggestions: 'that immediate steps be taken to increase the number and amount of collections at places of worship' and 'that a small sum be charged to the masters or mistresses of domestic servants on their admittance as in- or out-patients'. This second recommendation appears to have been ignored.

On the subject of possible economies the Financial Committee was outspoken. Domestic service was costing too much; in particular the number of laundry and charwomen who were brought into the Hospital and fed there: 'their power of work is not in proportion to their power of consumption'. The servants consumed 13 of the 23 lbs of butter bought each week: moreover the price of 1s.6d. per pound was too high. The

Hospital consumed 10,477 quarts of ale a year, at 44s. per barrel; this amounted to 201 quarts each week, of which the servants consumed 123 quarts. Three thousand quarts of small beer were also consumed each year. Ale at 36s. per barrel should be bought and a better system of issuing it should be devised. A fixed quantity of coal should be allowed to each ward, as in other hospitals, and the number of gas burners should be decreased. The Dispensary account had increased, although the number of patients had not. The report ended 'Your Committee in conclusion cannot help remarking on the serious want of some responsible head over the details of the Institution; on the very meagre definition that exists as to the duty of the several servants of the establishment and on the very independent way each one does or does not perform his duties.'

This report was received and approved by the Governors on 15 July.[1] Dr Paget, on behalf of the Drug Committee and the medical staff, agreed to try to avoid prescribing expensive drugs. Some two months later[2] it was reported that most of the recommendations had been complied with. The Committee's recommendations implied serious criticism of the Matron, Miss Bishop. The medical staff's request for changes in the nursing arrangements[3] also implied criticism of the Matron, who protested vigorously, but she submitted her resignation in March 1868.

In September[4] the Treasurer informed the Governors that the current account was overdrawn by £341, but there was a balance in hand of £484 in the Building Fund and £86 in the Samaritan Fund. Mr Dennis, Mr Turner and Mr Hattersley were appointed a Special Committee to ascertain the state of affairs. They found the net deficiency to be £990.16s.9d. The Governors[5] closed the Building Account and transferred the balance to the General Account.

Between June and September 1868, a committee to consider and revise the rules of the Hospital met many times. Their recommendations were accepted by the General Quarterly Court of 5 October 1868. Many obsolete rules were omitted. The most important change was the annual appointment of twelve Select Governors who would undertake to attend the Weekly Board and to visit the Hospital.

The response to the appeal for church collections was disappointing.[6] Two of fourteen Cambridge parishes had sermons and collections in 1866 and three in 1867. In the County, corresponding figures were, in 1866, 32 of 160 churches and, in 1867, 48. There had been an increase of only £87 in the income from church collections in 1867 compared with 1866. The Secretary had omitted to arrange the annual Charity sermon at Great St

Mary's! Further appeals to the clergy were more successful and in 1869 collections brought in £551; in 1870 this source provided only £473.[7] In December 1872,[8] only Humphry and Lilley attended the Improvement Committee. There was a note of despair in their proposal that a circular appeal be sent out 'but the Committee cannot anticipate any great increase of revenue to arrive therefrom'. The Secretary was to ascertain whether a 'Hospital Sunday' had been profitable in those towns in which it had been instituted.

In the Hospital year ending Michaelmas 1872, there was a notable rise in expenditure. A circular was prepared[9] explaining that the rise was due only in part to an increase in the number of patients and in the price of provisions. It was partly due to the necessity felt in this, as in other hospitals, of improving the dietary and adding to the comfort of the patients. This appeal met with slightly greater success and brought some new, and some increased, subscriptions. In 1874 an annual Hospital Sunday to be held in the town on the last Sunday in May was organised. The first such Sunday raised £258 in 21 churches and chapels.

These small improvements in the Hospital's financial status encouraged the Governors, in May 1875, to ask the Improvement Committee to discuss the means of raising funds for new buildings.[10] Its Chairman, Professor Humphry, drafted a circular and by the end of the year[11] this appeal had brought in £1,100. As new subscribers and also new subscriptions had been obtained the Committee thought that the time had come to start building.

The Building Fund continued to attract subscriptions, but the Hospital's financial position still seemed precarious. Since attempts to increase its income had had such limited success the Governors decided to concentrate on reducing expenditure and, in January 1877,[12] appointed a committee 'to enquire into the cause of the great increase in the expenditure of the Hospital'. This committee met six times between 5 January and 8 February; the members were Campion, Turner, Gotobed, Swan Hurrell and Cockerell. On 14 February they suggested that the Matron, Mrs M.E. Sale, might like to anticipate their report by resigning; she did so. On 28 February they drew the attention of the Physicians and Surgeons to the increase in the average length of stay of in-patients, which was considerably longer than in any one of various other hospitals for which they had obtained statistics. 'The Committee can imagine no other cause for this excess than a want of vigilance in discharging the in-patients . . . as soon as it may properly be done.'

In its report[13] the Committee was very critical of the Matron as a housekeeper, but felt that as she had now resigned it was unnecessary to consider her shortcomings in detail. The Weekly Board had failed to control the daily expenditure because no proper accounts had been kept, although there was a book for this purpose. The Committee recommended strict control of the issue of wines and spirits and provisions and planned to introduce a new system when the next Matron had been in office for a time. All the members of the Committee signed the report but Cockerell stated that he considered the recommendations 'inadequate to meet the severity of the case'. The report was received and adopted.[14]

Four Matrons, Miss Robertson, Miss Bishop, Miss Stanley and Mrs Sale, had proved inadequate for the job. It was the Hospital's good fortune next to appoint Miss Alice Fisher as Matron in August 1877. Her energy, ability and tact enabled her to reorganise the housekeeping and to reform the nursing. Her economies in the housekeeping won the support even of reactionary Governors who had opposed her appointment and despite the principles on which she was reorganising the nursing. In November 1878, she organised a bazaar in the Hospital which raised £1,020. Before long she was running the nursing school at a profit.

At the suggestion of the Committee for Raising Funds, the General Quarterly Court[15] approved the appointment of a Finance Committee to meet not less than once a month and 'to watch over the income and expenditure of the Hospital'. The original members of the new committee were the Revd H. Hall and Dr Campion, Gotobed, Knowles and Marshall. They met regularly and looked into possible economies in all parts of the Hospital. Humphry, attending the Committee by invitation,[16] suggested that brandy or wine should not be given to any patient for more than a week without the written authority of his Physician or Surgeon. British brandy at 13s.9d. per gallon should be used.

In March 1880,[17] after another appeal, the Finance Committee resolved to employ a Collector who would be paid two shillings in the pound for each new subscription, and one shilling in the pound on those old subscriptions for which he should be specially directed to apply. Mr Alfred Southwell started work on 29 April 1881, and had collected £180.10s. by 17 June, but he did not maintain his initial success and he resigned in February 1883.

Although the Finance Committee congratulated the Governors[18] on their economies, in September 1881,[19] the General Account was overdrawn by £116.4s.8d. By the following March[20] the position had improved, due 'in a great measure to the zeal and ability of Miss Fisher'. Yet by June 1883,[21] it was again necessary to sell stock to meet current expenses. These precarious swings of fortune continued. Probationers' fees brought in a substantial sum, but the income from subscriptions and dividends was inadequate. A committee on investments was set up in October 1884.[22] In January 1885, Mr F.C. Hutt was appointed Canvasser and Collector[23] but he was dismissed in May of the same year for failing to hand over the money every week. He was succeeded in October by Mr Arthur Rutter who resigned after one year when J. Stuart Hulder took his place until March 1888.

The crisis occasioned by the drainage disaster in 1893 led to a more systematic approach to fund raising. House-to-house collections (Fig. 28) were organised in Cambridge and Chesterton by Miss Miller and in the County by Mrs Townley. By June over £3,000 had been raised from all sources by the Drainage Fund.

The drive on the financial position continued and, in October 1897,[24] when the Finance Committee for the year was appointed, Mr Parker, Dr MacAlister and Mr Wherry were added to it to undertake yet another enquiry into the state of the Hospital's finances and with authority to call in an expert in Hospital management. This enlarged committee, known as the Special Finance Committee, resolved to call in Sir Henry Burdett who was willing to prepare a report 'gratuitously', charging about 50 guineas 'for certain clerkage expenses'. He actually charged less than £40. The bank agreed to allow the Hospital an overdraft of £366.0s.1d. without interest, pending the receipt of Burdett's report.

Burdett attended a meeting of the Special Finance Committee on 11 June and 'asked a large number of questions'. The Committee met again on 24 June to discuss his report. Sir Henry Burdett, as the author of standard reference books on hospital administration, is likely to have had considerable knowledge of the state of affairs at Addenbrooke's before he was formerly invited to advise the Governors. He was therefore in a position to provide a detailed report in little more than a week. The Governors referred their report back to the Special Finance Committee, with additional co-opted members. This committee met in July, August and September, approving on 30 September[25] their report on Burdett's report, to be printed and sent to all Governors. The members of the Special Committee were Besant, Clark, Peck, Waraker, Whitehead,

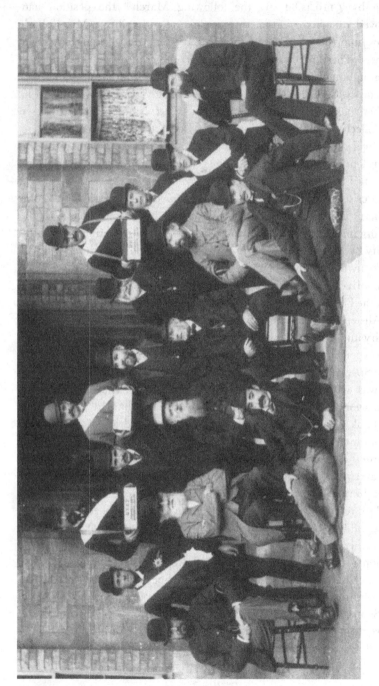

Fig. 28. Hospital group, 1891, believed to be collectors.
Reproduced by permission of the Cambridgeshire Collection.

Young, MacAlister, Parker and Wherry. Co-opted members were A.P. Humphry and Spalding. Adeane was away from Cambridge and unable to accept the invitation to join the Committee.

This Committee recommended accepting all of Burdett's recommendations with the exception of the appointment of a resident Superintendent, and this only on the grounds of expense. His recommendations in relation to nursing were no longer relevant as the Hospital had since introduced only one category of probationer.

Burdett's recommendations included radical changes in the administrative structure of the Hospital. A management committee consisting of eighteen Governors and a Chairman should be appointed annually. A Governor should annually be appointed Vice President of the Hospital; he would act as Chairman of the Committee of Management. This Committee should appoint from their number an executive sub-committee of twelve to meet weekly and a financial sub-committee of five members to meet as required.

A properly representative Selection Committee should be appointed to recommend to the General Committee suitable candidates to fill vacancies in the medical staff; canvassing for the votes of Governors should disqualify a candidate.

The Committee of Management should have authority to invest donations and legacies and to sell securities if this was necessary to make up for deficiencies in revenue.

Burdett's 'Uniform System' of accounts should be introduced as soon as possible. He also wrote: 'After a most exhaustive series of tests I am glad to be able to assure the Governors that if they err at all they err, and have erred for some years, not in the direction of over-expenditure but of under-expenditure.'[26] He went on to say that it was now generally admitted that a Hospital with invested property over five times its gross annual expenditure could consider the excess as a reserve available for building purposes.

There was considerable opposition to Burdett's recommendations. On 14 November 35 people attended the General Court, including Allbutt and Burdett. Fifteen voted for, and sixteen against, the proposal that the report should be adopted. The names are not recorded, but the grounds for the opposition are obvious. For many years the Governors running the Hospital had included a self-perpetuating group of local businessmen whose hostility to the University and to scientific, as distinct from practical, medicine was obstinate and unyielding. A poll was demanded and took place on 28 November when 145 Governors voted in favour of the report and 95 against it.

Further discussion followed. Eventually Mr Adeane and Mr Pemberton, both local landowners whose families had long been associated with the Hospital, proposed[27] that a committee be set up consisting of twelve Governors of the Hospital, four from the County, four from the Borough, and four from the University. These were to consider the administration and financial position of the Hospital and especially to consider the desirability of forming an advisory council, representative, as far as possible, of the County, the Borough and the University, to make recommendations to the General Court on all questions of the administration, finance and general policy of the Hospital. The Court accepted this proposal and elected:

For the County	Pemberton, Adeane, Knowlesly Thornton and A.P. Humphry·
For the Borough	Kett, S.L. Young, A.W. Smith and Joshua Taylor
For the University	Revd G.B. Finch, Revd A. Austin Leigh, Revd Dr Porter and Mr Hoy

This Committee's report was received by the General Quarterly Court on 1 January 1900, but discussion was deferred to an adjourned court meeting in the Guildhall on 22 January.

The new administrative system which was introduced as a result of this report was to serve the Hospital with no radical changes until 1948, and will be considered in some detail later (see p. 264).

There were other developments affecting the financial and administrative status of the Hospital during the last years of the nineteenth century which are worthy of mention. In 1897 the ladies of Cambridge who had organised house-to-house collections formed the Addenbrooke's Hospital Auxillary Association of Ladies. At about the same time a local Hospital Saturday Committee was formed, in imitation of similar committees in other parts of the country. The Hospital took steps to ensure that the two organisations were not in direct competition. On 4 February 1898, it was agreed that the Auxillary Association should confine itself to house-to-house collections and leave to the Hospital Saturday Committee collections in streets, places of work and public houses.

On the administrative side, in October 1880, Frederick Barlow, who had been Secretary since 1838, died. John Bonnett was elected his

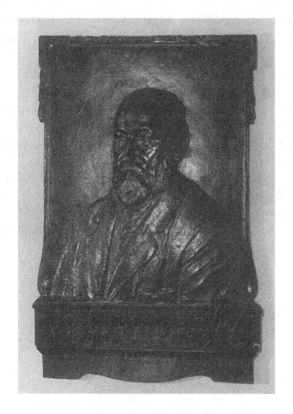

Fig. 29. Plaque in memory of John Bonnett. His mother built and
equipped the Clinical Laboratory.

successor. It was agreed that his appointment should be renewable
annually and that he should be paid £75 per annum. Bonnett was very
highly regarded and was re-elected annually until 1904 when Ellet, the
Superintendent, resigned. The short period of divided responsibility since
Ellet's appointment in 1900 had been an unhappy one. Bonnett, who
resigned to make possible the appointment of a full-time Secretary-
Superintendent, was later appointed legal adviser to the Hospital.

Also of interest is the sequence of events which ended the restriction on
investments to the low-yielding Government securities. In February
1899, the Finance Committee[28] discussed a letter from the Town Clerk,
Whitehead, who was also a member of this committee. The Local
Government Board had authorised the Corporation to raise a loan of

£17,260 for a period of ten years 'for the purpose of paving certain streets with wood'. The Committee recommended making this loan at 3% interest.

The next General Court[29] asked the Finance Committee, with Mr Parker, to consider the general question of reinvestment of capital. The Committee[30] recommended that a considerable amount of capital should be invested in other trustee stocks, as the interest on Consols would be reduced to $2\frac{1}{2}$% in 1903. The Court[31] agreed to the sale of £40,00 Consols and the transfer of the money to trustee investments.

The year ending Michaelmas 1900, found the Hospital with a greater determination than ever before to put its house in order by improved administration and by more systematic organisation of fund raising, relying on the support of a wider section of the community than heretofore.

~ 24 ~

The conditions of probationer nurses

Although the Board in 1887 had obliged Miss Brown to submit her resignation as Matron, their expressions of sympathy for her were sincere. The duties of the Matron had become so heavy and so diverse that only a very exceptional woman could be expected to carry them all out efficiently.

In June 1887, Miss Mary Newcombe Cureton was appointed Matron; there were nineteen applicants.[1] In August the committee set up to consider the Matron's duties recommended the appointment of a Matron's assistant who would take over some of the housekeeping responsibilities, would eat with the probationers and carve for them at supper, and would ensure that they were properly attended when ill.

The Committee later[2] drew up revised bye-laws on the Matron's duties. They are in some ways surprising in their emphasis.

> It shall be the duty of the Matron:
> – to see that the patients have a bath on admission when necessary.
> – to report the presence of any guests in the Hospital.
> – to report to the Weekly Board when any Relieving Officers refuse repayment of necessaries granted by this Institution on behalf of any Union to pauper patients.
> – to see that samples of Meat, Bread, Milk, Groceries and Provisions should be placed during each contract for inspection of the Governors and Resident Medical Officers.
> – to keep a book of the Visitors' names and produce same to the Weekly Board.

The duties of the Matron's assistant were as laid down when the post was created in 1887.

The Staff Nurses having complained that they were paid less than in other Hospitals, it was agreed in February 1889, that they be paid an additional £5 per annum and a grant of £1.5s.0d. per quarter 'for the purpose of purchasing their indoor nursing dress'. For some time, too, the lack of accommodation for sick nurses had been under discussion. A

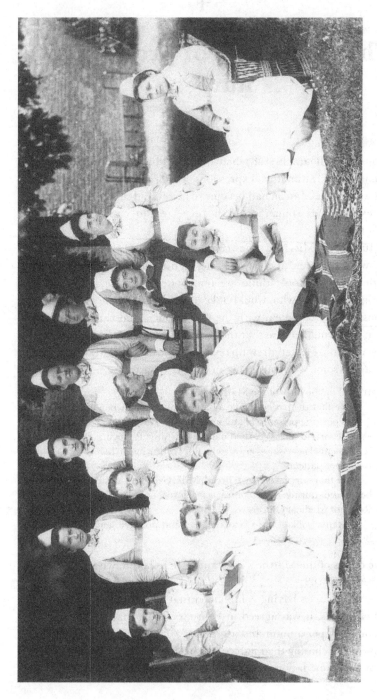

Fig. 30. Hospital night nurses, 1895. The central figure is believed to be the Matron, Miss Mary Cureton. Reproduced by permission of the Cambridgeshire Collection.

committee was set up to consider the matter.[3] It was eventually agreed that a building be put up adjoining the south end of the nurses' dormitory. The Matron also was dissatisfied with her salary. In March 1893, she informed the Board that she was applying for the post of Matron at the Worcester Hospital. The board offered to increase her salary to £90 per annum, the salary paid in Worcester, and she agreed to stay on.

Miss Cureton, if one may judge her by the testimonial given her by the Board when she applied for the post at Worcester, was an efficient Matron and a strong personality. She came into conflict with Miss Kelly, one of her Staff Nurses. This petty domestic discord is worthy of record only because, over a period of months, it divided the Governors into a party demanding Miss Kelly's resignation to uphold the authority of the Matron, a party demanding an enquiry into the Matron's conduct, and a party insisting that no further action should be taken.[4]

The feud unfortunately continued and, in July 1894, the Matron reported Miss Kelly for having Mr Stabb, the House Physician, in her room at 11.00 p.m.[5] Miss Kelly was given six weeks' leave. The disproportionate amount of time devoted by the Governors to such domestic trivia reminds one that the Hospital was still a very small community, and still discontented with pay and conditions.

The principal grievance was the sleeping accommodation – the cubicles were small and noisy. Probationers wrote to complain and Dr Alex Hill, who described himself as 'one who systematically fails to do his duty as a Select Governor' wrote to advocate an improvement in their accommodation; a committee was appointed to formulate a plan for so doing. They agreed that the accommodation consisting of four rooms with six cubicles each was unsatisfactory. They recommended dividing each room into four single rooms and building an extra storey.

The Committee on Probationers' Accommodation received, on 6 November 1894, a letter from Mr Burdett on the subject of the training of probationers. Henry Burdett was immensely influential in hospital reform. He quoted the Nursing Directory, which he edited: 'Addenbrooke's Hospital. Excellent training which only needs to be lengthened to three years for the standard to rank amongst the best in the Kingdom.' Fifty-seven provincial hospitals had already adopted a three-year training. In fact, the Addenbrooke's certificate had, until March 1893,[6] when the minimum training had been increased to two years, been given after only one year's training.

The Committee met several times during November and December

1894, and prepared a report.[7] The report made two main recommendations: the training period should be increased to three years and nurses should be relieved of much rough work by the appointment of seven ward maids. A proposal that this report be received and adopted was not put to the vote. An amendment that the Court adjourn for five weeks was carried.[8]

The Minutes of the committee meeting provide further details of their plans. There should in future be 36 probationers (six Special Probationers for one year, fourteen Special Probationers for three years' training, and sixteen Nurse Probationers for three years' training). The revised scale of fees recommended was:

	1st year	2nd year	3rd year
Special Probationers	£56	£28	£14
Nurse Probationers	£28	£12	nil

The Governors were reluctant to implement the full scheme and the members of the Committee emphasised its financial advantages.[9] The fees received from the probationers would amount to £1,000 a year, whilst their maintenance would cost the Hospital only about £750. The services of 36 probationers were equal to the services of at least 20 trained nurses, who would cost the Hospital at least £900. The training scheme would therefore bring the Hospital a profit of at least £1,000 a year.

The competition amongst hospital training schools was, they said, now very great. Addenbrooke's had hitherto held a high place in this competition. Unlike some hospitals it had maintained a full complement of probationers without paying salaries and without advertising. Since January there had been 212 applications in excess of the number of vacancies. 'If Addenbrooke's is not to be left in the rear it must move in accordance with the spirit of the age.' The Governors were nevertheless slow to act on the Committee's recommendations. This lack of progress may have been due in part to the Matron's prolonged sick leave from January 1896.[10] Much extra work fell on the highly regarded Georgiana Sanders, who had trained at Pendlebury Children's Hospital and was appointed Assistant Matron in March 1896.[11]

In February 1898,[12] a committee was at last set up 'to consider the payments for and duties of Special and Nurse Probationers'. The Committee reported the following week.[13] The Matron had provided comparative figures for several hospitals:

	Daily Average of Beds occupied	Total Nurses	Salaries and Wages	Received in Probationers fees
Addenbrooke's Hospital	108	45	1460	855
Radcliffe Infirmary, Oxford	99	38	1686	365
Queen's Hospital, Birmingham	115	45	2158	
Westminster Hospital, London	128	61	3185	
Royal Free Hospital, London	112	44	2591	188

From these figures it was evident that Addenbrooke's was not over-staffed and that the Hospital paid less in salaries than other hospitals and was the only teaching hospital to pay its probationers nothing. The Committee must have been content to let this exploitation continue as long as there were sufficient applicants willing to accept these terms. Their only positive proposal was that there should in future be only one class of probationer, who should pay a total of £60 for the three years. In November 1899,[14] a committee was established to consider the retiring age for nurses and the possibility of providing pensions. The Committee's report was presented to an unusually well-attended Weekly Board a fortnight later.[15] Enquiries addressed to six other hospitals showed that there was no uniform practice. At Addenbrooke's Hospital there was a prescribed retiring age – 65 – only for the Matron. As nurses were required to be in their wards from 8.00 a.m. to 9.00 p.m. the Committee felt that there should be a prescribed age limit after which no nurse should be allowed to undertake such heavy responsibilities. They recommended that nurses should produce birth certificates on appointment and should be allowed to retain office after the age of 60 only by special permission of the Board. The Hospital could not at present afford to pay pensions, but future provision should be made for a contributory scheme. The medical staff[16] thought it inexpedient to introduce a fixed retiring age or a pension scheme. However, the Board approved[17] a retirement age of 60 'in the case of nurses hereinafter appointed', but deferred the pension scheme for further consideration.

Action on the financially impracticable matter of providing pensions was precipitated by a letter from six probationers on Bowtell Ward.[18]

They complained that they were dissatisfied with their training – 'we are sure you are under the impression that we receive . . . the best of training. This is not the case.' They wished to make their complaint privately as they were deeply attached to the Hospital and 'should indeed regret if our complaint was the means of making any of its shortcomings public'. Another letter, signed by the remaining probationers, corroborated these statements.

An enquiry, at which the evidence was given 'without the slightest sign of animosity against any single individual', showed that there was no teaching in two of the surgical wards. The Sisters of these wards admitted that this was so and said that 'when they came they were engaged to nurse the sick patients and not to train the probationers'. It was agreed that the Sisters concerned should be asked to resign without any reflection being cast on their conduct, as they had been engaged before modern methods of training nurses had been adopted. Each Sister should be awarded a pension of £40. Rebecca and Mary Newman submitted their resignations as requested.

The Finance Committee[19] suggested that pensions could not be a charge on Hospital income; they thought a general pension fund should be established. It was recommended that this should be carried out. Donations and legacies so designated would be paid into the fund together with 5% of each nurse's salary and an equal contribution from the Hospital. After some discussion and minor amendments the scheme was approved[20] and referred to the Advisory Council which appointed a Sub-Committee to consider it. This Sub-Committee formulated bye-laws setting up a pension fund. The fund would maintain for each nurse a policy with the Royal National Pension Fund. The Advisory Council deferred further discussion but, in June 1901, circulated a letter from its Sub-Committee on pensions. They recommended a scheme which 'involved the minimum of burden' and tended 'to encourage thrift among the nurses'. The Addenbrooke's Pension Fund would take out and maintain under the Royal National Pension Fund for Nurses (R.N.P.F.N.) a policy for a pension of £10 per annum to commence at the age of 50 for any nurse under 40 years of age who in her own name took out a policy with the R.N.P.F.N. for not less than £10. The Quarterly Court[21] deferred further discussion on the grounds that there was no wish amongst the nursing staff for such a scheme.

The Hospital's reluctance to improve the conditions of service of probationers and to reduce their fees was dictated largely by financial stringency. Addenbrooke's Hospital compared so unfavourably in these respects with most other hospitals that it is not surprising that, by March 1901,[22] the Matron had to report a serious decline in the number of applicants for places in the Training School. She recommended reducing the fees and increasing the staff; she had at times been compelled to employ the same nurse on day and on night duty. A Probationers' Committee was set up to investigate the problem.

It was to be left to her successor to tackle these difficulties, for Miss Cureton, in July 1901, submitted her resignation; she 'did not feel equal to the work and worry of another winter here'. She was asked to consider withdrawing her resignation but would not do so. The Board[23] placed on record 'its deep appreciation of the many services rendered to the Hospital and its patients by Miss Cureton'.

~ 25 ~

The Hospital closes for reconstruction of the drains

Fever and drains

The Governors' enthusiasm for the reconstruction work of the 1860s was shared by the medical journalists. However, the New Building Committee, which in October 1866 was reappointed, but renamed the Repairing Committee, was for the next 30 years frequently preoccupied with problems of drainage.

In January 1866, the Manager of the Town Water Works had informed the Governors that in future the Hospital, which had previously paid 5 guineas a quarter for water, would have to pay for the quantity consumed, as measured by a meter on the supply pipe. This letter initiated an obsessive concern with measures to reduce consumption. The weekly consumption varied from 20,000 gallons to 33,000 gallons and explanations were sought for any abnormally high figures. Weekly records were kept. In February 1867, consumption ranged from 9000 to 16000 gallons. Burst pipes were frequent. The Repairing Committee called for a report by local plumbers,[1] sent it to Digby Wyatt and informed the Governors 'that the plumbing work of the Hospital is in a very bad state'. The problems were the results of a high but variable water pressure and were partially resolved by installing cisterns.

The Governors were able, for a while, to forget their plumbing difficulties and to turn their attention to fever wards.

A scheme to erect, in 1871, a detached building of two five-bed wards for patients with infectious diseases, was held up because the problem of infectious diseases was under consideration by the Government. The following year[2] it was resolved to purchase a hut or huts capable of receiving two patients and a nurse. No action was taken and other schemes were discussed. In October 1874,[3] a committee was appointed 'to consider whether any steps should be taken to provide more accommodation for the use of patients in the event of any infectious disorder

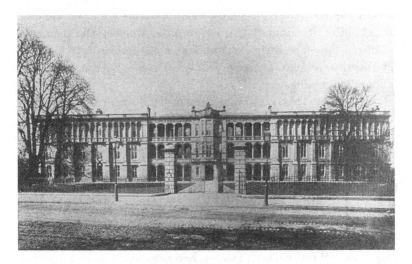

Fig. 31. Addenbrooke's Hospital, 1870.

occurring in the surgical wards'. The medical staff recommended the construction of a small ward for females on the ground floor on the site of the mortuary with a male ward on the floor above it. There was opposition to the plan by the Governors who justifiably felt that the Hospital could not afford any more buildings. In fact, a more ambitious extension was constructed with wards on three floors. It was completed by March 1878;[4] Fawcett was the architect. The ground floor provided two children's wards, named Townley and Alice (later renamed Alice Fisher Ward in memory of the Matron). The upper floor was a surgical ward and the middle floor was for contagious female cases. In the basement was a Turkish Bath which on two days in the week ladies could use at a charge of 2s.6d.[5]

The plumbing soon attracted attention once more. In February 1881, 50 pipes in the Hospital burst.[6] In October 1882, Bushell Anningson, the Medical Officer of Health, was asked to make a thorough examination of the sanitary conditions in the Hospital for a fee of 3 guineas.[7] The report was received on 24 January 1883, and it made depressing reading for it described an antiquated system, with some broken pipes. All the sewage of the Hospital was conveyed to the public sewer by a brick barrel drain, two feet in diameter, which passed under the centre of Bowtell Ward. It seemed probable that the burrowing of rats had established direct connections between this ward and the sewer. A committee appointed to consider the report, recommended that work costing £39.15s. should be carried out on the drains.[8] It is not recorded whether Dr Anningson considered the work adequate; the Governors, despite their financial difficulties, were more interested in plans for new buildings than the drains of the existing ones.

It was proposed to erect a building on the land acquired in 1861 from Corpus Christi College, 'to provide sleeping and other accommodation for 26 patients and nurses'.[9] Humphry would have preferred an extension of the existing structure rather than a separate building[10] but the Committee went ahead and approved the plans of the architect, Elbourn. The buildings were completed in March 1885, and the medical staff were invited to give their views on how the accommodation should be used. They recommended a number of changes which were approved. Collignon and Maynard Wards, called 'fever wards' but seldom used as such, were converted into children's wards. Fever cases were to be accommodated in the new wards on Tennis Court Road. One of the existing children's wards (Townley) was urgently required for ophthalmic outpatients. The other (Alice) should be restored to its originally intended use for women with venereal disease. Other minor changes were also approved.

In April 1886, the local manager of the South of England Telephone Company offered to place 'a set of telephones' at the disposal of the Hospital, free of charge. The offer was accepted.

The next building project was a ward for sick nurses in 1889.

In 1891 a committee[11] met to discuss the building of wards for infectious cases. On two occasions during the past 30 years isolation wards had been constructed but each time they had come to be used for general medical or surgical cases. The Building Committee[12] hoped that the new admission papers would discourage the admission of infectious diseases. They did not recommend any extension of the buildings as the Hospital funds 'are not in a flourishing condition'. It seems probable that although the infectious nature of the specific fevers was accepted, the contagiousness of wound infections was not.

Professor Latham had, for some time, been complaining about the insanitary state of the wards. Eventually, in 1892, the Governors appointed a committee to consider the matter.[13] The Committee ordered a complete plan of the drains to be prepared. The plan was sent to Rogers Field, a civil engineer with special experience of drainage. Field prepared a report which was discussed. The Committee at the next Quarterly Court accepted Mr Field's advice 'that nothing but an entire reconstruction of the system of drainage would suffice to place the Hospital beyond danger from a sanitary point of view', although this would involve closing the Hospital entirely for some weeks.

The Committee, now referred to as the Committee on Drainage, met frequently. They decided that no arrangements could be made to accommodate medical in-patients.[14] Surgical in-patients could be accommodated in the new Medical School building in Downing Street. The billiard room of Grove Lodge (Humphry's house) might accommodate four severe cases, and the room above it three less severe cases.[15] The Vice Chancellor conveyed the Senate's approval of the use of the Medical School buildings during the Christmas vacation. Mr Eaden Lilley offered his house in Fitzwilliam Street and the Governors decided to use it to accommodate nurses and servants.[16] The adaptation of the Medical School building was arranged by a hospital committee appointed for this purpose, in negotiation with Mr A.E. Shipley of Christ's College, Secretary of the Museums and Lecture Rooms Syndicate.

The Hospital had to bear the cost of these adaptations in addition to the cost of reconstructing the drainage system, for which Kerridge & Shaw's estimate of £2,705 was accepted.[17] Borough, County and University all responded to an appeal for funds. The Hospital was closed on 26 December and out-patients, accidents and urgent surgical cases were accepted at 'The temporary Hospital at Downing Street'.

The opportunity provided by the empty hospital enabled the Governors to refloor Bowtell, Albert and Griffiths Wards with teak. Dr MacAlister made himself responsible for raising the necessary funds.[18] A further improvement carried out at this time was the installation in the kitchen of a 'gas cooking arrangement' on the advice of Mr Wood of the kitchen of Trinity College.

Meanwhile the work on the drainage system made satisfactory progress although the condition of the drains had been found to be even worse than had been suspected. 'The whole area was honey-combed with old drains . . . in the centre of the kitchen an old cesspool was found with two drains, one of which was under the larder.'[19] In the middle of April the Outpatient Department and two wards were re-opened. During the period of four months whilst the Hospital was completely closed there had been 3126 attendances at the temporary Out-patient Department in Downing

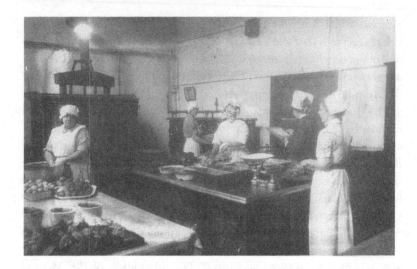

Fig. 32. The Diet Kitchen c.1895. The second figure from right is
thought to be the Matron, Miss Mary Cureton.

Street, and many urgent cases had been admitted. The Governors
ordered that the 'Temporary Hospital' should be restored to its original
state to the satisfaction of the Museum Syndicate.[20]

Rogers Field advised the Governors on structural defects apart from the
drainage. The gas-fittings, he said, urgently needed repair, but the
Committee did not welcome his suggestion that electric light be
installed.[21] He also found several of the hearths to be in a dangerous state.

All this work was completed by the beginning of June, but the
contractors remained responsible for the drainage for six months after its
completion and were obliged under their contract to make good a few
small defects which became apparent during this period. The public
response to special appeals had been so good that of the total cost, £4,701,
the Hospital had to pay only £1,053 out of capital.

The Surgical Out-patient Department, Nurses' Home and operating theatre

A few months after returning from the temporary accommodation to the
Hospital, the Committee, with Sir George Humphry as Chairman, met to
discuss the extension of the Surgical Out-patient Department, towards

the cost of which Humphry had contributed £500.[22] Also urgently needed was improvement in the accommodation for probationers. Fawcett's plans for the Out-patient extension were much criticised, and these and the plans for the extension of the Nurses' Home were shown to Keith Young, an associate of Burdett. Burdett and Young visited Cambridge, inspected the buildings, and conferred with Fawcett and submitted a detailed report. They recommended erecting a new building as a Nurses' Home and using the existing building for servants and ward maids. Fawcett's plans, revised in accordance with these suggestions, were accepted.[23] They included the construction of a room for the Ophthalmic Department. Humphry wrote that he would prefer his donation to be used for bringing the operating room 'when freed from the Out-patients . . . into a condition suited to modern requirements'. The tender of £198 for the Out-patient extensions from Messrs Coulson & Lofts was accepted. In June the Special General Court[24] accepted the tender of £3,392 from Kerridge & Shaw for the new Nurses' Home and appointed a Committee to supervise the building.

Humphry's comments on the state of the operating theatre were expressed more specifically by the meetings of the surgical staff which submitted a report to the Governors in February 1896.[25] A Committee was appointed;[26] it sought the advice of Keith Young who recommended a terrazzo floor, tiled walls, and an anaesthetic room. The latter and a staff room could be constructed by annexing Mary Ward. The total cost would be about £1,000. The Committee's report was accepted.[27] In November 1896,[28] the Secretary was asked to obtain an estimate for lighting the Hospital by electricity. After considerable correspondence it was decided[29] to accept the estimate of Bailey, Grundy & Barrett for installing electricity to the Out-patients' Department only (including the Eye Room) for £19.1s.[30]

At this stage the generosity of Alexander Peckover, landowner and banker at Wisbech, induced the Governors to name the new Nurses' Home the Peckover Building.[31] He had contributed largely towards its cost. The plans for the operating theatre were approved 'at a cost not exceeding £1,000';[32] at the same Court it was announced that Peckover had given £1,000 for the operating theatre, 'because the financial position of the Hospital is so serious'. Peckover's gift was certainly timely. The estimate for the theatre, including electric light, was £1,545.10s.8d. not including the architect's fee and instrument cases[33] and the eventual cost was £1,987.19s.2d. The theatre was completed by the end of 1898. The

Operating Theatre Committee met on 8 March 1897 to consider a letter from Keith Young, pointing out that the existing system of heating water for the theatre in kettles on an open fire would not be possible in the new theatre. He sensibly suggested that when the heating system for the theatre was being installed the opportunity should be taken of providing an adequate supply of hot water for the whole hospital. This suggestion was rejected after heating experts from London had advised that the cost would be high.[34]

Discussion of a possible hot water supply drew the Governors attention to the problem of the Hospital laundry. This was still a hand laundry. Eight laundry maids in succession had come to the Hospital in apparently robust health and had broken down and been obliged to leave.[35] The existing practice of airing linen in the wards at night occupied too much of the nurses' time and was unhealthy and a fire risk.

A Committee was set up in August 1897[36] to consider the proposed steam laundry. The Chairman was Mr W.P. Spalding. He, accompanied by the Matron and Miss A.P. MacAlister attended the Laundry Exhibition at the Agricultural Hall in London. They also visited hospitals and laundries in London, Liverpool, Ipswich and elsewhere. They recommended[37] installing a steam laundry which would also provide hot water, heating and cooking pressure from the laundry boiler, and would include drying closets. The recommendation was accepted by the Weekly Meeting but the Quarterly Court[38] referred the report back to the Committee. Their two principal objections: the possibility that the laundry would be unacceptably noisy and a restricted covenant on the proposed site. Both were proved to be unfounded. The Committee accordingly resubmitted its recommendations, pointing out that the steam laundry would save at least £78 per annum. It would cost £1,250, which as at present invested, brought in £31 per annum in interest. The report was approved in March.[39]

The Hospital was still largely gas-lit when the Cambridge Electric Supply Company, whose manager, J.H. Barker, was a member of the Hospital's Advisory Council, wrote[40] offering to supply the Hospital with electricity at 4d. per unit and 1d. per unit as rent for the wires and fittings which they would install free. For several weeks the advantages and disadvantages of electricity and gas were argued. Mr Barker thought that 'the fumes given off by gas are most undesirable in sick rooms'. After visits to other hospitals and more correspondence the installation of electricity was approved;[41] largely on financial grounds; the Committee recommended that the gas system should be retained for use in emergencies.

The supply of hot water provided by an obsolete boiler in the basement was inadequate and a Hot Water Committee, of which Dr Besant was the Chairman, met on a number of occasions during the first half of 1902, before preparing its report.[42] They found the hot water system to be so inefficient that water had to be heated in kettles in ward kitchens for hot baths. The Committee had found it necessary to extend their investigations to the heating system. Wards and rooms were inadequately heated by open fireplaces, and corridors and staircases were virtually unheated. Coal fires involved much work and were dirty and, as the Hospital could store only six tons, coal had to be delivered two or three times each week. The Committee was in favour of a central heating system which would burn coke to the value of £80 annually in place of the present consumption of coal using over £300 per annum.

The Quarterly Court of 30 June[43] adopted the Committee's report on hot water supply and heating, despite an attempt to defer a decision and the Committee was authorised to carry out the work at a total expense not to exceed £1,400.

Some six weeks later the Governors[44] received a letter signed by Bradley, Humphry, Griffiths, Deighton, Lloyd Jones and Wright expressing the opinion that to heat the wards with hot water pipes and radiators would be 'prejudicial to the health and convalescence of the patients and to the health of the nursing staff'. The medical staff protested that they had not been officially informed and consulted.

The Committee[45] considered this letter. The contract for the heating system had already been signed on the authority of the Quarterly Court of 30 June and when Bradley, Griffiths, MacAlister and Wherry had been present. The Committee replied that they had shared the misgivings expressed in the letter, but had taken advice and had been assured that their fears were groundless.

The next weekly meeting[46] discussed the medical staff's letter, which was supported by a strongly worded letter from Allbutt: 'This time when the Hospital is so poor that the Scientific Departments on which the highest efficiency of the therapeutics of the Institution depends are starved, it seems to me ill chosen for expensive and doubtful experiments, alterations, made without proper and expert assistance.'

For once Allbutt and Latham were in agreement, for a conference between the Hot Water Committee and the medical staff on 24 August received a letter from Latham '. . . I trust I have been misinformed for I can hardly believe that such a proposal whether considered from a financial or sanitary point of view or as regards even the comfort of the patients, could be entertained for a single moment by anyone at all conversant with hospital requirements.'

The conference failed to reach agreement but on 10 October, soon after the fire had become the main preoccupation of the Governors and medical staff, the Hot Water Committee gave the contractors, Messrs Renton Gibbs, permission to start work. The junior medical staff made a final protest[47] when they asked that radiators should not be placed in the private sitting room so that they would not 'have to endure the discomfort attending the proposed system'. Radiators were installed but fireplaces were retained.

The Hospital fire

At 1.45 p.m. on 1 October 1902,[48] fire broke out in the roof over Victoria Ward. Marion Still, a maid in that ward, had discovered the fire. She told a nurse and H.A. Farrow, the Under-Porter, climbed the ladder to the trap-door with a hose whilst the fire brigade was sent for. The fire was soon under control but not before it had caused considerable damage. The roof over Victoria Ward and the adjoining corridor had been completely destroyed. The walls, floor and contents of Victoria Ward had been damaged and the ceiling of Hatton Ward had been damaged by water. No-one had been injured. All the property destroyed was insured with the Sun Fire Office.

Committees were set up, one to supervise the repairs (known as the Fire Committee)[49] and another to enquire into the cause of the fire.[50] This was certainly never established. Workmen using naked candles had been working on the installation of pipes near the point of origin of the fire, but the Committee decided that the fire had probably started in a beam which partially supported a chimney stack.[51] This report on the cause of the fire did not satisfy all the Governors and the Court[52] referred it back to the Weekly Board to make further enquiries, but MacAlister, the architect, later reported that he had found other flues in which 'timbers were within dangerous proximity to the insides of flues'.[53] They had now been removed.

The Press was normally admitted to the Quarterly Courts but not to Committee meetings. The Court on 11 November[52] took the report of the Fire Committee as read, then requested the Press to withdraw. The Fire Committee's report was then received. The £1,828 compensation from the Fire Office would pay for all needed repairs and also for the installation of a lift and two external staircases. The Fire Committee was authorised to carry out the proposed work provided no more was obtained from the Fire Office. The Press was then re-admitted. The Governors had been over-optimistic for the seven tenders for the work ranged from £2,236 to £2,690. MacAlister persuaded Mr Sindell, who had submitted the lowest tender, to reduce it to £1,740.

More heating problems

The Hospital's biggest problem after the repair of the fire damage was once again the heating system, which caused as much anxiety as the increasing inadequacy of the children's ward. The installation of the new heating system was completed by December 1903. The Works Sub-Committee[54] was concerned that the new boiler consumed one ton of coke daily and had to be stoked every hour.

In April 1904,[55] the medical staff and the Works Sub-Committee were together appointed a committee to consider the heating of the Hospital, especially from the points of view of health and economy. The boiler was now burning 14 or 15 cwt of coal daily and only the sides of the wards were adequately heated. The heating of other parts of the Hospital was inadequate; the radiators were often defective, difficult to regulate and difficult to clean. New fire places were authorised to replace the old type in Victoria, Hatton and Albert Wards.

There were many meetings but no firm conclusions were reached and, in March 1905, the Court[56] appointed a Committee to consider the cost and efficiency of the heating apparatus and whether a return to the old system would not be more economical and more efficient. This Committee[57] met several times and consulted Renton Gibbs, who had designed and constructed the heating system. The essential recommendations in the long report[58] were:

1. More expert stoking.
2. Use of coke.
3. Repair and modernisation of ward fireplaces.

It is clear that no satisfactory solution to the Hospital's heating problems had been achieved. When the difficulty of heating the theatres was again discussed in December 1906,[59] J.B. Lock and Horace Darwin suggested double-glazing the large skylights.

The children's wards

The medical staff had long been complaining about the condition of the children's wards (see Fig. 23, p. 158). The Sanitary Inspector's report on these wards in December 1903[60] found the drains defective and the floors 'rough, pervious and quite unsuitable'. Steam from the laundry in the basement made the walls wet. The fever wards were much too near. The children were removed, but, after the drains had been put right, the medical staff agreed only reluctantly to allow the children to return.[61] 'They do not think these wards can be considered as made satisfactory for present occupation.'

However, when the General Committee in the same year[62] proposed that the children's wards be closed at an early date, on the grounds that they were unsuitable and expensive to run and that the accommodation was needed for administrative purposes, the medical staff protested at the 'uncertainty (of) the efficiency of the Hospital'.[63] The allocation of children's beds in other wards was arranged.

More fires

On 6 January 1906, a fire broke out in the roof of Mary Ward, the anaesthetic room and the staircase and corridor near Victoria Ward.[64] It caused damage which cost £781 to repair. The Sun Fire Office settled this claim.[65] The fire was once again blamed on a defective flue but the cause remained uncertain. A further fire in the Sister's room in Bowtell Ward in February 1907 fortunately did little damage.

The decade from 1894, after the Hospital had survived the drainage catastrophe which so nearly forced it to close down, was perhaps the most unsatisfactory in its long history. Shortage of funds was in part responsible for the difficulties but the Hospital's malaise had no single cause. Much money was wasted on ill-advised schemes entered into without sufficient consultation or planning. Sir Philip Panton,[66] who, it has already been mentioned, was a House Surgeon in Addenbrooke's in 1904, wrote: 'Addenbrooke's in those days was a mere shadow of its present competence. Then it was passing through a period of eclipse when this famous institution had forgotten its tradition and lost its soul, regained in the fine modern hospital as it exists today.'

Reforms and modernisation

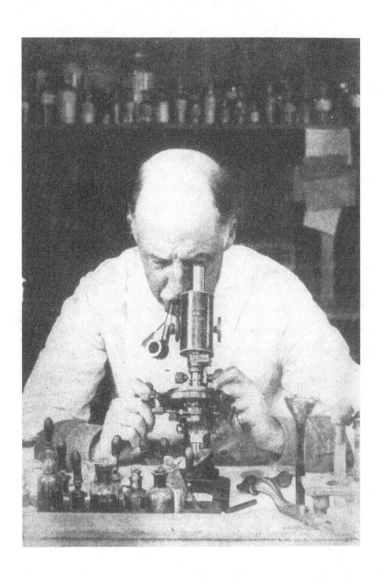

~ 26 ~

Medical teaching at Cambridge

The development of medical teaching at Cambridge University began to play a significant part in the history of the Hospital in the late 1800s.

Henry VIII had established a Regius Professorship in Physic as well as in Divinity, Civil Law, Hebrew and Greek in 1540, which should have ensured a viable school of medicine in Cambridge, but in fact the faculty slumbered until the nineteenth century and those responsible for it 'were much inclined to treat their posts as sinecures'. Between 1500 and 1856 there were only, on average, four Cambridge medical graduates per year.[1]

The eighteenth century, when Addenbrooke's was founded, was the least satisfactory period for the University and it was a time in which the Medical School was held in 'justified contempt'.[2] In some years only two or three students entered upon the medical course[3] and, although dissections were carried out, it is not known how frequently. Some cadavers at least came from the London resurrection men for, in March 1768, a body in the dissecting room of Charles Collignon, Professor of Anatomy, was identified as that of Laurence Sterne, author of *Tristram Shandy*, who had been buried in London a few days earlier.

Before John Haviland became Regius Professor in 1817 a candidate for the M.B. had only to reside for nine terms, retain his name on the books for five years, witness two dissections, and keep a single Act.[2] The 'most that the Regius Professors did in the way of lecturing was the delivery at the end of the formal physic Act of a "determination" or speech in Latin on the subject, a duty which did not occur more than four times a year'.[1] Haviland gave regular courses of 50 lectures annually in pathology and the practice of medicine[2] and persuaded the Senate to pass in February 1829 a Grace which recast the medical curriculum and examinations and laid the foundations for the future school. It was also during Haviland's Regius Professorship in 1842 that Paget initiated clinical examinations in the final M.B. These were the first to be held in the United Kingdom and are now universal. A few years before this Addenbrooke's appears to have become a recognised School of Medicine.

There was a connection between the Medical School and the Hospital from its earliest days. The Physicians Plumptre, Collignon, Pennington and Harwood were all professors in the Medical School and Glynn is known to have lectured regularly.

There is no mention of pupils or apprentices in the original rules of the Hospital but the first record of instruction given at the Hospital to a medical student is found in a letter written in 1843 by Dr Frederic Thackeray, informing the Governors of his 'connexion of half a century with Addenbrooke's Hospital as a pupil, Surgeon, and Physician';[4] we know that he and his brothers were pupils of Thomas Thackeray and helped him both in his practice and in his hospital work. It is therefore probable that other surgeons' pupils were also admitted to the hospital, but that the arrangement between such apprentices and their masters was regarded as a private one which did not usually concern the Governors.

Occasionally the Governors did intervene however, as in May 1839, when Mr Lestourgeon's pupil, Mr Lee, was alleged to be guilty of misconduct and Mr Lestourgeon was asked to inform him that he must not in future enter the gardens or visit the Hospital except at the requisite hours.

The apprentices of the Apothecary, a full-time officer of the Hospital, were in a different category and the first was admitted in 1824. The House Surgeon too was allowed to have one apprentice residing in the Hospital in the first half of the nineteenth century and in 1840 this youth's annual premium was £80, half of which went to the Hospital and half to the House Surgeon.[4]

By 1839 the Hospital appears to have been recognised as a School of Medicine because on 22 November the report of a special meeting of the Auditors was concluded as follows: 'The increased expenditure has been occasioned by the introduction into the Hospital, two years ago, of twenty-two additional beds, by which very important benefits have been derived, in affording the opportunity of relieving a great many more cases than could otherwise have been attended to and in placing the Hospital upon the footing of a recognised School of Medicine.'

It seems likely that the practice of taking young men into the Hospital was becoming more widespread because in 1840[5] Mr Lestourgeon gave notice that at the next Court he would 'bring forward the subject of admitting to the practice of the Hospital the pupils of the Medical gentlemen connected with that Institution'. The Court of 28 December agreed that such pupils should be subject to the same regulations, made that year, as the Apothecary's apprentice[4] but, on 29 March 1841, approved special regulations which extended the permission to attend the Hospital to medical students other than the private pupils of the staff so long as they were recommended by one of the Medical Officers.

Another of these regulations stated that the names of the pupils were to be entered monthly into a book kept by the Secretary. This Register of Pupils has fortunately survived and shows between one and ten names monthly until March 1843. Some names appear for only one or two months. Most of these men were undergraduates but some were local apprentices.

On 7 December 1842, Dr Thackeray on behalf of the medical staff informed the Weekly Board that they wished 'to establish a system of Clinical lectures for practical instruction of the pupils in Medicine and Surgery and to require from them the payment of a certain fee as is usual in similar institutions'.

The scheme was accepted and, on 27 March 1843, a Code of Rules for Clinical Lectures was adopted. Now, in addition to attending the wards during the visits of the Physicians and Surgeons, the pupils were to receive one medical and one surgical lecture per week during full term, and one lecture, alternately medical and surgical, every week during the residence of the year. The lectures were to be delivered in the Board Room, and a fee of 8 guineas for six months, 10 guineas for twelve months, or 15 guineas for perpetual attendance was to be paid by each pupil to the Medical Officers 'on his admission to the practice and lectures of the hospital'. Pupils needed the recommendation of one of the Physicians and one of the Surgeons for admission, and were allowed to visit the patients between 9 a.m. and 2 p.m. on weekdays.

Only two pupils signed on for the Michaelmas term 1843, but there were six in 1844, including Francis Galton, five in 1845, eight in 1846, and eight in 1847, including Timothy Holmes. The number of new signatures in any one year allows no reliable estimate to be made of the total attendance, as a large proportion of pupils paid the full 'perpetual' or 'unlimited' fee. The practice of re-entering their names every month had been discontinued. The largest entry was 106 in 1847. The number of new signatures increased slowly and irregularly, reaching fifteen by 1860. The pupils included many men who later became well known, for example T. Clifford Allbutt in 1857.

By 1860 it was the declared policy of the Governors[6] that the 'Hospital should both satisfy the continually increasing need of the poor and afford suitable practice for the Medical classes of the University'.

The students who signed on for the lectures were entitled to work in the wards between 9 a.m. and 2 p.m. on weekdays, and their presence must have influenced both staff and patients. The lectures were given in the Board Room until 1869 when the Male Convalescent Room was used for this purpose.[7] Later they were again given in the Board Room.

By 1879 the number of students was, as we have seen, in the region of 50 and some of the Governors were beginning to resent their presence, which brought considerable financial benefits to the medical staff, but none to the Hospital. The Secretary was asked to write to a number of other hospitals asking what proportion of lecture fees went to the teachers and what to the Institution.[8] No further action was taken at that time but the matter was raised again eleven years later[9] when the Board noted that the attendance of medical students caused additional expenditure of Hospital funds; whilst they realised that the association with the Medical School was of advantage to the Hospital and to the patients, it should not 'entail a charge on eleemosynary funds'. They recommended an admission fee of £2 for each student, from 1 January onwards. A committee set up to consider the matter decided on an alternative arrangement under which the medical staff would pay £10 per annum to the Hospital to meet any expenses occasioned by the presence of the students.[10] However, the Weekly Board declared itself unsatisfied with this arrangement[11] and a copy of the resolution was to be sent to each of the medical officers.

Sir George Paget died on 29 January 1892, and Thomas Clifford Allbutt became Regius Professor of Physic on 8 March 1892. It had since 1785 been the custom for an Addenbrooke's physician to be appointed to this position and there were three in residence; however, 'to have appointed any one of them would have aroused fierce antagonism with the other two, while to have appointed any of them would have been distasteful to considerable, if different, sections of the University; so it is not surprising that it was hoped that the choice would fall elsewhere'.[2]

Allbutt had made his name in Leeds, although he had studied at Cambridge, one of his contemporaries at Caius being Peter Walwork Latham, who was now one of Addenbrooke's Physicians. Langdon-Brown[2] says of Latham 'His contribution to the Medical School may be summarised as throwing a spanner into the works whenever occasion offered.' Allbutt was not given a place at Addenbrooke's when he first came to Cambridge and he remained in that anomalous state for eight years, although negotiations between the University and the Hospital were vigorously pursued.

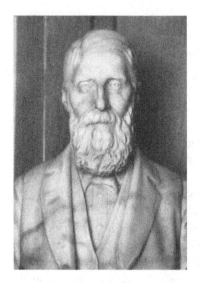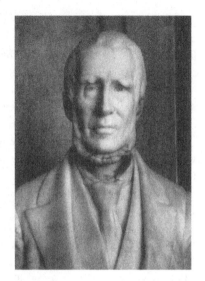

Fig. 33. Marble busts of (a) Sir G.M. Humphry and (b) Sir G.E.
Paget, now in the Clinical School Library.

In 1895[12] the Hospital received a letter from the Vice Chancellor of the
University asking for a conference to be held 'with a view to establishing a
closer and more regular connexion between the Hospital and the University Teachers in the Department of Medicine.'

A Committee, consisting of Dr P.W. Latham, Dr E. Carver, Dr W.H.
Besant, Dr T. Waraker, Dr W. Cockerell, Mr J.E.L. Whitehead, Mr J.
Hamblin Smith, and Mr Edmund H. Parker, was approved[13] to consider
the relations now existing between the Hospital and the University
Medical School. On 1 May 1895, they agreed a report that summarised
the history and present position.

In addition to some of the points already related, the report says that
once the Regulations had been approved in 1843 the members of the
medical staff had been left to carry them out, and during the past 50 years
the Governors had been consulted only on trivial changes. Subsequent to
the Code being established Certificates of Attendance on the practice of
the Hospital were recognised by the University, the Royal Colleges of
Physicians and Surgeons, the Society of Apothecaries in London, and
other Licensing bodies.

The rapid growth of the Medical School in the University had been
accompanied by a great increase in the number of students attending the

Hospital practice and lectures. Hence in 1841 there were nineteen entries on the Register, in 1844 six, in 1854 three, in 1864 twenty, in 1874 thirty-four, in 1884 sixty, and in 1894 eighty-nine.

The instruction now given to the students was similar to that prescribed in 1843. Clinical lectures in medicine were still partly given in the wards and partly in the Board Room; clinical lectures in surgery were given in the wards and the operating theatre.

The fees paid by the pupils were wholly paid to the Medical Officers who had the power to alter the amounts without reference to the Governors.

Although no formal relations had ever been established between the University Medical School and the Hospital, there was a connection because (a) all the members of the staff except one were members of the University, some being Professors and Teachers, (b) all the students attending the hospital were members of the University and students in the Medical School, and (c) some of the patients, who were paid a small remuneration from the University Chest, were utilised in the University Medical and Surgical examinations.

The report was signed by the members of the committee and accepted by the General Quarterly Court of 7 May 1895.

Further discussions, meetings, and conferences with the Vice Chancellor and his colleagues produced the following Regulations in a report by a further committee that was accepted by a Special General Court on 17 June 1896.

REGULATIONS

I. That permission may be granted to certain persons, approved by the Governors, but not members of the Hospital Staff, to deliver Lectures in Medicine or Surgery in the Board Room of the Hospital, or in some other room approved by the Select Governors.

II. That the Lecturers shall deliver lectures at such times and under such arrangements as may be agreed upon between them and the Medical Staff of the Hospital, with the approval of the Select Governors.

III. That for the illustration of his Lectures the Lecturer may refer to cases among the In-patients or Out-patients of the Hospital, and may show to his pupils in the room assigned for his use such of the In-patients and Out-patients as are able and willing to appear, provided that in each instance the Medical Officer in charge of the case assents thereto.

IV. That the Lecturer may, with the consent of the Medical Officer in charge, examine such of the cases in the wards as he may desire to refer to, but shall not exercise any control over the treatment.

V. That no constraint of any kind shall be put either upon an Out-patient or upon an In-patient, who may be unwilling to submit to the examination of the Lecturer.

If the foregoing Regulations be approved by the Governors, the Committee will propose that permission to deliver Lectures in the Hospital be granted to Professor T. CLIFFORD ALLBUTT and Professor Sir G.M. HUMPHRY.

> J. HAMBLIN SMITH (Chairman)
> P.W. LATHAM, Senior Physician
> E. CARVER, Consulting Surgeon
> T. WARAKER
> W.H. BESANT
> EDMUND H. PARKER
> HUGH PORTER
> J.E.L. WHITEHEAD
> DONALD MACALISTER'

Humphry had been lecturing in the Hospital for years but this was a development for Allbutt who previously had only been allowed to act as a stand-in for MacAlister.

Allbutt seems to have been kept out of Addenbrooke's partly by the medical staff, Latham prominent among them and being credited with saying that Allbutt would only enter the wards over his dead body,[2] and partly by the Governors. 'One cause of the indifferent success of the negotiations was an impression in the minds of many Governors that there are "existing rights" on the part of the Honorary Medical Staff which prevent the Governors from making such an arrangement with the University as they consider desirable for the good of the Hospital. Another cause was the feeling among them that no return is made by the University adequate to the advantages afforded to it by the Hospital.'[14]

However when Latham resigned from the staff in 1899 an arrangement was soon arrived at between the Hospital and the University. Grace 3 of 15 March 1900, confirming a report of the Council of Senate,[15] stated:

> There shall be paid to the Treasurer of the Hospital out of the University Chest, the yearly sum of £300, such payment to continue so long as the provisions hereinafter contained on the part of the Governors are observed, namely:
>
> (i) That the Governors, on the application in writing of the Vice-Chancellor, elect the Regius Professor of Physic to be a Physician, and the Professor of Surgery, if any, to be a Surgeon of the Hospital; such respective Professor to hold office during the tenure of his Professorship.
>
> (ii) That the Governors, on application in writing of such Physician or Surgeon respectively, assign to him a proportionate share of the beds in his

department corresponding to the number of Physicians or Surgeons in such respective department.

(iii) That if either of the said Professors shall not desire to have charge of beds, all proper and reasonable facilities be afforded to him for lecturing either in the Wards or in the Board Room as may be desirable.

(iv) That all proper facilities be provided at the Hospital for conducting the University Examinations in Clinical Medicine and Clinical Surgery, any expenses incurred in the conduct of such Examinations being paid by the University as heretofore.

Neither of the said Professors shall receive any share of the fees paid by the students.

In addition, an advisory council to the Hospital was set up consisting of fifteen governors – five from the Borough, five from the County, and five from the University – all to be elected in General Court, and five to retire each year.[16]

Cole[16] says: 'This small link with the university in teaching and administration was perhaps the most enduring legacy left by George Paget and George Humphry from the nineteenth century but Humphry's hope that Addenbrooke's might become a clinical school for undergraduates persisted.'

Allbutt's path in the Hospital had not run smoothly. In 1901 he reported that he had returned home from a vacation 'Some little time ago' to find that the room for clinical research, in which he regularly lectured, 'had been given up to the Matron without any communication with me and with the formal consent of the Professor of Pathology who had been but just appointed and knew nothing of the needs of clinical research as there carried on nor indeed of any circumstances of the case.' £50 worth of apparatus had been thrown into the street. Since then he had apparently been making do with the Board Room but 'I can have no instruments there as I had before, no pathological specimens either large or microscopic, no blackboard, no diagrams and no continuous investigations.

'Moreover interruptions occur on both sides. I interfere with other users of the room and I am subject myself to interruptions.'[17,18]

A Committee was set up to consider the matter and, although Allbutt did not get his room over the porch back, the Physicians were allotted Paget Ward for a lecture room.[19] Thirteen years later Allbutt was to recount the story at the opening of the John Bonnett Clinical Laboratory[20] and to explain that the old Board looked upon their work in the laboratory as an intrusion of University methods on practical medicine, whereas now, he supposed, there was hardly any large or important hospital without a clinical laboratory.

~ 27 ~

Discontent among the medical staff

The resident medical staff

During the last decade of the nineteenth century the number of applicants for the posts of House Physician and House Surgeon declined, first to ten or twelve, then to three or four. The work was undoubtedly very heavy. Mr Tabbs, appointed House Surgeon in June 1892, lived at Humphry's house whilst the Hospital was closed for the reconstruction of the drainage. In 1894[1] he was granted a year's leave on medical grounds; he died two months later.[2] He was succeeded by Charles Todd who resigned in October and spent the winter abroad also on medical grounds. Only three applications for the post were received.

A committee was set up to consider the appointment of an Assistant House Surgeon.[3] A proposal that an Assistant House Surgeon be appointed with board and lodging but no salary was defeated and the Committee adjourned,[4] but an appointment on these terms was approved by the Governors in June 1896.[5] R.W. Jameson, apparently the only applicant, was appointed. The surgical staff paid the Hospital £25 as a contribution towards the cost of his board and lodging. His principal duties were 'to administer anaesthetics, to keep a register of the surgical cases treated and to assist generally'.

Arthur Burton was one of only four applicants for the post of House Physician in 1895.[6] His health failed and he went to South Africa whence he wrote[7] that although his health had improved 'he did not think that his strength would be equal to the duties of House Physician at Addenbrooke's for several months'. He practised in South Africa and later in Cromer, Norfolk.

The Hospital's financial difficulties were imposing an unusually heavy load on the resident staff. R.E. Delbruck, who was the only candidate for the position of Assistant House Surgeon in January 1898, resigned after two months 'to apply for a better appointment' but he in turn was succeeded in June by Percy William Sargeant[7] (later Sir Percy Sargeant) who held the post until the end of the year.

The surgical appointments continued to attract few applications, but the House Physician's post was more popular. The seven applicants in December 1898 included a woman for the first time. Dr G.S. Haines, later Physician to the Hospital, was appointed.[8] Relations between the resident staff and the Governors were often strained. The Governors rejected a request to pay a locum during holidays although this was normal practice in other hospitals.[9]

In 1901 the recently appointed Advisory Council included in its annual report a memorandum from the honorary staff on the resident staff.[10] The residents were appointed for an indefinite period. The House Physician (H.P.) and the House Surgeon (H.S.) were each paid £65 per annum and the Assistant H.S. nothing; the Honorary Surgeons paid £25 to the Hospital as a contribution to the cost of the latter's board and lodging. For some years the H.P. and H.S. posts were filled by able men who accepted a salary below that paid by comparable hospitals, as they could become members of the University and the hospital work left them sufficient time to read for their examinations. The hospital work had now increased to such an extent that it was impossible to find the time to study for a degree. The Addenbrooke's appointments had therefore ceased to have any special attraction and Addenbrooke's was competing with other provincial hospitals for young men who were in any case in short supply because of the Boer War. It was difficult to fill any of the posts and impossible to fill the Assistant H.S. vacancy.

The staff recommendation was endorsed by the Advisory Council and approved by the General Court. Selection Committees should prefer candidates who were already graduates in medicine and surgery. The H.P. should be elected for one year at £50 per annum. The Senior H.S. should be elected for six months at £50 per annum; the Junior H.S. should be elected for six months at £30 per annum and, if approved, be promoted to the H.S. post at the end of this period.

Appointments were made according to this system for the second half of 1902 onwards. The names and the numbers of unsuccessful candidates were not recorded in 1903 but, in March 1904, there were four applicants for the post of Assistant H.S. P.N. Panton was elected[11] and six months later he was promoted to Senior H.S.[12]

Philip Noel Panton (1877–1950) later became Director of the Bacteriological and Biochemical and Clinical Laboratories at the London Hospital. Some of his comments about Addenbrooke's from his autobiography have already been reported.

The Hospital Minute Book records that Francis Gayner, the House Physician, developed appendicitis in July 1905, but went to London for the proposed operation. In September 1905,[13] the only application for the post of Assistant H.S. was withdrawn. In October 1905, further advertising brought in one applicant[14] who resigned after three months. The salary of the Assistant H.S. was increased to £50 per annum. The medical staff recommended a candidate who declined the appointment.[15] The difficulties experienced in securing resident staff continued and the increase in the salary of the H.P. and H.S. to £65[16] brought about no improvement. However, by 1907 it was at least possible to fill the vacancies. In November of that year it was agreed that resident Medical Officers 'upon their arrival to take up their duties should attend before the Committee and that a charge together with a copy of the Rules and Regulations should be handed to each of them by the Chairman'.[17] The 'charge'[18] was in fact an exhortation . . . 'you are strictly required to be circumspect in your conduct while you remain in the important office to which you have been appointed, and to endeavour (to the utmost of your power) by judicious, considerate and kindly treatment to relieve the suffering of the patients in the Hospital to the greatest possible extent'. Is it reasonable to suggest that the wording of the 'charge' implies a lack of confidence in the resident staff, and reflects on the quality of the applicants?

The posts remained difficult to fill, but the Governors were reluctant to accept the proposal that there should be two House Surgeons of equal standing, each paid £65 per annum, but after there had once again been no applications for the Assistant H.S. post they agreed to this plan but reduced the salary to £60.[19] Two weeks' advertising in the journals brought in only one application for the newly named post in January 1910.[20]

In August 1910, the residents' request that a small reference library be provided was endorsed rather half-heartedly by the medical staff[21] because of 'the facilities there are in Cambridge for consulting books'. The Governors[22] accepted the proposal for a library, but rejected the Finance Committee's recommendation that an annual grant be made towards it.

In November 1910, the overworked residents asked the Governors to increase their salaries to £100 per annum, 'As we hold University degrees we can command higher salaries elsewhere.'[23] On 12 December a further letter from the residents demanded immediate action. Woodham Rogers, the H.P., resigned on 28 December. On the same day the Governors[24] increased the salaries of all three posts to £80 per annum, but the increases would apply only to future residents.

There were usually few or no candidates when appointments were vacant in 1911 and 1912, but on occasions there was a reasonable field: eight applied for the post of Second H.S. in October 1911,[25] five in April 1913, when Charles Budd was appointed House Physician.[26] A year later the only applicant for this post was considered too inexperienced; the post was re-advertised at a salary of £100 per annum;[27] there were only two applicants.

The outbreak of war in August 1914 found the Hospital still struggling with junior staff shortages, a situation further aggravated by the war itself, and which was managed with help from senior staff and medical students.

The visiting medical staff

After the death of Paget in January 1892, Sir Andrew Clark, P.R.C.P., was approached by Dr Alex Hill, Master of Downing College, on behalf of some members of the Medical Faculty, but he declined their invitation to accept the Regius Chair. The Chair was then offered to T.C. Allbutt of Leeds, who, after some hesitation, agreed to accept it.[28]

Since the opening of the Hospital it had been customary to appoint one of its Physicians to the Regius Professorship. Latham undoubtedly expected to be appointed; his undergraduate career had been outstandingly brilliant and his reputation was sound. Donald MacAlister also hoped for the appointment. His wife later wrote:[29] 'It was generally expected that he would succeed Sir George, having been his deputy for so long and having practically been the professor in all but name.' MacAlister accepted his disappointment with dignity; Latham, on the contrary, opposed Allbutt vindictively, and successfully organised the support of the majority of his colleagues in excluding Allbutt from the Hospital. On 5 October 1892,[30] the Weekly Board, on the proposition of the President of Queens' College, appointed a committee 'to confer with the medical staff as to the possibility of associating Dr Allbutt, the Regius Professor of Physic, with the work of the Hospital'. After conferring with the staff, the Committee reported that they could make no satisfactory recommendations.

The refusal of the staff to allow Allbutt charge of beds or out-patients

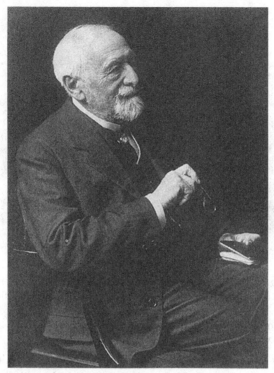

Fig. 34. Sir Clifford Allbutt, Regius Professor of Physic and
Honorary Physician to Addenbrooke's.

had serious consequences for the development of clinical teaching and also
inevitably led to a deterioration of the relations between the University
and the Hospital. It has been stated that Allbutt was totally excluded
from the Hospital until 1900.[31] This is not strictly true. Allbutt acted as
MacAlister's deputy during the latter's summer holidays in 1896 and
1897.[32,33] On the latter occasion Allbutt was referred to as 'Clinical
Lecturer to the Hospital'.

In February 1899, Latham resigned. In a long letter[34] he explained that
he approved of the rule prevailing in all London hospitals providing for
retirement at the age of 65. 'If at that age a physician is actively engaged in
private practice, he requires all his energy successfully to treat his private
patients; if he is without private practice or has only a few patients it is not
right that hospital patients should be under the care of one whose help is
not valued by those who can exercise selection as to their medical
advisers.'

Latham's resignation made possible an agreement between the Univer-

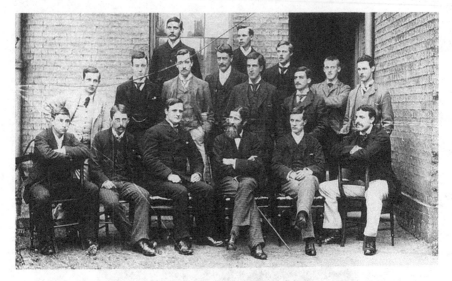

Fig. 35. Hospital group about Sir George Humphry, May 1892.
Reproduced by permission of the Cambridgeshire Collection.

sity and the Hospital[35] and the Governors duly received an application
from the Vice Chancellor which resulted in Allbutt being appointed
Honorary Physician on 23 April 1900.[36] The following day Allbutt wrote
to the Advisory Council. He was, he wrote, already well supplied with
patients for teaching purposes, and he did not propose to ask for the
charge of beds.

On 1 October 1894, Sir George Humphry resigned as Surgeon, an
appointment he had held for 52 years. His services to the Hospital and to
the Medical School had been immense. As a teacher whose lectures and
writings were soundly based in physiology and pathology he had
influenced more than a generation of Cambridge medical students, many
of whom became surgeons of distinction. Unfortunately those of his
former pupils who succeeded him at Cambridge were not of his calibre.
They were slow to accept new concepts: aseptic techniques came late to
Cambridge.

The vacancy on the surgical staff created by Humphry's resignation
was filled by the election of Frederick Deighton[37] who had been Assistant
Surgeon since 1891.

Frederick Deighton (1854–1924), the son of a Cambridge general
practitioner, was a medical graduate of Peterhouse, Cambridge, and of St
George's Hospital, where he held junior appointments in general
surgery, ophthalmology and orthopaedics. He worked also at the Hospi-

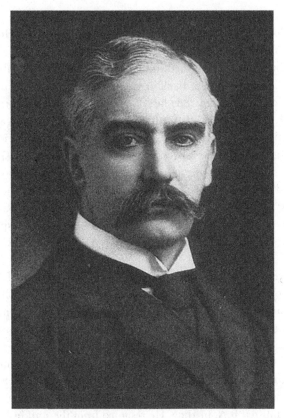

Fig. 36. Frederick Deighton, Honorary Surgeon to Addenbrooke's,
1891–1921.

tal for Diseases of the Throat, Golden Square. In 1883 he returned to
Cambridge to take over the practice of his father who had died in an
accident. He continued in general practice after his election to the
Hospital staff. He established an Ear, Nose and Throat Department, and
on Douty's premature retirement took over the Gynaecological Department and remained in charge of the latter for two years after he retired as
Honorary Surgeon in 1919. His successor as a Surgeon praised his
versatility and his gentle and meticulously careful surgical technique.

The vacancy left by Deighton's promotion in 1894 was filled by the
election of Joseph Griffiths as Assistant Surgeon.[38] Griffiths became full
Surgeon the following year when Carver retired and E.H. Douty was
elected Assistant Surgeon and Surgeon in charge of the Gynaecological
Department.[39]

Edward Douty (1861–1911) was a man of great ability and the loss of his services when pulmonary tuberculosis forced him to resign in 1897 was a serious blow to the development of surgery at Cambridge. He gained first class honours in Part I of the Natural Sciences Tripos in 1884. His father, a schoolmaster, then died suddenly and Douty left Cambridge to look after his family affairs. Back in Cambridge in 1885, he supported himself by coaching. From 1887 he was a Demonstrator of anatomy. He qualified M.R.C.S., L.R.C.P., in 1888 and the following year was House Surgeon at the Middlesex Hospital. He began practice at Cambridge with Hyde Hills in Bridge Street. After tuberculosis ended his professional life at Cambridge he spent some years in a sanatorium and then settled at Cannes, and also had rooms in Paris. He was M.D. Lausanne, 1901, M.D. Paris, 1904, and M.R.C.P. London, 1904. In 1906 he was F.R.C.S. He practised in Cannes where he held appointments to private hospitals. In 1909 he married the daughter of Sir Frederick Wills. He died at Cannes in 1911.

The Governors obviously anticipated that the election of Douty's successor would be keenly contested, for they arranged for a poll, should one be demanded. One was called for and took place on 16 November. All the candidates were local general practitioners and one Hubert Higgins was elected. He had qualified M.R.C.S., L.R.C.P., from St George's Hospital in 1888 and, after holding junior surgical appointments there, had been House Surgeon to Addenbrooke's Hospital from March 1890 to February 1892. In 1890 he had become a member of King's College and had been admitted B.A. in 1893. He resigned from the staff in 1903.

The vacancy for a Physician created by Latham's retirement was filled by the promotion of L. Humphry. At the same meeting of the Governors in March 1899,[40] Lloyd Jones was elected Assistant Physician.

Ernest Lloyd Jones (1862–1942) was born at Bowden, Cheshire, and educated at Manchester Grammar School whence he won a scholarship to Downing College. He qualified M.B., B.Chir. from St Bartholomew's Hospital in 1888 and proceeded M.D. in 1891. In 1894 he was awarded a B.M.A. research scholarship and returned to Cambridge to work as a Demonstrator of pathology under C.S. Roy. He also acted as Clinical Pathologist to the Hospital. He retired as Senior Physician in 1927. He had a gentle, quiet manner and was very successful in practice which he continued until 1940. His wide interests included geology; he was an acknowledged authority on the foraminifora on which he was writing a book at the time of his death.

MacAlister resigned as Physician in March 1902, on account of his

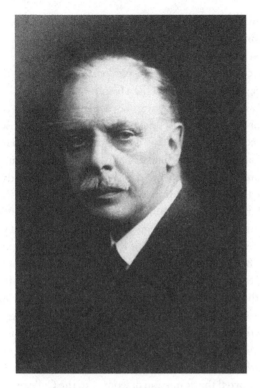

Fig. 37. John Aldren Wright, Pathologist and Addenbrooke's first
Dermatologist. By courtesy of Mrs M.A. Radley.

health, but he hoped he would be allowed to lecture from time to time in
his capacity as Linacre Reader in Physic.[41] The vacancy left by MacAlister's retirement was filled by the unopposed election in June 1902 of J.
Aldren Wright as Assistant Physician.[42]

John Aldren Wright (1865–1942) was born at Halton, Cheshire, and
came to Cambridge as a non-collegiate student, later joining Sidney
Sussex College. He qualified M.B., B.Chir. from St Mary's Hospital in
1894. He was forced by ill health to abandon his ambition to become a
medical missionary and in 1897 he started general practice at Histon. He
qualified M.D. in 1902 and M.R.C.P. in 1911. From 1905 he was
Pathologist to the Hospital as well as Physician; as Pathologist he assisted
the Professor of Pathology to carry out post-mortem examinations.
During the 1914–1918 war he was a Major on the staff of the First Eastern
General Hospital and combined these duties with his work at Addenbrooke's Hospital. After his retirement from the Hospital in 1930 he spent

eight months in a mission hospital in Syria before returning to continue to practice in Cambridge.

The election of Howard Marsh as Professor of Surgery in 1903 was followed, in accordance with the Hospital's agreement with the University, by his election as Surgeon to the Hospital.[43]

Howard Marsh (1839–1915) was born in Norfolk. In 1856 he was apprenticed for two years to his uncle John Marsh of Clerkenwell, and in 1858 he entered St Bartholomew's Hospital as a student. He qualified L.S.A., M.R.C.S., in 1861. He held appointments as House Surgeon at his own hospital and at Great Ormond Street Hospital. His advancement was rapid. In 1866 he was admitted F.R.C.S. In 1868 he was Chloroformist to St Bartholomew's Hospital, where the following year he became Demonstrator of anatomy and Surgical Registrar. In 1868 he was elected Assistant Surgeon to the Hospital for Sick Children, Great Ormond Street, and in 1873 Assistant Surgeon to St Bartholomew's Hospital where he became full Surgeon only in 1891. However he was appointed Surgeon in Charge of the Orthopaedic Department in 1878. He became known particularly for his orthopaedic work. His Hunterian lectures before the Royal College of Surgeons in 1889 were entitled 'Tuberculosis in Some of its Surgical Aspects'. These, and his other writings, show his conservatism in surgical theory and practice. In public affairs he was more liberal and he strongly supported the admission of women to the College of Surgeons.

Since the death of G.M. Humphry in 1896, the Chair of Surgery had been suspended. The Chair was poorly endowed and offered few attractions to a man of the calibre the University would wish to appoint. However, Marsh had examined in Cambridge and felt that there might be an opening there for him, so he let it be known that he would be willing to accept the Chair should it be offered to him.[44] He was fully aware that many colleges were opposed to any clinical teaching for medical students at Cambridge, particularly when this involved students extending their stay at Cambridge for one or two terms, as it had at times under Humphry. Marsh was a popular and tactful man and he accepted the situation, confining his work to organising the examinations and surgery, and to teaching physical signs in the principles of surgery at an elementary level. Marsh moved into 10 Scroope Terrace in December 1903, but for a year or two he retained his rooms in London as he was President of the Metropolitan Branch of the B.M.A., and, until 1908, a member of the Council of the Royal College of Surgeons.

In 1907 Marsh was elected Master of Downing College. He was very active in University affairs until his death. He spoke to the Senate on 21 February 1914, emphasising the University's need for research laboratories, but a recent historian[45] claims that Marsh himself was never able fully to accept the germ theory of disease.

The resignation of Higgins in 1903 was followed by the election of Arthur Cooke as Assistant Surgeon.

Arthur Cooke (1868–1933) was born in Bradford, Yorkshire, the son of a wool merchant, and educated at Giggleswick School and New College, Oxford, where he was a prominent athlete and footballer. He qualified B.M., B.Chir. in 1895 from the London Hospital where he was House Surgeon. He was also Clinical Assistant at Moorfields. In 1895 he moved to Cambridge, joining the general practice of W.W. Wingate. He became F.R.C.S. in 1898. He became full Surgeon to Addenbrooke's Hospital in 1917, and in 1919 also took charge of the Ophthalmic Department. He published little but he was a popular and successful Surgeon.

In March 1905, Professor Bradbury resigned as Physician under the twelve-year rule and offered himself for re-election. He was duly re-elected[46] for a further twelve years, but not without some protest, for he was already in his sixty-fourth year. The General Court rejected an amendment making the election subject to the effect of any future bye-laws. Nevertheless the necessity for a statutory age of retirement was one of two problems which continued to cause the Governors some concern. For some years Bradbury had been taking an annual holiday from 1 July to 30 September, leaving his in-patients in the care of Lloyd Jones. Lloyd Jones eventually found this too much for him and in 1911 was allowed to delegate his out-patient work to Haynes, a general practitioner, who was also an Honorary anaesthetist.[47]

The other problem was the tendency – in consequence of the increasing numbers of patients – for many out-patients to be left to the care of House Physicians and House Surgeons and never seen by the Honorary Staff. Complaints to this effect were received.[48] The House Committee[49] had recently resolved that honorary staff should not call on Resident Medical Officers to act as their deputies, but the General Court[50] conceded that they might do so for short periods in an emergency. The Court agreed also to the appointment of a Clinical Assistant to help with ophthalmic out-patients.

The honorary staff complained in March 1908 that they were dissatisfied with their representation on the General Committee.[51] Continued complaints and a claim that four of the active staff should be ex-officio members[52] led to the appointment, in April 1909,[53] of a Special Committee to confer with the medical staff. The Special Committee's recommendation that honorary medical, surgical and dental staff should have the right to attend meetings of the General Court, but not to vote[54] was declined by the staff.[55]

~28~

The building of the Clinical Laboratory

Although the staff were authorised from 1766 onwards to carry out a post-mortem examination whenever the cause of death was in doubt, no records of early autopsies have survived. Some teaching in pathology was provided by Charles Collignon as part of his annual course of anatomy lectures.[1] From 1819 John Haviland included pathology in his lectures on medicine,[2] and H.J.H. Bond lectured on pathology until 1872. Paget did not continue this course but J.B. Bradbury lectured on pathology every Easter term from 1873 to 1884, when C.S. Roy, the recently appointed Professor of Pathology, took over the teaching in this subject.

It was not until the last decades of the century that techniques of cutting and staining histological sections for microscopy became sufficiently sophisticated to provide reliable information concerning the accuracy of diagnosis.[3,4]

At Addenbrooke's Hospital autopsies were usually carried out by the House Surgeon or House Physician until 1885. After 1888 they were performed by a person nominated by the medical staff and paid £40 per annum, out of students' fees.[5] Under this arrangement autopsies had been carried out successively by Professor Roy, Dr Griffiths, Dr Lloyd Jones, Professor Kanthack and from 1899 by Professor Woodhead, assisted until 1905 by Dr Strangeways and then by Dr Aldren Wright.

Long before it could usefully be applied to histology, the microscope was widely used as a diagnostic tool in what became known as clinical microscopy. Hughes Bennett of Edinburgh in 1841 was the first in Britain to teach the use of the microscope in this way. The range of investigations which could be undertaken gradually increased; the cells of the blood, urinary deposits, ringworm fungi and cells scraped from the cut surfaces of tumours could all be usefully examined by 1880. The chemistry of the blood and urine and other body fluids became of increasing practical importance to the clinician during the second half of the nineteenth century, but even by 1900 the number of investigations available in routine hospital practice was still very limited.

Until about 1880 such bacteriological work as was practicable was still within the capacity of the interested clinician who knew how to use a microscope, but during the 1880s staining and culture techniques were developed and increasingly large numbers of pathogenic organisms were identified. Many physicians and surgeons appreciated the need for special laboratories, but hospital governors seldom considered it to be any part of their business to establish laboratories to investigate disease.[6] By 1878 there was only one London hospital with an efficient clinical laboratory.

The important annual meeting of the British Medical Association at Cambridge in August 1880 aroused great interest in the laboratory investigation of disease and led to the formation in that year of the Cambridge Medical Society, at the early meetings of which this modern approach to medicine was particularly emphasised.[7] G.M. Humphry, the Professor of anatomy from 1866 to 1883, was also a morbid anatomist of some distinction. From 1876 to 1878 his Demonstrator of anatomy was Charles Creighton (1847–1927), a pathologist by inclination and training, who continued to work in Cambridge for three years after his demonstratorship terminated, and who was incidentally the first Secretary of the Cambridge Medical Society. It seems justifiable to assume that such clinical pathology as was carried out was at first based on the Department of Anatomy.

The Chair of Pathology was established in 1883 and Charles Smart Roy (1854–1897) was elected the first Professor in 1884. Roy, who was essentially an experimental pathologist, was single-handed until 1886 when Joseph Griffiths, later to be so closely associated with the Hospital, came to Cambridge as his assistant. Griffiths resigned the following year and a demonstratorship of pathology was established and was held first by Almroth Wright, then from December 1887 to April 1888 by H.D. Rolleston, and from May 1888 to October 1890 by J.G. Adami. During these early years the Department of Pathology occupied rooms in Fawcett's building. Those working in the Department included Charles Sherrington, J. Graham Brown, E. Lloyd Jones and William Hunter. In 1888 the Department moved to the Jacksonian Laboratory, vacated by the Department of Chemistry. In 1892 Roy suffered a nervous breakdown and Alfredo Antunes Kanthack (1863–1898) began to act as his deputy, unofficially at first, but officially from 1895. When Roy died in 1897 Kanthack was elected his successor.

Kanthack helped the Hospital staff set up and maintain a small clinical laboratory in the room which later became the Matron's sitting room.[5]

After Kanthack's premature death in 1898 the laboratory facilities available to the Hospital declined until Allbutt and Humphry jointly provided £100 per annum for three years to establish a service. Graham Smith helped to provide this, and it was only when his increased University teaching commitments prevented him from continuing it that the Governors began to accept the need, but not their obligation to pay, for the service.

In December 1902,[8] the Advisory Council received a letter from Humphry informing them that Graham Smith had been appointed 'Clinical Pathologist to the Staff' for 1903; 'this is only an extension of what has already been done to facilitate the pathological work of the Hospital'.

In their report to the Governors on 6 April 1908, the medical staff recommended the appointment of an Honorary Consulting Pathologist with general supervisory responsibilities, of a Pathologist to undertake post-mortem examinations, and of a Clinical Pathologist 'to undertake the examination of material taken from the patients in the wards'. All remunerations were to be paid from students' fees; the service was therefore to be paid for by the medical staff, between whom these fees would otherwise have been divided. The Governors failure to appreciate the importance of pathology is well illustrated by their referral of this report to the House Sub-Committee, which deferred a decision because the report recommended that the porter should attend post-mortem examinations, but did not state how much of the porter's time should be so occupied.

Four months later the Governors,[9] rather grudgingly, accepted the report, insisting that Clause 6 (chemicals and utensils required by the pathologist in the interests of the patients should be provided by the Dispensary) be accepted for one year only in the first instance. In August[10] the Governors accepted these staff nominations: Honorary Consulting Pathologist, Professor Sims Woodhead; Pathologist, Dr Aldren Wright; and Clinical Pathologist, Dr W. Malden.

German Sims Woodhead (1855–1921), an Edinburgh graduate, had worked in Vienna and Berlin and then returned to Edinburgh as assistant to W.S. Greenfield. He was one of the pioneers of bacteriology in Britain and took a particular interest in tuberculosis. In 1890 he went to London as first Director of the Clinical Laboratories organised jointly by the Royal Colleges of Physicians and Surgeons. He succeeded Kanthack as Professor of Pathology at Cambridge in 1899. He organised the Depart-

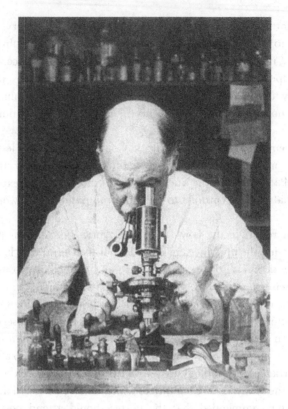

Fig. 38. Walter Malden (1858–1918). First Clinical Pathologist.

ment of Pathology in the new Medical School opened in 1904. In association with Varrier Jones he organised the Tuberculosis Colony at Bourn and later at Papworth.

John Aldren Wright (1865–1942) graduated M.B., B.Chir. in 1894 from Sidney Sussex College, Cambridge, and St Mary's Hospital. He soon entered general practice at Histon, and was in 1902 elected Assistant Physician, and in 1908 also Pathologist to Addenbrooke's Hospital. He was the first Physician to take a clinic exclusively for dermatological patients.

Walter Malden (1858–1918) also was a Cambridge graduate and was M.B. from Trinity College and St Bartholomew's Hospital in 1886. He practised in Kent for some years before returning to Cambridge in 1903 to practise in Lensfield Road and to undertake some research. He began to work as a Demonstrator for Woodhead. After his appointment as Clinical Pathologist to the Hospital in 1908 he continued in practice. He also founded and edited the 'Medical World', which became the organ of the Medico-Political Union. From 1915 to 1918 he was Chairman of the *Cambridge Chronicle*.

The pathology services for the Hospital organised in 1908 remained more or less unchanged until 1914. All obituaries of Malden refer to the charm of his personality. He used this charm to good effect in persuading Mrs Bonnett, mother of John Bonnett who had been Secretary to the Hospital for many years, to offer to build, equip and endow a Clinical Laboratory. In June 1912,[11] the Governors accepted her offer.

The medical staff had all signed a report explaining why they considered clinical pathology so important. The Clinical Pathologist should be highly trained and should give the greater part of his time to the work. 'In most hospitals provision is made for this important work by the governors of the hospital.' 'Owing to lack of Hospital funds the staff have for years endeavoured to supply the deficiency by their own contributions. For about 25 years they have paid £40 per annum to a pathologist. Some 12 years ago they built and equipped at a cost of £400 a laboratory in connection with the post mortem room and supplied a small honorarium of £30 a year to the Clinical Pathologist.' These arrangements, they said, had been quite inadequate. Moreover, they relied on assistance obtained 'in a fortuitous and more or less casual way' through the kindness of the Professor of Pathology and those working in his department. 'The Clinical Pathologist at present occupies a room at the Pharmacological Department, which at any time he may have to vacate.'

The attitude of the Governors towards pathology changed now that they were to have this service provided at no cost to the Hospital funds. Mrs Bonnett offered £3,000 to build and equip the Laboratory, £350 per annum for maintenance during her lifetime, and an endowment to provide a similar sum after her death. Mrs Bonnett's solicitor proposed that a Board of Managers of the John Bonnett Memorial Fund be appointed, to have control over the income and expenditure and general management of the Laboratory. The Pathologist's salary would be £250 per annum. The appointment was to be vested in a committee consisting of three managers and three members of the Hospital staff. The building should be in the hands of the Hospital Building Committee, but the plans must be approved by the Managers and by Mrs Bonnett.

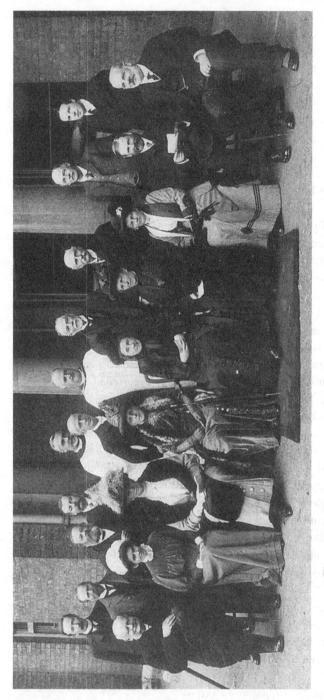

Fig. 39. The Laying of the John Bonnett Memorial Stone by Mrs Bonnett on 28 April 1913.

The Governors deferred further discussion, but asked the Chairman to inform Mrs Bonnett's solicitors that the terms of this draft scheme were not in agreement with the general scheme for the management of the Hospital.[12] The Governors felt that the control of the Laboratory and of the Fund should be in their hands. On the other hand Mrs Bonnett, on the advice of Dr Malden, wanted to ensure 'that the management of the Laboratory was in the hands of persons with sufficient technical knowledge'.[13] After further discussion it was agreed that separate accounts should be kept for the Laboratory and that an Advisory Sub-Committee should be appointed.

Plans for the new building in which Mrs Bonnett had been persuaded to include a mortuary and a chapel, to be maintained by the general Hospital funds, were approved by her, by Sims Woodhead and by the Governors.[14] The tender of Rattee and Kett was accepted.[15] After some hesitation Mrs Bonnett agreed to lay the foundation stone at a private ceremony in April 1913 (Fig. 39).

Meanwhile the Governors had, on 14 October, elected a Clinical Laboratory Sub-Committee consisting of two lay members of the General Committee, two members of the medical staff, the Regius Professor of Physic and the Professor of Pathology.[16]

In December 1913, Dr Malden was appointed Clinical Pathologist.[17] The Sub-Committee drew up regulations on his duties and responsibilities, and their recommendations were approved, with minor amendments, by the Governors.[18] The Clinical Pathologist was to be Director of the Laboratory, responsible to the Sub-Committee. He was to attend every weekday from 10.30 a.m. to 1.00 p.m. and to supply a locum if he was absent. He was 'to keep a register in which he should enter his report on each specimen, with the time at which it was received and the time at which the report was ready'. An abstract of this register was to be kept by the Secretary-Superintendent for the information of the General Committee. The Clinical Pathologist was to be allowed to carry out his own investigations in the Laboratory 'provided they be not allowed to interfere with the work of the Hospital and provided he keep an account of any material used'.

The Laboratory was opened on Friday 13 February, by Sir Clifford Allbutt in the presence of a large company of medical representatives of University, Town and County, who had been entertained to luncheon at Downing College by Mrs Bonnett. A reporter for a local newspaper was given a conducted tour a few days before the ceremony and was clearly impressed and had described in great detail what he saw: 'as fine and completely equipped a laboratory for this enormously increasing branch of work as can be found anywhere'.[19] The architect was Mr Pick of Liston. The mortuary chapel had been beautifully designed by a Miss Falcon. Mrs Bonnett, as a woman, could not be present at the luncheon but Dr Malden replied to the toast to the memory of John Bonnett on her behalf.

~ 29 ~

The founding of the Cambridge and District Workers' Hospital Fund

The Committee on the Administration and Finances of the Hospital presented a 20-page report to the General Court on 1 January 1900, but discussion was deferred to the adjourned court held at the Guildhall on 22 January. This Court expressed its general approval of the report and proceeded to discuss its recommendations.

The Committee could make only one recommendation which might reduce expenditure. This was that all tenders should be advertised for and be open. They noted that the patients' diet had improved in recent years but this was an economy as it tended to shorten the average stay in Hospital. They noted also that Addenbrooke's was the only teaching hospital not paying its probationers.

They found that some 15% of in-patients were from outside the County and for this and other reasons suggested that an organised system of collections was essential. This could be achieved only with the services of a Superintendent. Their second recommendation therefore was to appoint a Superintendent to be responsible for all hospital affairs except those within the spheres of the Hospital staff or the Matron. His main task would be to organise the collection of funds and to help the Treasurer. They thought that 'the services of a competent retired naval or military officer could probably be obtained for about £150 a year'. Peckover, the Lord Lieutenant, who was unable to attend the Court, had promised to give £400 to cover the Superintendent's salary for two years.

The Court then discussed the financial implications of the relationship between the University and the Hospital. The medical staff had agreed to relinquish to the Hospital 25% of the money they received from the students if the Hospital would enter into certain arrangements with the University. A proposal had been suggested.

The medical staff was in approval with this provided that the Hospital staff could be readjusted as vacancies occurred, so that there should ultimately be: two Physicians and two Surgeons in charge of beds in the adult wards, and two Assistant Physicians and two Assistant Surgeons in charge of the out-patients and the children's wards; and, when practicable, an Ophthalmic Surgeon and a Gynaecologist.

They suggested that:

1 The next vacancy for a Physician be not filled but a second Assistant Physician be appointed instead.
2 The next vacancy but one for a Physician be not filled by a new appointment unless the Regius Professor of Physic did not desire to undertake the charge of beds.
3/4 Similar arrangements for the surgical side.

The Committee recommended that this memorandum from the medical staff be referred to them for further consideration.

The Committee then reported their conclusions on the vital question of an alteration to an executive committee. Almost every hospital in the country had such a committee but under the George III Act it was *extra vires* for Addenbrooke's. The nearest approach to an executive committee would be an Advisory Council which could make recommendations on all matters outside the province of the Select Governors. The Council should, they thought, take on the duties of the Finance Committee. 'They should also examine the testimonials of candidates for vacancies on the honorary staff and to report to the Governors which candidate or candidates they considered best qualified to fill the appointment.' The Council should meet at least once a quarter. It should have fifteen members representing equally Town, County and University.

These were the most important recommendations in the report.

All the recommendations were approved. The Committee was asked to consider including a member of the honorary staff on the Advisory Council. This they unanimously declined to do.[1] The Quarterly Court on 19 March approved the Committee's more detailed recommendations.

Members of the Advisory Council were to be elected by the Governors in General Court, having previously been nominated by those Governors in the interests they were to represent. One fifth of the Governors should retire annually on the last Monday in October.

At any meeting of the Council with reference to a vacancy on the honorary staff, nine members should form a quorum but in all other cases a quorum should be seven. The Council should summon a Special

General Court when vacancies occurred not only on the honorary staff but also in the posts of House Physician and House Surgeon, Dispenser, Secretary, Superintendent and Matron.

The recommendations in the original report relating to the Medical School were accepted including the medical staff's recommendation. A significant paragraph was added to allow the Governors to replace any Professor in charge of beds 'who has become disqualified for such charge by age, ill health or other serious impediment' – a necessary precaution at a time when there was no compulsory age of retirement for professors.

The Advisory Council* took over the responsibilities[3] of the former Finance Committee. In September the so-called Uniform System of Accounts was introduced. In December[4] they noted expenditure had exceeded ordinary income by £1,086. The principal increase in expenditure had been on patients, but the number of in-patients had been 117 more than in the previous year. In September 1901, the Hospital appointed professional accountants (Messrs Blackburn & Co. of Bradford) for the first time, as auditors at ten guineas per annum.[5]

In December 1902,[6] the death of E.J. Mortlock was reported. He had been Treasurer since 1859. Until the appointment of a Superintendent, he had himself kept the books. He had often allowed interest-free overdrafts from his bank. E.H. Parker was elected his successor.[7]

Parker had immediately to consider the Advisory Council's report on the finances of the Hospital. The deficiency of the past year was £2,112.12s.9d.[8] In the past such deficiencies had been made good by bequests and donations. The Council did not advise containing the Hospital's work but felt that appeals should be addressed to a wider circle, coinciding more closely with the area served, which extended well beyond the County. Although attempts were made to reduce expenditure, by Michaelmas 1903, the General Account was £3,450 overdrawn. Fortunately the Treasurer had just received a legacy of £5,263 under the will of Mrs Pyne of Royston.

However, the inadequacy of the income was a continuing problem. A new appeal was planned but further discussion of it was postponed[9] until the new Secretary had taken up his appointment. The Finance Committee warned the Governors the following April[10] that, if economies were not made, the number of beds must be reduced. The total number of occupied beds must never be allowed to exceed 148.

* In 1903 they and the Weekly Board were replaced by a General Committee re-constituted under Act of Parliament.[2]

This warning was heeded and it was reported in November 1905[11] that expenditure in the past quarter had been reduced by about £1,000 compared with the corresponding quarter the previous year. Unfortunately the income for the quarter had fallen by £300.

In an attempt to encourage legacies it was agreed that the executors of a will bringing the Hospital £100 or more might be appointed as Honorary Governors.[12] The appeal which had for so long been under discussion was launched in November 1905. 'An Urgent Appeal for additional income of £2,500' was printed and was circulated widely. Leading articles appeared in *The Times* and *The Standard*.

In October 1906,[13] a committee was formed to be called 'Addenbrooke's League of Mercy' to organise the collection of subscriptions in co-operation with the existing organisations. The Committee was influential and represented Town, County and University, and its members also included the President and Vice President of the County Organisation Fund and the Addenbrooke's Ladies Auxillary Association. Addenbrooke's League of Mercy soon received a letter of protest from the League of Mercy in London and changed its name.

A public meeting at the Guildhall on 20 October was addressed by Sidney Holland, Sir Robert Ball, Mr T.F. Rawlinson, K.C., M.P., and Mr S.O. Buckmaster, K.C., M.P., and Mr Spalding. The resolutions put to the meeting were:

1 That this meeting recognises the urgent necessity for largely increased support of the Hospital and pledges itself to endeavour to obtain it.

2 That a representative committee be appointed to give effect to the foregoing resolution, with power to add to its members.

Promises received at the meeting ('cards filled in') amounted to:
£190.15s.0d. in donations
£54.12s.0d. in new subscriptions
£65.0s.0d. increased subscriptions
but advertising and printing costs had amounted to £54.9s.7d.

The appeal did not achieve its aims (by the end of 1908 it had brought in £1,560 most of which consisted of donations and only a small proportion of which consisted of subscriptions). In December 1907[14] a Special Committee was appointed to consider the financial position. This Committee, like its predecessors, carefully reviewed the Hospital's expenditure but made no radical proposals. They wondered whether the Hospital was not doing work which fell within the province of the Education Authority. They suggested that a Special Committee would co-ordinate fund raising.[15] To help in this work a lady typist was engaged at 14s. per week, 'paid from a private source'.

In April 1910, Lord Peckover gave two cheques for £500, one for the upkeep of the Peckover Buildings and the operating theatre, and one for the Convalescent Home. There was no significant improvement in the financial position and a special sub-committee was appointed the following month[16] to confer with the medical staff 'on the several pressing needs of the Hospital'.

Cambridge and District Workers' Hospital Fund

In June 1910 was founded the organisation which was to give Adden-brooke's Hospital regular financial support for a number of years. The principles of the Fund were that members paid their small subscriptions to a representative in each place of work (factory, shop or office). The Secretary of the Fund was E.J. Papworth, an employee of the Great Northern Railway Company. The Chairman was W.J. Dyball, employed by Matthew, a grocer of Trinity Street.

In July 1910, the Secretary and the Treasurer and four committee members were received by the Governors[17] as they wished to ask that the Hospital's medicines and dressings charge of 3d. should be omitted for the regularly subscribing members. This was eventually agreed.[18] The Fund already received contributions from employees of 54 Cambridge firms and expected to collect £500 in its first year. In fact the collection amounted to £622. During the next year £629 was collected of which £477 was paid to the Hospital. Small sums were paid to the nurses' homes and the Surgical Aid Society. The Fund collected over £1,000 for the first time in 1921.

King Edward VII Memorial Fund

In August 1910,[19] Mr Spalding, the Mayor, proposed that a memorial to Edward VII should take the form of 'substantial assistance towards the establishment of a children's ward and the provision of a new Out-patients' Department.' This proposal was adopted[20] and the appeal was launched. By April it had proved so successful that the appeal was closed, having raised about £11,000. The Hospital also had available the Harris Norman Bequest of £4,960, and £3,000 collected by the Ladies Committee. It was estimated that the children's ward and the Out-patient Department would cost between £14,000 and £20,000.

~ 30 ~

Patients before the First World War

The treatment of tuberculosis

Tuberculosis was extremely common in nineteenth-century Britain. Its growth was favoured by poverty and overcrowded living conditions. In 1865 the infectivity of the disease was proved by Jean-Antoine Villemin who inoculated it in animals. The Tubercle bacillus was discovered by Robert Koch in 1885. Treatment had traditionally been by close confinement in conditions which can only have hastened its progression. Many of the great clinical observers of the eighteenth and nineteenth centuries became aware of the therapeutic benefit of fresh air. George Boddington (1799–1882) opened the first open air sanatorium, at Sutton Coldfield in 1840. Gradually the importance of rest and fresh air was generally recognised. Early in the present century Local Authorities in Britain began to set up free dispensaries for the diagnosis of tuberculosis, and sanatoria for its treatment.

In May 1900,[1] the possibility of converting the colonnade for the open air treatment of tuberculosis was discussed. Mrs Maud Peart's offer to pay the entire cost of the conversion of the colonnade outside Griffith Ward was accepted.[2] Mr Sedley Taylor paid for the similar conversion of the colonnade outside Hatton Ward. The open air treatment gave results 'which exceeded all expectations'.

In 1910 the Medical Officer of Health prepared a memorandum on the possible anti-tuberculosis scheme and the General Committee agreed to meet the Borough Public Health Committee to discuss it,[3] but the meeting was abandoned when the medical staff reported they considered it inadvisable to admit cases of advanced phthisis.[4]

Lloyd George's National Insurance Act made particular provision for the treatment of tuberculosis and the Public Health (Prevention and Treatment of Diseases) Act, 1913, inaugurated the effective development of the tuberculosis services.

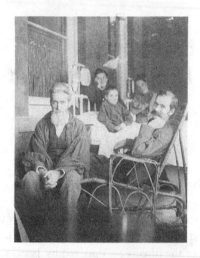

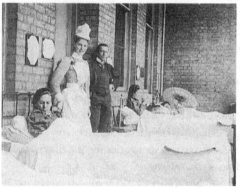

Fig. 40. Griffith Ward (top) and Hatton Ward (bottom)
Colonnades being used as open air wards, 1900. By courtesy of the
late Dr G.S. Haynes.

In February 1914, Dr Moss-Blundell, Medical Officer of Health for
Huntingdonshire, asked if the Hospital would provide beds for patients
with tuberculosis. The medical staff submitted their proposals to the
General Committee.[5] They recommended admitting suitable cases at 2
guineas weekly. Cases considered suitable were: cases of a doubtful nature
for observation and diagnosis; cases requiring immediate treatment on
account of complications; up to two male and two female early cases for
treatment on the colonnade; and a limited number of cases of surgical
tuberculosis. This report was referred to a special meeting of the General
Committee.

Meanwhile Cambridgeshire County Council had approached the Hospital asking if part of the Out-patient Department might be used at certain times as a T.B. Dispensary and if some beds could be used for cases under observation. A special committee considered their request and recommended that the County Council should be granted the facilities they required, including four beds in the general wards of the hospital, if the medical staff would give their assurance that the reception of tuberculous patients 'would not endanger the well-being of ordinary patients'. The medical staff gave this assurance.

Payments for medicine and dressings

In June 1902,[6] the Advisory Council considered introducing a charge for medicine and dressings. Since 1898 the London hospitals had charged 3d. per dressing and 3d. for a two weeks' supply of medicine. Guy's Hospital had had no difficulties in operating the same system since 1883. School children and the really poor were not charged. During the past seven years the average number of out-patients seen at Addenbrooke's Hospital had been 5,211 (excluding dental patients). The expenditure on out-patient medicine and dressings in the year ending 30 September 1901 was in excess of £1,000. The London Hospital system would bring in at Addenbrooke's about £250 per annum. The Advisory Council recommended that it should be introduced.

The next Quarterly Court[7] modified these proposals and agreed that out-patients should be charged 3d. per visit for medicine and dressings, and not 3d. per item. Notices were prepared for the Out-patient Department.[8] Tickets had to be purchased on arrival and later given to the Dispenser for medicines or to the Sister for dressings. The money collected had to be carefully accounted for and the Matron had to report regularly to the Weekly Board. Later the collection of dressings' money was entrusted to the House Surgeon.[9] The Matron was requested to send to the charity organisations the names of patients who claimed that they could not afford to pay. By 27 December,[10] that is to say, after about eight weeks, the charge had brought in only £12.8s.3d. and collecting it had proved particularly difficult.

The British Medical Association (B.M.A.) Hospitals' Committee organised a conference in 1906 to discuss 'abuses which are generally considered to exist in the administration of medical charities'. Names of patients about whose ability to pay there was some doubt, were referred to the local Secretary of the Charity Organisation Society. The latter wrote to the House Sub-Committee in April 1907,[11] pointing out that the great increase in the number of out-patients unable to pay was the result of the efforts of school nurses and health visitors. The medical inspection of school children became mandatory under the Education Act, 1907.

It was the growing problem of assessing patients' ability to pay which led the medical staff to recommend the appointment of an almoner.[12] Mrs Keynes, the Secretary of the Cambridge Branch of the Charity Organisation Society, would be willing to provide a trained almoner if the Hospital would contribute £25–£30 per annum. The number of school children referred to hospital continued to increase and the Governors arranged to discuss the problem with Education Authorities.[13] In November 1910,[14] numbers were still rising but no almoner had been appointed.

The Royal Surgical Aid Society wrote in 1914 to ask the Hospital whether there was a need for a Cambridge branch. After much discussion Mrs Keynes of the Charity Organisation Society (C.O.S.) offered to deal with all those cases needing appliances. Eventually[15] a Cambridge City Surgical Aid Society was set up under C.O.S. auspices.

Paying patients

The occasional admission of paying patients had been accepted for some years, but only in cases in which urgent treatment was required and could not otherwise be obtained. It is a tribute to the improvement in the Hospital's facilities and the advances in treatment that requests for admission became increasingly common in the early years of the present century.

In 1904[16] the General Committee resolved that, before more paying patients were admitted, a Sub-Committee should discuss the situation with the medical staff. Some patients, such as the wife of a chemist's manager whom Aldren Wright wanted to admit,[17] were too prosperous to be admitted as ordinary patients but could not afford nursing home charges. This lady was admitted for a charge of 15s. a week. It prompted the General Committee to ask the Bye-laws Committee to provide rules for the admission of paying patients. Bonnett thought: 'the question of receiving paying patients bristles with difficulties'.[18] Allbutt's views, expressed in a card to the General Committee, were very different: 'I don't know why we make difficulties about taking in paying patients.'[19]

Registration

The question of keeping a register of all patients was discussed in 1906 and a sub-committee was set up to consider the Secretary's report on a visit he had recently made to Birmingham Hospital, and the broader problems of out-patient administration. The General Committee adopted the majority of the Sub-Committee's recommendations.[20] The principle of registering casualties and out-patients by the Secretary or his deputy was agreed. A book with a removable case was substituted for the paper which the patient had previously retained during his period of treatment and the book containing the records should be kept in the Hospital under lock and key, with the patient only receiving a card. Those recommendations which were not accepted are revealing: one of them stated 'That as the male patients who attend are generally out of work and women patients frequently have housework to do, women and babies should as a rule be seen first.'

~ 31 ~

The reorganisation of the nurses

On 3 September 1901, the Select Governors considered the 31 applications for the post of Matron. Four candidates were called for interview
the following week. Miss Margaret Morgan, who obtained eleven votes,
was appointed. It is interesting that the runner-up, who obtained five
votes, was Alicia Lloyd Still, later to become Matron of St Thomas'
Hospital and a leading figure in British nursing.

Miss Morgan lost little time in making her presence felt. She recommended various improvements in the housekeeping arrangements, which
were accepted.[1] The suggestion that additional probationers be taken on
was also approved[2] but she was obliged to report in April 1902[3] that she
had been unable to fill the vacancies and that the nursing staff, far from
increasing from 36 to 40, had fallen to 34, although she had accepted every
candidate. She was authorised[4] to engage three additional nurses from
amongst the probationers completing their training and to pay them £20
per annum and to accept two probationers without premium.

The atmosphere in the Hospital in the early years of the century seems
not to have been a happy one. There was, for example, a feud between the
Matron and the House Surgeon, whom she claimed was undermining her
authority. A committee was unable to substantiate her complaints[5] and
no action was taken.

The unsatisfactory state of the working conditions of the nursing staff
was brought to the notice of the Governors in June 1902[6] in a letter from
W.M. Fawcett but, before action could be taken on his suggestion that a
committee be appointed to investigate the problem, the Superintendent
told the Governors[7] that he had been requested 'on behalf of a considerable number of the nursing staff' to inform them of the strong feeling of
dissatisfaction and unhappiness among the nurses and to ask for an
enquiry. The following day[8] the nurses' complaints were heard, but they
were not recorded in the Minutes. The Governors met yet again on 4 July[9]
and resolved that the Matron be requested to draw up rules for the

nursing staff and submit them to the Governors. They recommended that she should, if possible, be provided with an office.

A committee consisting of Miss Hargood, the Revd A.C. Allen, and the Revd C.W.A. Brooke, was appointed to confer with the Sisters. The next Weekly Meeting on 9 July set up another committee, of which also Mr Allen and Miss Hargood were members, to interview the Matron. Both committees were appointed[10] to consider the question of an office for the Matron and to consider the rules applicable to the nursing staff.

By the end of August[11] 'Regulations for the Guidance of Sisters' was received by the Governors. These regulations were finally approved the following week;[12] they give a very clear picture of the life of a Sister and little indication that the regulations had any purpose other than to tighten the discipline. The hours of work remained exceedingly onerous; her only hours off duty were from 2.30 to 5.30, or from 5.30 to 8.30 daily, and 'whenever possible' a half day a week and alternate Sundays. It seems that conditions for nurses of all grades were unusually harsh at Addenbrooke's at that time.

In March 1903, the Matron reported that difficulty in obtaining probationers was increasing. She received many applications for entry forms but so few entries that she was unable 'to weed out those who are unsuitable'. This problem was referred to the Select Governors and the Medical Officers.[13] The Matron had been compelled to fill the gaps owing to the shortage of probationers by engaging nurses from the Home for Nurses in Fitzwillian Street (see Appendix 1) at a greatly increased cost to the Hospital.

By the end of April[14] six such nurses were being employed at £25 per annum each. On 14 May, the Select Governors and the Medical Officers held the first of a series of meetings at which the probationer problem was discussed at length. The Matron had ascertained that Addenbrooke's was the only hospital paying no salary to nurses in training and expecting them to provide their own uniforms. They considered[15] the shortage of probationers was due to the failure to modernise the system of training introduced many years before. The grievances of the Sisters they found to have resulted from actions the Matron had been obliged to take because of the shortage of nurses. Of the six probationers who had left, none had done so for reasons 'connected to the management of the nursing department'.

The Governors at the Quarterly Court[16] accepted this rather reassuring report and approved a recommendation that the existing system of payment of a premium should be continued.

During the next year the reorganisation of probationer training was actively discussed. In May 1904, the Probationers' Committee agreed its report which was then adopted by the General Court.[17] The 'New System' involved taking fifteen probationers in August or September each year. They would pay a premium and take a three-year course. In the first and second years they would 'acquire the art of nursing and obtain an elementary knowledge of medicine and surgery through systematic lectures'. In the third year, they would 'occupy positions of responsibility under the supervision of the sisters'. The practical details of operating this scheme would be in the hands of the Education of Nurses Committee, consisting of the honorary medical staff and the Matron.

On 15 August 1904, Miss Morgan resigned as Matron.[18] Her reasons for doing so were not recorded. She had had to face a great deal of criticism, but the parsimony of the Governors, in particular their reluctance to abandon the premiums for probationers, had presented her with staffing problems which were probably insoluble, and all the charges against her, including that of ordering probationers in charge of infectious cases to take on other work as well, seemed to have been unwise decisions forced on her by severe staff shortages.

The General Committee took the opportunity of redefining the Matron's duties.[19] She was to be between 30 and 45 years of age and was to retire at 60. She was to be assisted by a working housekeeper responsible to her.

There were 58 applications for the post of Matron. Miss Susan M. Adams of the David Lewis Hospital, Liverpool, was appointed.[20]

Early in April 1905, Miss Adams was found dead at Oakington, some three hours after she had left the Hospital for a Sunday morning cycle ride. Her three months as Matron cannot have been easy. She had had to face the continued complaints of the Governors at the large number of extra Staff Nurses employed. The new system of probationer training had brought more applicants but these were still in their first year. Moreover she had opposed the General Committee's plan to appoint a housekeeper. She offered to do the housekeeping herself with a Miss Spencer as her assistant.[21] Miss Spencer was also Theatre Sister and Home Sister. Despite these differences of opinion the General Committee was able to write to her family[22] 'in a short time . . . She had won in a remarkable degree the esteem and confidence of the staff'.

Alice Blomfield of the East End Mothers' Home was elected Matron on 1 May 1905.[23] Understandably she was very soon asked to report on the present nursing arrangements and give her suggestions for future staffing.[24] She thought the present staff just adequate for the routine work of the Hospital, but it did not allow for such contingencies as holidays and sick leave. She asked for seven Sisters (at present six), thirteen Staff Nurses as at present, and 27 probationers (at present 25). She said that this level of staffing had been introduced at other hospitals in 1896. Such an increase would require additional accommodation and therefore capital expenditure, the prospect of which was particularly unwelcome at a time when the question of probationers' premiums, still an important source of income, was again under discussion:[25] most provincial hospitals had abolished them and some even paid salaries.

The Sub-Committee finally agreed to abolish premiums and to pay a salary of £5 for the first year, £12 (later reduced to £10) for the second, and £15 for the third year, and to supply the materials for uniform dresses and caps. Candidates for the normal three-year training were to be between 24 and 33 years of age. Any candidate above or below these ages or who did not bind herself for the full three-year course would be required to pay a fee.[26] It was agreed also that the number of probationers should be increased to 27.

The accommodation problem was partially solved by the fact that the leases of three houses in Addenbrooke's Place were due to expire.

The General Committee on 6 November, resolved that the new nursing scheme should come into force on 1 January 1906. To this scheme, as outlined above, two further recommendations had been added as a result of the Secretary's visit to Birmingham General Hospital: the appointment of a housekeeper who was a trained nurse, and the appointment of a Theatre Sister capable of undertaking massage work and who could act as Assistant Matron.[27]

The many recommendations accepted during the reorganisation of the nursing arrangements were incorporated in new Standing Orders for Probationers.[28] Their timetable was still rigorous: Breakfast 6.30 a.m., Wards 7.00 a.m., Dinner 1.30 p.m. or 2.15 p.m., Wards 2.00 p.m. or 2.45 p.m., Tea 5.00 p.m. or 5.30 p.m., Prayers and Supper 8.30 p.m., Bed 10.30 p.m. The General Rules applicable to probationers contain few surprises but Rule 7 forbade nurses to go out with members of the University without special permission from the Matron. Curiously there is no mention of any similar restriction on going out with other men.

The new scheme was introduced on 1 January 1906, according to plan, and was immediately successful in attracting applications from intending probationers. During the second half of January and the first week of February, 200 applications were received.[29]

In 1906 Miss Macintyre of Glasgow was appointed the first Sister in Charge of Out-patients' and Massage.[30] The Out-patient Department had always been treated from the nursing point of view as an appendage of Bowtell Ward.

Despite the new schemes and the undoubted competance of Miss Blomfield as Matron, all was not well with the nursing at Addenbrooke's and, in December 1907, the House Committee set up a special committee 'to look into the question of nursing'.[31] The members were Mrs Austin Leigh, Mrs Finch, Mrs Mansfield, and Mrs Peart. This Nursing Committee prepared a report which was referred to the medical staff for their comments. They replied that they were 'dissatisfied with the general nursing arrangements throughout the Hospital'.[32] The reasons for their dissatisfaction are not clear.

Miss Blomfield resigned in March 1908, to take up her appointment as Matron of Queen Charlotte's Hospital, and she later wrote to the General Committee complaining that she had not received their support.[33]

The emphasis of the report of the Special Committee on the nursing was on more precise definitions of spheres of responsibility. Miss Spencer, Assistant Matron and Housekeeper, resigned on 13 April,[34] two weeks before the Report on Nursing was presented to the General Committee. The malaise that had affected nursing at Addenbrooke's for so long appears to have resulted from divided responsibilities, conflicts over seniority and clashes of personality.

The principal recommendations of the Special Committee were as follows:

> The Matron shall be responsible to the General Committee for 1. The Nursing. 2. The Housekeeping. 3. The Laundry. The Matron shall be assisted by (a) Nursing Sisters, and (b) a Sister Housekeeper. The Nursing Sisters shall be responsible under the supervision of the Matron for the nursing in the wards under their charge respectively. The Sister Housekeeper shall be responsible, under the supervision of the Matron, for the kitchen and provisions departments, for the female domestic servants and for the laundry. (Sister Housekeeper need not be a certified nurse.)
>
> The Sister Housekeeper shall take seniority with the Nursing Sisters according to the date of their appointments.

These and other recommendations were approved.

On 28 May 1908, Miss Mary Gertrude Montgomery of St Thomas'

Hospital was elected Matron. There were 43 applicants. Miss Montgomery was a forceful personality and must be given much credit for the improvement in nursing affairs during the next few years, though the new structure of nursing administration probably played its part.

By January 1909, there were 42 probationers. In May 1909,[35] Miss Lloyd Still, Matron of the Brompton Hospital was invited to become the first external nursing examiner. Later that year Miss Montgomery was appointed Principal Matron of the East Anglian Division of the Territorial Army Nursing Service.[36] In October 1911, the Hospital agreed to supply the War Office with six nurses should war break out.[37]

The Minutes have little to record on nursing matters during Miss Montgomery's term of office, other than appointments; nurses trained at Addenbrooke's were now securing senior appointments in important hospitals throughout the country. Unfortunately for Addenbrooke's Miss Montgomery resigned in July 1913, as she had been appointed Lady Superintendent of the Middlesex Hospital.[38] She had been Matron for five years. The members of the General Committee presented her with a Welsh dresser.

The building of the new Out-patient Department

The decade preceding the outbreak of the First World War was notable for administrative reforms but there was little structural change.

In 1906 telephones were installed throughout the Hospital at a cost of £168.14s.0d. which was paid by Mr Sedley Taylor.[1]

In 1911 a Building Committee was appointed.[2] Several different schemes were proposed. The most urgent need was for extensions to the Out-patient Department and the construction of a children's ward; it had at one time been thought to build them together in a new building called the 'Victoria Memorial Wing'[3] but over the years the schemes had separated. Also required were new boilers and a new boiler house, a new electric lift, improved sanitary arrangements for the wards, and more accommodation for the nurses.

The plans were discussed in May 1912, at a Special Meeting of the General Committee[4] attended by Mr S. Perkins Pick, F.R.I.B.A. The Hospital had available more than £18,000: £13,102 in the Memorial Fund, £3,000 raised by the Ladies Guild and £2,000 from the Norman bequest. The new Out-patient Department was to be built at right angles to the main building in the south west corner of the grounds, taking in the sites of two houses in Trumpington Street to which the main entrance could open. The children's ward would be built on top of the existing building. Colonel Harding, the Chairman of the Building Committee, suggested that it might be wise to defer the building of the Out-patient Department for a year as the National Insurance Act might reduce the contributions of the Workers' Hospital Fund and might also affect the number of out-patients. He reminded the Governors that the extra accommodation would increase the maintenance costs by £1,400 per annum. The plans were approved but it was decided to delay for a year the construction of the Out-patient Department, although the Memorial Fund had been raised primarily for this purpose.

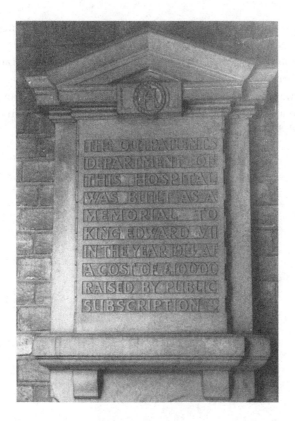

Fig. 41. Memorial plaque on the Out-patient Department.

In June 1912, as has already been mentioned, Mrs Bonnett offered to erect, equip and endow a Clinical Laboratory in memory of her son.[5] Work was quickly put in hand.

The other building schemes were making less satisfactory progress.[6] It was decided to go ahead with rather less ambitious children's wards and a new boiler house and the ward sanitary annexes on the North West side of the Hospital.

The General Quarterly Court[7] in May 1913 authorised the General Committee to spend from the General Funds what was necessary to build the new Out-patient Department. The General Committee on 21 April 1913 approved the Building Committee's plan for a new Out-patient Department at £3,000. Colonel Harding's motion that only the X-ray Room be built was carried by seven votes to four, although some

Governors considered the existing departments 'a source of danger'. The General Committee with the support of the Finance Committee overruled this decision and ordered the House Committee to sign the contract before 1 December.[8]

There was much wrangling in the Finance and Building Committees at the outbreak of war that the work on the Out-patient Department was continued, but the Department came into use in June 1915.

Two World Wars

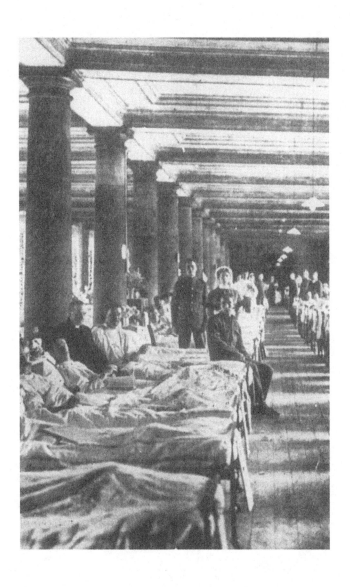

~ 33 ~

The First World War

The outbreak of war in August 1914 found many of the medical staff already committed to serve on the staff of the First Eastern General Hospital and some of the nursing staff were consigned to this Hospital or to other nursing units. Addenbrooke's Hospital provided many of the members of the staff of the First Eastern General Hospital and the two hospitals were closely associated throughout the war.

An extraordinary situation had been allowed to develop and on 17 August the House Sub-Committee heard that the entire medical staff had been mobilised. An immediate appeal to the War Office brought the answer that the Commanding Officer (C.O.) of the Eastern General Hospital had discretionary powers, and indeed Griffiths, Senior Surgeon to Addenbrooke's, and C.O. of the Eastern General Hospital, played a large part in maintaining the medical staffing of both institutions throughout the war.

When Haldane, in 1907, in his army reforms, replaced the old Volunteers by the Territorials, Keogh, the Director General of Medical Services, reorganised the Medical Services of the Auxiliary Forces. Keogh held a meeting at Downing College and soon afterwards Cambridge was selected as one of the Units which would constitute the First Eastern General Hospital.[1]

There had been two Units with the old Volunteer Force at Cambridge. There was the Cambridge University Rifles Volunteer Corps (4th Battalion, Suffolk Regiment), of which Griffiths and Roderick, both members of the staff of Addenbrooke's Hospital, were the Medical Officers, and there was the 3rd Volunteer Battalion of the Suffolk Regiment, of which Apthorp-Webb, a successful Cambridge general practitioner, was Medical Officer. Griffiths was appointed Colonel in Command of the new General Hospital and Apthorp-Webb was appointed Registrar. Roderick was placed in command of the medical section of the Cambridge University Officers' Training Corps which was instituted as a section of a Field Ambulance for the training of cadets.

From 1908 Griffiths began to enlist men for the staff of the Hospital and

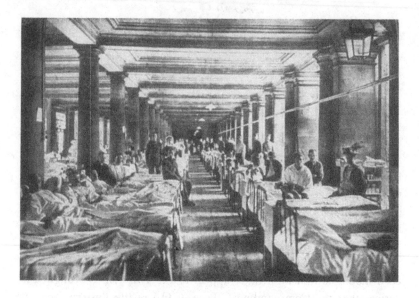

Fig. 42. Beds of the First Eastern General Hospital in Trinity
College Cloisters. Photo by J. Palmer Clarke. Reproduced by
permission of the Cambridgeshire Collection.

the Unit was soon complete, even to its complement of buglers. Each year
the Unit went for summer training to camps at Colchester, Netley or
Shorncliffe. Winter training included lectures on anatomy and physiology by the Commanding Officer and on First Aid by the Registrar.

Mobilisation orders were received by the Unit on 5 August 1914, only a
few days after their return from camp at Shorncliffe and on the same day
quarters were found in the New Museums. The men were billeted in part
of the old Physiology Laboratory, then being renovated for Dr F.G.
Hopkins.[2] The offices of the Unit were located in the Drawing Office of the
Engineering Laboratory, but the Headquarters was soon transferred to
the south west corner of New Court, Trinity College. The first beds were
made available in the Leys School on 14 August, and on 20 August
Deighton carried out the first operation there.

During the few weeks that the Unit occupied the buildings at the Leys
School 171 patients were admitted. The patients were then transferred to
Neville's Court, Trinity College, which had been equipped as an open air
hospital of 250 beds. The first casualties from France were admitted on 31
August.

The accommodation in Neville's Court was gradually increased and wooden floors were laid because the paving stones of the cloisters were uneven. Food for patients and staff was prepared in the Judge's Kitchen in the Master's Lodge. Tents for orderlies were erected on the lawns to the south of the Wren Library. As further beds were required 250 more were provided in a marquee in the paddocks beyond the river.

The original intention to use school premises for beds[3] was rejected in favour of open air hospitals and, in September 1914, a contract was signed for the construction of temporary buildings on the cricket grounds of Clare College and King's College, to the south of Burrell's Walk, and within a year there was a small hutted town with a total bed complement, including Neville's Court, of over 1,500.

At the outbreak of war many medical students joined the Forces. Those who remained at Cambridge were enlisted in the Medical Unit of the Officer's Training Corps[4] and attended lectures on First Aid, ambulance work and hygiene. Some, after ward experience in London hospitals, went to Red Cross hospitals as dressers, others joined the Royal Army Medical Corps (R.A.M.C.) as orderlies but were soon sent back to their medical studies. Some became 'Probationary Surgeons' in small naval vessels. The open air hospital in Cambridge employed as dressers students who had passed their 2nd M.B. examination on anatomy and physiology; they wore R.A.M.C. officers' uniforms without badges of rank.

In October 1915, the Hospital contained a record number of 1528 beds.[5] In March 1916, the *Gazette* published some interesting statistics. Since 16 August 1914, 21 201 patients had been admitted, including 10 502 men and six officers of the Expeditionary Force, 10 043 men and 106 officers of the Home Forces, and 351 Belgians. During the month of February 1916 alone, there had been 1042 admissions.

During May and June 1916, Dr Malden, the Editor of the *Gazette*, complained of the lack of material which was perhaps due to the continuing pressure of work at the Hospital. A visit by the King was recorded in August the same year and by Rudyard Kipling in November. The Hospital continued its war duties until 1920.

Meanwhile the affairs of Addenbrooke's Hospital and those of the Eastern General Hospital had continued to be very closely linked. As early as 17 August 1914, Addenbrooke's had offered the War Office 60 beds for wounded soldiers.[6] In May 1915, Colonel Griffiths, with the approval of the Governors, commandeered Albert and Griffiths Wards; the War Office would pay 4s. per head per day and would provide beds and bedding. These wards were regarded as an extension of the Eastern

General Hospital. In October 1915, Bowtell Ward also was taken over by the Eastern General Hospital, bringing the total of military beds to 100.[7]

In September 1916,[8] the War Office asked the Hospital to make two or three beds available for paraplegics, who, 'knowing they have a comparatively short time to live, have a very strong desire to return as near as is practicable to their own home localities'. Griffiths, at the request of the House Sub-Committee, made available one bed in each of the three military wards.

The treatment of war pensioners at Government expense was to make important contributions to the financial support of the Hospital after the War. The first request to admit such patients was made in June 1917, by the Huntingdon Local Committee under the Naval and Military War Pensioners Act. It was agreed that pensioners would be accepted at 4s. per day. In July[9] it was agreed with the Bedfordshire Local Committee to accept their pensioners on the same terms, and at 6d. a day for ordinary out-patients or 1s.8d. per day as out-patients with electrical treatment and massage.

In March 1918,[10] the Governors agreed, on the request of the War Office, that 25 of the military beds should be used for pensioners. The Governors insisted however that payment should be made at the top rate of 7s. per day because the Hospital had an X-Ray Department, a Bacteriological Laboratory and also provided massage. After some correspondence the Ministry and the Local Committees all agreed to pay this top rate.

After the end of the war, the Governors were anxious to have the military beds withdrawn ward by ward or entirely, and not one or two at a time. In January, 1919, the average daily number of unoccupied military beds was 20. Griffiths was asked to fill the beds or to release them.[11] When the last soldiers were withdrawn on 3 March 1919, it was recorded that 2,885 had been admitted since May 1915. Under the arrangements with the War Pensions' Committee another ward with 36 beds was set aside for discharged soldiers.

~ 34 ~

Building after the Great War

The new Out-patient Department, which was built onto and superceded the old Out-patient Department, came into use in June 1915. The old Out-patient Department was converted into a modern Pharmacy and Surgical Dressings Stores, while the old Pharmacy became Recovery Rooms for the Out-patient Operating Theatre.[1]

At about the same period, 1913–1915, work was completed on two more of the hospital's long-needed improvement schemes: the children's wards and the boiler house.

The childrens' wards were a problem because of the associated drains.[2,3] A number of schemes had been considered and eventually a 25-bed ward was erected in the North Wing, on the third floor over Albert Ward, together with new sanitary annexes. It was completed just after the outbreak of the 1914–1918 war. Both annexes on the same side were also remodelled.[1] During the Great War this 'new' ward at the top of the hospital was to become known as Tipperary, from the words of the popular song that the soldiers marched forth to, because it was a 'long, long way' for the soldier patients to go.[4]

An electric lift was also installed about this period,[5] paid for by two of the Hospital's benefactors, Mrs Almeric Paget, who contributed £750, and Lord Peckover (especially known for donating towards the Peckover Nurses' Home in 1895), who contributed £250. The Hospital already had a hand-powered balanced lift, 6 feet long by 4 feet wide; it had been installed in the well of the northerly main staircase as part of the repairs paid for by the compensation for the 1902 fire; outside staircases at each end of the hospital were put in at the same time.[6]

The only item on the list of building requirements reported by the Committee in 1911[7] that had not yet been at least partially dealt with now was additional accommodation for nurses. The cost of adding a storey to the Nurses' Home had been considered in 1913[8] and postponed at the time as being too expensive. It had been considered again in 1919[9] when an extension was estimated at £7,750 and it was decided that the money in hand from the Geldart Trust Fund would cover it.

However, the Joint Demobilisation Board of the British Red Cross Society and St John's Ambulance Association gave the hospital a cheque for £3,500 in 1920[10] with the provision that it should be used only for building purposes. The next month a further £1,000 was received from the County Red Cross Society and in August it was learned that the hospital was to get £6,000 from the War Memorial Committee[11] – it had asked for £20,000.[12]

The Red Cross started to press for contracts to be completed on the building work that was to be carried out with its £3,500 and threatened to withdraw the money if they were not.[13] They were eventually sent details[14] of the new £15,000–£16,000 Nurses' Home, part of a £26,000 scheme drawn up by the architect Mr T.H. Lyon of Corpus Christi, which covered increased accommodation for nurses and new accommodation for domestic staff.[15] That part of the scheme involving the Nurses' Home was to be proceeded with. It was to be a new building providing 50 bedrooms, sitting rooms, a class room and writing room, and was to absorb the old Nurses' Home 'consisting mainly of cubicles and now occupied by some half dozen nurses and a large proportion of the domestic staff'.

The Secretary of the County War Memorial Fund was also sent details of the new Nurses' Home[16] as being the building to be erected with the Fund's £6,000.

A tender of £11,694 from Messrs Saint was accepted in May 1923[17] and, although the work was interrupted in August 1924 by the strike of building workers, the new block was completed that year.

With the completion of the Nurses' Home the General Committee turned its attention to the provision of a Servants' Home.

In 1922[18] numbers 12–14 Fitzwilliam Street had been purchased from Peterhouse for £3,000 from the Geldart Bequest. Numbers 13 and 14 were soon scheduled to be demolished to make way for the £10,000 Servants' Home in Mr Lyon's scheme. The Hospital was not able to proceed however until it gained possession of these houses, one of which was occupied by a tenant under the Rent Restriction Act, and a further seventeen years' lease on the other being held by the Cambridge Nursing Association.

By October 1924,[19] the Hospital had obtained possession of the properties required and, in April 1925,[20] work on the Servants' Home was approved, although by this time the Home was to be a conversion of numbers 13 and 14 Fitzwilliam Street, instead of a completely new building, and to cost only £1,250. There was to be accommodation for 34.

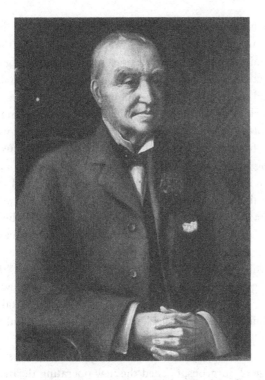

Fig. 43. T. Musgrave Francis, Chairman of the Central
Committee, 1923–1931.

In 1919[21] improvements to the operating theatre were said to be one of
the needs of the Hospital, and in 1922[22] the medical staff had reported
that the theatre accommodation was obsolete and totally inadequate, and
had suggested that two new theatres should be built on the top floor above
the present theatre which could then be used only for septic cases.

Work on the two new operating theatres was part of a tender for
£14,514 from Messrs Henry Martin Ltd, accepted by the General
Quarterly Court in 1926.[23] It was said at this time that the builders,
although ready to start work, had been prevented from doing so by the
General Strike. However, by May 1927[24] the work was well in hand. The
Chairman at this meeting received authority for the space previously
occupied by the theatre on the second floor to be used, with Mary and
Turton Wards, to provide three 8-bed wards for Maternity cases. This
work was to cost £2,600.

Although there was at this time a wave of public opinion in favour of
building a maternity home, and a special sub-committee had been
appointed to look into the possibility of providing premises, these

maternity beds were for hospital cases. In August 1927,[25] at the General Quarterly Court, Mr T. Musgrave Francis, Chairman of the General Committee, said: 'However desirable preventive medicine might be it was not the object for which the hospital was founded . . .' and 'curative treatment had the first claim on the committee'.

A new block to go in the front of the Hospital was planned, and a photograph of a sketch of it appeared in the local paper.[26] It was to be in line with the front of the Out-patient Department, connected with the main building by a corridor. On the ground floor were to be a new board room, lecture room, general offices and porter's lodge, and on the first floor two wards for children. It was thought the 'children would enjoy being near the street and that passersby would enjoy seeing the children'.

It was to be part of a £37,400 scheme which also included a new ward over Victoria (eventually built and completed in 1930 as Musgrave Ward) and which would add a further 82 beds to the hospital (the current number being 190) and practically 'do away with the waiting list altogether'. A year later[27] however, no action had been taken as the wisdom of building a new block in front of the Hospital had been questioned.

On 1 June 1928, Sir Berkeley Moynihan of Leeds, the President of the Royal College of Surgeons, opened the new operating theatres and the Maternity Wards. In his speech[28] he said that the future of medicine was 'with the general practitioners, because surgery had reached near to its goal'.

The operating theatres were built partly with the balance of funds from an old building fund, and partly from some realised investments. The same building scheme included sanitary annexes to the South Wards postponed in 1914 because of the War and some improvements to the kitchen and Victoria Ward.

Meanwhile ambitious plans to enlarge the Hospital had been taking shape and neighbouring properties purchased as they came on the market. Between 1921 and 1926 the Hospital had purchased numbers 5, 9, 10, 12–14 and rented number 17 Fitzwilliam Street. It had also bought numbers 28 and 29 Trumpington Street.[29] In June 1928 Lady Darwin proposed to the General Committee, 'That before further alterations and additions are made to the Hospital, this Committee consider the question of the removal of the Hospital to a relatively inexpensive site with room for further expansion.'[30] Her motion was defeated by fifteen votes to six but before many more years had passed she was shown to be the most forward-thinking member of the Committee.

In 1928[31] the General Committee received a letter from the staff reminding them of the urgent need for more female surgical beds, and in October of that year tenders for a new ward on the third floor over Victoria were invited[32] and one for £6,696 from Messrs Coulson was accepted a few months later.[33] The work was completed in 1930 at a final cost of £6,273.[34] It was a surgical ward for women, contained 27 beds, and was called Musgrave after Mr T. Musgrave Francis, Chairman of the Hospital General Committee[35] since 1923. The building of Musgrave Ward corrected the balance of the Hospital which had looked rather lopsided since Tipperary was built.

The pressure on the funds and on the limited space remained heavy and schemes intended to make the best use of both were put forward in quick succession, the priority varying. Wards for paying patients, a new children's ward, new septic wards, an enlarged X-Ray Department and accommodation for Massage, Dental and Artificial Sunlight Departments were all required. An appeal for £90,000 for the extension of the Hospital was launched and between 1929 and 1934 raised £86,000;[36] the cost of certain of the extensions and improvements to the Hospital carried out during this period were defrayed from this fund. (The appeal was closed after a handsome legacy of nearly £32,000 was received from Mrs E.A. Goode.)

Extensions to the Peckover Nurses' Home were approved and built in 1930 for £11,998. This made 59 bedrooms for nurses, together with a sitting room for Sisters and quarters for the Matron, compared with only 39 bedrooms for nurses when the Home was first built.[36]

Two years later[37] it was agreed to enlarge the Servants' Home at 13 and 14 Fitzwilliam Street by the erection of a four-storey block, to include 23 new bedrooms, 3 bathrooms and a dining room at the Tennis Court Road end of the hospital.[38] It was completed in 1933 and the cost, inclusive of furnishing, was £6,610.

Further building in 1933 raised a third storey to Nurses' Home no. 2, giving accommodation for 22 more nurses.[36] This meant that both the nurses' homes now had four floors. In addition, an office for the Maintenance Fund was erected in the grounds of the Hospital with direct entrance from Trumpington Street.

Meanwhile, in 1931, minor changes which gave the Hospital its long familiar facade were approved[39] at an estimated cost of £750 from the general funds. The front was remodelled by taking in the balcony portion on each side of the main entrance door to provide an almoner's room, telephone room, porter's dining room and staff room. In the same year the

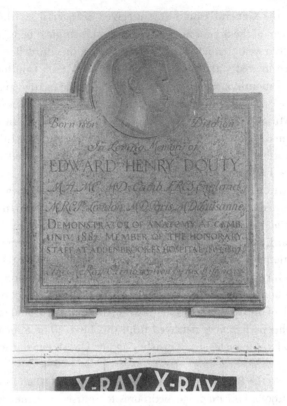

Fig. 44. Memorial plaque to Dr Douty.

Hospital had received an anonymous gift of £6,000 to enlarge the X-Ray Department.[40] A new X-Ray Department at the back of the building right against Tennis Court Road had originally been part of the £90,000 enlargement scheme but it was not considered ideal as it should have been nearer the Out-patient Department. With the extra funds, however, an entirely isolated wing could be devoted to radiology to the south of the Out-patient Department.

The new 23-room clinic took a year to construct and was named after Dr Edward H. Douty, 1861–1911, a Surgeon on the honorary staff between 1895 and 1897. All previous X-Ray work had been carried out in one room. The anonymous donor was his Wills tobacco heiress wife.

The block designed in 1927 for the front of the Hospital, but which did not materialise, had a Lecture Room, Board Room and offices planned for the ground floor. These were eventually obtained by a conversion of

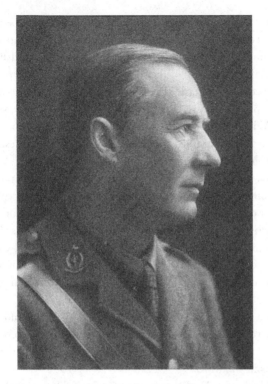

Fig. 45. Arthur Cooke (1868–1933), Surgeon to Addenbrooke's
1903–1933, Surgeon in charge of Ophthalmic Department
1919–1933.

Bowtell Ward,[41] while the old Board Room, Lecture Room and Matron's
bedroom were converted into eye wards.

The eye wards, which were on the first floor of the hospital, contained
thirteen beds, and were opened in June 1932 by Mrs Arthur Cooke, wife of
the Honorary Surgeon in charge. They consisted of three wards, each
fitted with specially dark blinds, and had their own up-to-date operating
theatre.[42] Previously in-patients had had to go in the ordinary wards
'which could not be darkened because of the large number of other
patients'.

The night after the opening, ten patients were to be admitted for
operations. Mr Cooke said that they had lost less than 1% of eyes operated
on since the development, during the last few years, by Dr Whittle, of a
culture test 'to see that the eye was free of germs'. Before the test they had
lost 9% of eyes operated on.

Meanwhile two new blocks had been planned and were being built.

The first, comprised of children's wards on the ground floor and accommodation for paying patients on the first and second floors, was approved for the north side of the Hospital, at right angles to the main building, at a cost of £27,342.[43] It was opened by the Duke and Duchess of York in July 1932, in the presence of guards of honour of the Boys Brigade, Voluntary Aid Detachments, smartly attired Sisters and nurses, and a cheering crowd of thousands.[44] The band of the Cambridgeshire Regiment played the National Anthem.

Thirty beds were available in the private wards, six in the men's ward, six in the women's and eighteen in single rooms. They were for those whose income did not exceed £350 per annum for single persons, or £500 p.a. for a married couple, and another £50 on top of these was allowed for each dependant. The maintenance charge, including drugs, was 10s.6d. per day in a ward or 12s. per day in a single room, and professional fees for medical and surgical treatment were reduced to one-third of those usually charged.

The private wards do not seem to have been in such demand as the eye wards and X-ray clinic because when they were visited by a reporter from the local newspaper a week after first admitting patients there were only eight patients in the wards.[45]

A Septic Block with X-ray, massage, dentistry, ultraviolet light, male and female septic and other wards, and accommodation for the resident Medical Officers had been provisionally approved in 1929 at an estimated £31,000 in place of the isolation block and a neighbouring block between it and the Hospital which were to be pulled down.[46] Later, however, this plan was modified to utilise part of the old building and a tender from John Brignell of Newmarket Road for £22,690.10s. was accepted.[47]

On the ground floor there was improved accommodation for the Dental Department, an up-to-date Orthopaedic Department, rooms for massage and light treatment, a linen sewing room, stationery store and Chaplain's room; on each of the first and second floors there was a main 'septic' ward with 18 beds (including four single observation wards) and a five-bed venereal disease ward; and on the third floor there were eight bedrooms for resident medical staff, a sitting room, bathrooms, etc.[48]

After this new south east block was opened in February 1934, the first floor women's ward was named Goode Ward after Mr and Mrs J.M. Goode,[49] and the small ward was named Thackeray after the former Honorary Physician. The second floor men's ward was named Bowtell in place of the former ward on the ground floor of the main building, and the

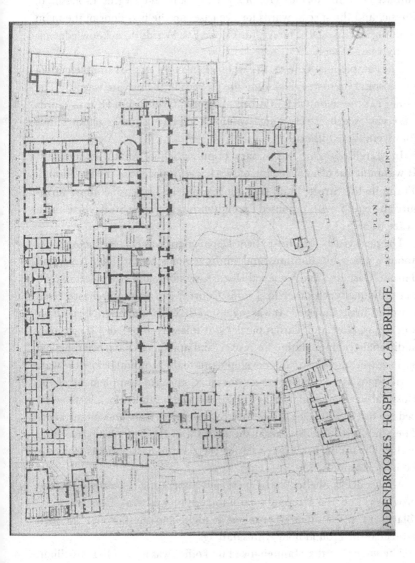

ADDENBROOKES HOSPITAL · CAMBRIDGE · SCALE 16 FEET = AN INCH

PLAN

Fig. 46. Photograph of a tracing of a plan of Addenbrooke's
Hospital, *c*.1934.

small ward was named Paget after the former Honorary Physician and Regius Professor of Physic.

An observation ward on the third floor of the main building was called Allbutt after the former Honorary Physician and Regius Professor of Physic, and the special wards for eye cases on the first floor of the main building were called 'The Arthur Cooke Eye Wards' to acknowledge his many years of service.[50]

The completion of the south east block brought the bed complement of the hospital up to 312, including the 30 beds in the private wards.[36] The same year the colonnades of Albert, Victoria, Griffith and Hatton Wards were enclosed by steel-framed windows, replacing the venetian blinds that were there hitherto.[51]

In March 1935, the Preliminary Training School for Nurses opened.[51] It was built out of a conversion of two houses adjacent to the Hospital in Trumpington Street,[52] and cost approximately £2,500 including furniture and equipment. It housed the eight probationers, a Staff Nurse and a Sister tutor.[53]

The next year[54] the Out-patient Department was enlarged at a cost of about £3,000 by additions and improvements to the Ear, Nose and Throat, Casualty, and Venereal Diseases sections, and two pieces of land that adjoined each other in Tennis Court Road were purchased from Corpus Christi College.[55] It was suggested that this land might be used for a new Ear, Nose and Throat block[56] but this was costed at £15,500 plus additional accommodation for nurses, and appears to have been shelved as there were no other major developments to the Hospital before the war.

In 1939, as a war emergency measure, the bed complement of the Hospital was increased from 316 to 364 and responsibility for a further 100 beds to be placed in the University Examination Halls was undertaken. These additional beds were at the disposal of the Emergency Hospital Service for use in Air Raids and for the reception of patients from the London Hospitals.[57]

An Air Raid Shelter and Emergency Operating Theatre were also provided, and the Hospital's radium supply was sunk in a borehole. 'Black-out' precautions were taken at night and the Borough Council protected the ground floor with sandbags.

The same year the Maintenance Fund office was moved to Fitzwilliam House and its former premises were used by the Council as a First Aid Post. The General Committee asked to be relieved of financial obligations with regard to the Home of Recovery at Hunstanton as it was thought this would not be used for the duration of the War.

The following year, 1940, surface air raid shelters for the staff were provided and a Cleansing Unit was erected in front of the Hospital to clean gas-contaminated casualties before admission.[58] Also, heat storage cookers were installed in the main kitchen of the hospital to provide alternative facilities should the public utility services be disrupted by air raids.

The University Examination Halls were opened up as an annexe of 101 beds on 17 June, and were in continuous use in addition to the main Hospital's 364 beds. The Leys School was taken over on 1 October with a view to being administered as an additional annexe of 375 beds, and the appropriate alterations and adaptations were carried out. It was opened in 1941[59] and at the end of the year there were 358 beds in commission at Addenbrooke's, 100 at the University Examination Halls, and 348 at the Leys.

In June 1941, a Fracture Department (Grade A) as laid down in a Ministry of Health Scheme, was set up at the Leys School and more than 100 beds there used for patients requiring orthopaedic and fracture treatment. An Out-patient and X-Ray Department were later to be established in connection with it.

A Massage Department was opened at the Leys too and some of Addenbrooke's out-patients received their treatment here, which relieved the congestion at the main hospital.

The Leys School also took over the functions of Griffith Ward, and the ward of 30 beds vacated in the Hospital was to be reserved as a resuscitation unit for air raid casualties and other severely injured patients.

In February 1942,[60] the total number of beds in use became 811, the Leys School now having 353.

The General Committee began to worry about the accommodation for in-patients and ancillary departments when the war ended and the annexes returned to their pre-war uses. However, the Ministry of Health, together with the Nuffield Provincial Hospitals Trust, had begun a survey of hospital services in the country in order to form a post-war hospital policy.

In 1944 an architect was asked to submit a scheme for the post-war utilisation of existing hospital sites and also of a possible new site in Tennis Court Road.[61] Steps were taken to purchase numbers 21 and 22 Trumpington Street to allow for the extension of the Medical Out-patient Department,[62] and to obtain possession of the gardens of numbers 4–8 and 17 Trumpington Street so that huts could be built to accommodate patients after the closure of the Leys School.[63] The air raid shelter adjoining the covered way to the Nurses' Home was to be converted for offices, and additions were planned to the John Bonnett Clinical Laboratory.

Two conferences with Ministry of Health officials[64] were held regarding alternative accommodation for the Hospital when the Leys School annexe was handed back to the school authorities, planned for 8 November 1945,[65] and the use of part of the American Hospital at Wimpole Park was discussed but turned down by the County Council and Hospital representatives as impractical. The possibility of using the County Hospital in Mill Road was explored. Meanwhile the 100 beds in the Examination Halls were still available.

Several requirements were to be put before the Ministry for urgent attention.

1 A hut for the Radio Therapeutic Centre was needed on the Addenbrooke's site and it would not be possible to remove the Centre from the Leys until such a hut had been provided.

2 The conversion of three houses in Trumpington Street (28, 29 and (sic) 20) into nurses' quarters was planned.

3 It was proposed to convert the Decontamination Unit into an Out-patient Department for the fracture clinic, and to convert rooms over the garages next to Kellet Lodge for the purposes of the Occupational Therapy Department.

4 An additional floor to the Pathological Laboratories, and a new ward of 22 beds on top of the private wing, were planned.

5 Additional accommodation for out-patients and clerical staff were required.

6 Unless learning that permanent buildings would be erected within the next year or two, the Hospital would have to press for temporary huts for the accommodation of patients, nurses, kitchen and dining room.

The General Purposes Committee also decided to ask the University to allow the Hospital the use of the Examination Halls for as long as possible, and agreed that there was need for additional accommodation for the Preliminary Training School. The Chairman was requested to approach Mrs Pemberton about the possible use of the Trumpington Hall Red Cross Hospital as a Convalescent Home.

After consulting members of the honorary staff the General Purposes

Committee then came to the conclusion that as a short-term policy the County Hospital should be asked to take over the abnormal maternity work at present dealt with at Addenbrooke's.[66]

The next month the Ministry of Health promised to provide a prefabricated hut for a Radio Therapeutic Centre,[67] and to consider making Owlstone Croft at Newnham available for the accommodation of nurses. The Matron reported the premises 'would be admirably suited for adaptation as a Preliminary Training School and would also house 25–30 Nurses when the Leys School closes', and the purchase of Owlstone Croft was eventually agreed for £12,500.[68]

The Leys reverted back to school use as planned in November 1945.[69] While it had been an Addenbrooke's annexe, 19,922 in-patients had been treated there and 3,312 evacuees had been housed. The Examination Halls were handed back the following year, on 28 February 1946, when Addenbrooke's bed complement was reduced from a wartime peak of 811 down to 357. Its pre-war complement had been 316; the increase had been made by crowding extra beds into the wards.

In March 1946, it was decided to approach the Ministry of Health for authority to proceed with the addition of the further storey to the Pathological Laboratories and the adaptation of 27, 28 and 29 Trumpington Street[70] for the accommodation of the resident medical staff, dietician-housekeepers and lady cooks.

On 21 January 1947, a meeting of the Joint Advisory Committee of the University and the Hospital heard that the population of Addenbrooke's catchment area was 339,000 and the area could provide 4,000 beds for all purposes but the number of first class beds was limited and there was urgent need for more. There was no room on the established sites except for the extensions already planned and it was proposed and unanimously agreed that a new site be developed to meet the needs of the Medical School, the teaching hospital and hospital services. It was thought 1500 beds might be required.

Various possible sites on the Pemberton Estate were discussed and later negotiations for the purchase of one at Trumpington were begun,[71] the Ministry was to be asked for consent to the purchase. Work on the existing hospital site would amount to £175,000–£200,000, it was said. The architects for the work on both the sites had been chosen.

In November[72] the Ministry agreed in principle to the purchase of the new site of about 60 acres and the Hospital was asked to draw up a scheme of minimum requirements for the current hospital.

~ 35 ~

The Addenbrooke's Hospital Maintenance Fund

In 1912 and 1913 annual expenditure exceeded income[1] but the balance was adjusted and after the outbreak of war in 1914 the position was again reasonably satisfactory. However, the war brought difficulties and there were[2] increasing costs of commodities including drugs and cleaning materials and an increased consumption of fuel to stoke the new heating and hot water system. Expenditure, and behind it income, rose steadily.

The trend continued and the Hospital's reserves began to fall. By July of 1928[3] it had been decided that the present method of maintaining the Hospital must be improved. A report of the Hospital's four contributing bodies, the Workers' Hospital Fund, the Friendly Societies Council, the County Organisation and the Auxiliary Fund, was reviewed and the General Committee agreed to set up a Special Committee consisting of four independent members of the General Committee and representatives of each contributing body to look for the best approach.

A few months later, in November,[4] it was suggested to the General Committee that the only practical means of raising the income of the Hospital was to set up a contributory scheme with a paid organiser, which should be under the management of the Hospital. This idea came from a meeting of the Vice Presidents of the County Organisation Fund.

At the same time a letter was received from the Cambridge and District Workers' Hospital Fund to say that their Committee did not feel that any useful purpose would be served by their representatives attending the Special Committee in future. They disapproved of a contributory scheme but would support any scheme which replaced the voluntary one should the latter fail. But until it had been proved a failure they reserved the right to take any course they considered best for the interests of their members. They also thought that an official should be appointed to canvas for subscriptions from the middle and upper classes: 'a large field for increased revenue'.

Further consideration of a contributory scheme was postponed for a year.

In 1929,[5] in November, the idea of a contributory scheme was brought forward again and the General Committee set up a Sub-Committee 'to investigate contributory schemes generally, with a view to determining what kind of contributory scheme would suit this hospital,' were it to be decided later to establish one.

The Sub-Committee decided after three conferences with representatives of the Workers' Hospital Fund that a contributory scheme should be established; the date for the commencement of this scheme was to be 1 October 1931. From that date a maintenance charge would be levied on all patients who had not joined the scheme, and letters of recommendation should cease to be operative.

The General Committee sent a draft of the proposed scheme to the committee of the Workers' Hospital Fund.[6] The scheme was to take the place of the Workers' Hospital Fund and of the County and Auxiliary Associations, and was to be similar to those which had proved such a success at Oxford, Ipswich and West Suffolk (the Secretary of the Radcliffe Infirmary at Oxford, Mr Sanctuary, had visited in November 1928 and explained the scheme in operation there). The Sub-Committee had decided that the scheme was to be managed by a Special Committee of the Hospital consisting of nine people: the Chairman of the General Committee, four of the Hospital General Committee, and four appointed by the Executive Committee elected by the contributors and, like the present committee, of the Workers' Hospital Fund. This Special Committee was to undertake the collection of all weekly contributions and adapt and extend the organisation of the present Workers' Hospital Fund to meet the new circumstances. Weekly contributions were to be not less than 2d. An income limit of contributors was to be fixed, a paid organiser of the scheme was to be appointed and also a paid Almoner for the Hospital.

The Workers' Hospital Fund did not approve of the proposed scheme. A letter from the Secretary[7] told the General Committee that to say his Committee had been astonished by the report and its contents was to put it mildly. On receiving this letter the Contributory Scheme Sub-Committee met with representatives of the Workers' Hospital Fund to learn more about their objections to the scheme. These were:[8] the loss of identity which the Fund would suffer by the name proposed – 'The Addenbrooke's Hospital Contributory Scheme' – the constitution of the Committee proposed to manage the scheme, and the failure to take into account other activities of the Fund such as convalescence, grants for surgical appliances, etc.

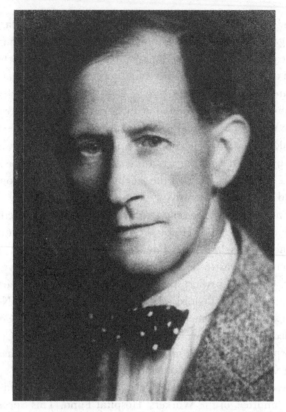

Fig. 47. Albert T. Potter, Chairman of the Addenbrooke's
Hospital Maintenance Fund, April 1937–November 1940.

Several changes were agreed: the title of the scheme, for example, was
now to be 'Addenbrooke's Hospital Contributory Scheme (formerly the
Cambridge and District Workers' Hospital Fund)', and the Executive
Committee was to be appointed on lines suggested earlier by the Workers'
Hospital Fund in which eighteen of the Committee were to be elected
from subscribers. Also there was to be an Advisory Committee consisting
of four members appointed by the Workers' Hospital Fund and four by
the General Committee, together with the General Committee Chairman. Ninety per cent of the total net collection was to be handed over to
the Hospital and the balance was to be retained by the Executive
Committee.

The Workers' Hospital Fund made further minor objections, so in the
name of the scheme 'incorporating' replaced 'formerly' and it was decided
that the Executive Committee should undertake the provision of the

Convalescent Home and of Home Nursing with their 10%.[9] This was in keeping with the objects of the Workers' Hospital Fund.[10]

Further discussions followed on the subject of management of the scheme. Some of the General Committee thought the Hospital should be in control and that 95% of the money should go to the Hospital.[11] Mr Talbot Peel wrote:

> I am most anxious that the Committee, while recognising the pioneer and indefatigable labour of the Workers' Association, will adhere to its previous decision that the new Scheme shall be in the hands of its own Committee, with the Chairman of the Hospital as Chairman.
>
> The new contributions will be the life blood of the Hospital and the whole policy of the Hospital as to medical service, nursing, food, benefits, will be in the hands of those who control this fund . . .

In February[12] the General Committee decided to divide the administration of the scheme into two sections, A and B, the Workers' Hospital Fund having the entire responsibility for operating the 'A' or Cambridge section of the scheme, and the Hospital for operating the County section. There was also to be a Contributory Scheme Committee on which the medical staff and the Workers' Hospital Fund were to be represented as well as the General Committee. At the first meeting of this Committee, held on 28 April,[13] Mr R.H. Parker was elected Chairman and three sub-committees were appointed to draw up general rules. There was also to be a paid organiser of 'B' Section, Major Wallington, who was organising Secretary of the Building Fund Appeal Committee.

The rules of the contributory scheme were basically:[14] that contributors were not entitled to benefits unless their income was below £5–£7 per week, depending on marriage status and number of dependants; the minimum contribution was 2d. per week. Benefits were treatment and maintenance at Addenbrooke's Hospital, maintenance at hospitals with which Addenbrooke's had an arrangement, and possibly assistance towards maintenance at other hospitals, and also maintenance or help towards it at a Home of Recovery if necessary. To apply for treatment the Contribution Card had to be presented and certificates signed by the contributor's doctor and Hospital Aid Committee or Centre Secretary. Non-contributors had to pay for treatment and maintenance unless they were indigent poor.

In July[15] the General Committee decided, on the recommendation of the Contributory Scheme Committee, to delineate the geographical area the Addenbrooke's scheme was to cover, and to negotiate with neighbouring hospitals so that they did not collect in each others' areas, but agreed to pay at fixed rates should their contributors find themselves in any of the other hospitals. It was, however, part of the agreement that individuals should be able to join a contributory scheme for an area other than that in which they were living.

It was important to have an agreement with neighbouring hospitals because their officials sometimes wrote complaining of encroachment on their areas.[16]

In November the response to the appeal for funds for enlargement of the Hospital was reported.[17] £82,644 had already been collected, the target being £90,000. The first moves of this appeal had been made only two years before when a Special Committee was instituted by the Lord Lieutenant as the President of the Hospital.[18] They had done well.

The Contributory Scheme was now working but the Workers' Hospital Fund (now Contributory Scheme 'A' Section) were still not happy.[19] They complained to the General Committee in January 1932 that the Contributory Scheme Committee had agreed to accept certain members at 1d. per member per week, less 15%, 'and in consideration of this glaring breach of the Constitution, this Committee cannot now feel themselves bound by any agreement previously reached'.

The Contributory Scheme Committee were asked to report on the matter to the General Committee. They replied[20] that they had made a special arrangement with the March and District Workers' Hospital Fund for members of their Fund coming to Addenbrooke's who would not require full benefits. They had not altered the rules of the Contributory Scheme.

The Workers' Hospital Fund[21] Committee were not mollified and gave notice that their year's agreement with the General Committee should terminate on 30 September 1932; at the Contributory Scheme Committee meeting of 9 March representatives of 'A' Section did not attend.[22]

The stormy passage of the Contributory Scheme continued. In April[23] the General Committee heard from the Assistant Secretary of the Huntingdon County Hospital, on behalf of the Governing Boards of his own and six other hospitals with areas adjoining that of Addenbrooke's, that 'very great anxiety is felt concerning what has been done', and a conference was requested to consider the collections of money in border-line districts. However, boundaries had been agreed and reciprocal payments arranged with five other hospitals, and one of those included above.

The same meeting heard that the Society of the Cambridge and County Friendly Societies Council, who represented over 25 000 members and had been negotiating with the General Committee regarding the Contributory Scheme,[21] had approached the Charity Commission with the proposal that the Workers' Hospital Fund take over the whole of the Contributory Scheme 'For the sake of economy and efficiency'. The General Committee decided to try to see the Charity Commission themselves.

A fortnight later[24] the General Committee heard from the Workers' Hospital Fund that they were still hoping to take over administration of both sections of the scheme. They said that between 1910 and 1931 they had raised £55,626; their grievances included the 'grossly extravagant' employment of two secretaries, one for each section of the scheme, and the contention that the system of representation in the 'B' Section was not democratic.

Huntingdon Hospital too was still complaining about the new scheme. Its letter on behalf of Addenbrooke's neighbours was received in May.[25] The Contributory Scheme Committee's reply to its earlier letter 'confirms the opinion, already expressed, that your Committee does not realise the extent to which their neighbours feel aggrieved'. On 31 May a Special Meeting of the General Committee conferred with representatives of the other hospitals and Contributory Scheme Chairman Mr Parker assured them that no centres in connection with the scheme had been established except in places for which patients were in the habit of coming to Addenbrooke's Hospital.

A revised constitution to the scheme was proposed to come into effect on 1 October 1932, in which overall responsibility was vested in the Contributory Scheme Committee. This was to consist of representatives of the General Committee, honorary medical and surgical staff, 'A' Section and 'B' Section; the Committee of 'A' Section was to be elected annually by contributors; and the Committee of 'B' Section was to consist of fifteen persons elected annually by representatives of the Hospital Aid Committees, two Contributory Scheme Committee members who were representatives of the General Committee, and the Contributory Scheme Committee Chairman. Decisions of the Contributory Scheme Committee were to be subject to confirmation by the General Committee.[26]

At the General Committee meeting of 19 July it was resolved that the Committee of 'A' Section should be asked if they were prepared to continue as part of the organisation under the revised scheme.

The Workers' Hospital Fund Committee unanimously decided[27] 'that they cannot in conformity with their rules, or in keeping with the object of their fund, recommend their members to continue as part of the Contributory Scheme under the New Constitution . . .' and asked to be allowed either to administer the scheme over the whole of the Hospital's area or to administer Section 'A' in a scheme in which all eligible persons were permitted freedom of choice as to where they paid their contributions. Failing one of these alternatives being accepted they would recommend members to contract out of the Contributory Scheme. The same General Committee meeting that heard this decided that income limits for eligibility be lowered to £4–£6 and 'all persons eligible for insurance under the National Health Insurance Act' be included as eligible.

Temporarily the prospect for an agreement looked bleak, however a new scheme was proposed[28] and a conference between the dissenting bodies[29] was held at the Hospital in September and arrived at an agreement.

There was to be a new scheme set up called the Addenbrooke's Hospital Maintenance Fund (incorporating Cambridge and District Workers' Hospital Fund and Addenbrooke's Hospital Contributory Scheme). It was to come into force on 1 October and executive powers were to be delegated by the General Committee to a Maintenance Fund Committee consisting of eighteen representatives of the members, nine representatives of the General Committee, and three representatives of the honorary medical and surgical staff. Meanwhile a provisional Maintenance Fund Committee consisting of six members of the Workers' Hospital Fund, six members of 'B' Section, two members of the honorary medical staff, and six members of the General Committee was set up to carry on until March 1933.

Clerical staff of the Workers' Hospital Fund and Contributory Scheme were to be retained as staff of the Maintenance Fund[30] and E.J. Papworth, Honorary Secretary of the Workers' Hospital Fund, and Major Wallington, paid organiser of 'B' Section, were to be Joint Organisers. (The next year Mr Papworth resigned but was retained in an advisory capacity. He had been Honorary Secretary of the Cambridge and District Workers' Hospital Fund for 21 years.[31] Major Wallington remained for a further three years.)[32]

In February[33] the General Committee agreed some G.P.s should be circularised about the new arrangements since many were said to be confused about the eligibility of non-members for treatment. They were to be told such people would be asked to pay according to their means but were not harshly assessed by the Almoner.

Meanwhile the Maintenance Fund, notwithstanding its birth pangs, got off to a good start and collected £29,000 in 1933.[34] It also managed to make mutual arrangements with some other hospitals[35] and was in a scheme involving the London Hospitals.[36]

The Maintenance Fund had run only a few years, however, before, in December 1936, the Hospital was in difficulties again, and Mr Parker, the banker, wrote that a 'somewhat large deficit (was) incurred by the Hospital last year,'[37] and 'I do feel that the procedure of the various Committees of the Hospital is lacking in some respects.'

In May the following year[38] it was reported that the deficit between ordinary income and ordinary expenditure was likely to be £3,500 in 1937, and to increase in subsequent years owing to the rising cost of commodities and to the commitments of the Hospital. The General Committee was recommended to limit extraordinary expenditure until the finances were on a sounder basis.

In August 1940,[39] the Maintenance Fund Committee recommended an increase in subscriptions from 2d. to 3d. per week for members of 18 years and over as from 1 October of that year. During 1939 the Maintenance Fund had collected £36,587.9s.4d.

The weekly contribution was raised again in 1944,[40] this time from 3d. to 4d., and income limits went up to £420 for the general wards, and £420 for the private wards for a single person, with £550 for a married couple.

In 1947[41] the Hospital had to ask the Ministry for financial help to tide it over until the National Health Service became operative. Addenbrooke's borrowing limit at the bank had had to be increased to £60,000.

The last annual report of the Maintenance Fund, in April 1948,[42] revealed it had raised £764,628 for the hospital since 1931.

~ 36 ~

The medical staff, 1914 to 1948

In 1915 a Special Committee was set up to consider the revision of the bye-laws with reference to the rearrangement of the honorary medical and surgical staff. Their report was received by the General Committee of 22 February and adopted subject to minor amendments, the principal changes being as follows:

1. The numbers of Physicians and Surgeons, Assistant Physicians and Assistant Surgeons, Dental Surgeons and Anaesthetists were to be determined by the General Committee, subject to confirmation by a General Court, instead of there being only one Physician, two Assistant Physicians, one Surgeon, two Assistant Surgeons and two Dentists in addition to the Regius Professor of Physic and Professor of Surgery who were elected because of their office.[1]

2. The Special Departments were defined as the Ophthalmic, Gynaecological, Ear and Throat, Orthopaedic, Skin, X-Ray and Electrical Departments. The General Committee had the discretionary power to place one or more of them in the charge of a member of the existing staff or, after consultation with the staff and subject to confirmation by the Quarterly Court, to 'elect an additional member of the Staff and appoint him as Assistant Physician or Assistant Surgeon as the case may be in that special department'.

3. 'Subject to the provision of bye-law 10 (which related to the proportionate allotment of beds to the Professors of Physic and Surgery) the beds for patients in the Hospital and the charge of the Out-patients shall be from time to time assigned to members of the staff by the General Committee after consultation with the Staff.' Previously the Physicians and Surgeons had charge of the adult beds and the Assistant Physicians and Surgeons had charge of out-patients and of children's beds.[1]

4. Staff were to retire at the end of the year in which they attained the age of 60 but appointments could also be terminated by a two-thirds majority of the General Committee. There was however a temporary provision that the retiring age should be suspended for those appointed before 1 January 1915 as previously the retiring age had been 65.[1]

5. Assistant Physicians and Assistant Surgeons were to have the title of Physician or Surgeon after ten years.

6. The honorary medical and surgical staff was to consist of the Honorary Consulting Physicians and Surgeons, the Physicians, the Surgeons, the Assistant Physicians, the Assistant Surgeons, the Dental Surgeons, and the Anaesthetists but the Dental Surgeons and Anaesthetists were to be summoned to staff meetings only when matters concerning their respective departments were to be under consideration.

A Special Committee was set up[2] to consider what steps should be taken as a result of the changes in the bye-laws and it was decided that Drs Lloyd Jones and Aldren Wright be made Honorary Physicians and Mr Arthur Cooke an Honorary Surgeon; Mr Deighton, Dr Griffiths and Dr Aldren Wright were to continue in charge of the Gynaecological, Orthopaedic and Skin Departments respectively; Dr Shillington Scales was, subject to confirmation by the Quarterly Court, to be appointed an Honorary Assistant Physician and to have charge of the X-Ray and Electrical Department (see next chapter); applications were to be invited by advertisement for Honorary Assistant Surgeons to have charge of the Ear, Nose and Throat (E.N.T.) Department and the Ophthalmic Department.[3] Some of the Special Departments were to have beds assigned to them after the new appointments had been made.

The staff recommendation that Mr W.H. Bowen should be appointed Honorary Assistant Surgeon in charge of the E.N.T. Department was accepted the next month.[4] He had been assisting in it for some years with Mr Deighton in charge. The staff also expressed their hope that further changes in the staff would be deferred until after the war because the field of candidates was at present limited.

In March 1917, the honorary staff proposed that a Standing Committee should be elected to consider the qualifications of candidates to the staff, but this suggestion was rejected by the General Committee as 'contrary to the spirit of the scheme by which the hospital is governed'. However, Allbutt continued to favour the scheme and such was his authority that the General Committee discussed the matter again[5] and eventually approved that such a committee should act in an advisory capacity to them.[6] It was to consist of the Chairman, the Vice Chairman and six elected members of the General Committee, the Mayor, the Regius Professor of Physic and four elected members of the honorary staff.

After the war had ended, in 1919, a Special Committee that was considering staff vacancies recommended the election of an Assistant

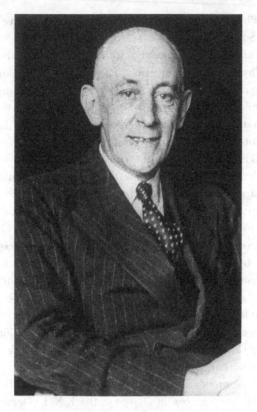

Fig. 48. J.R.C. Canney, gynaecologist.

Surgeon as Mr Deighton would be retiring at the end of the year, as an Assistant Physician to fill the vacancy caused by the retirement of Professor Bradbury. Drs Haynes and Roderick were selected to be Honorary Assistant Physician and Honorary Assistant Surgeon[7] to out-patients, and it was agreed to accede to Dr Shillington Scales' request that he be designated Honorary Physician in charge of the X-Ray and Electrical Department – previously he had been called Honorary Assistant Physician in Charge (four years) and Medical Officer in Charge (six years).

As Deighton was due to retire on 31 December after 25 years service at the Hospital, the views of the staff were taken on the possible appointment of a Surgeon in charge of the Gynaecological Department.[8] The staff thought it would be best to ask Deighton to stay on for the present and to provide him with an assistant who could eventually succeed him. As a result Dr J.R.C. Canney (Fig. 48), one of the Honorary Anaesthetists, was appointed Honorary Assistant Surgeon to the Department[9] and Deighton was asked to stay on for another two years. Dr Laurence Humphry, Senior Honorary Physician, died in 1920.[10] His death caused a vacancy on the staff and Dr J.F. Gaskell was appointed[11] to the post of Honorary Assistant Physician. A year later[12] it was decided he should succeed Aldren Wright[13] as Honorary Pathologist.

The hospital biochemical work was carried out until the Autumn of 1920 by Mr Clark Kennedy, a Fellow of Corpus Christi College. When he accepted a post in London the General Committee advertised for an Honorary Biochemist who would be provided with a laboratory in the Hospital but would be at liberty to undertake private work and research. Dr C.G.L. Wolf of Southacre, Latham Road, Cambridge, was appointed for a year as from 1 January 1921.[14] He was to remain for the next seventeen years.

The John Bonnett Clinical Laboratory had been built in 1913 with £3,000 from Mrs Bonnett who had also endowed the Laboratory with £10,000, the income from which was for maintaining the buildings and paying the remuneration of a Pathologist or any other persons employed in connection with the Laboratory.

The first Pathologist had been Dr Walter Malden who had helped Mrs Bonnett arrange the benefaction. He died in 1918 and was succeeded by Dr A.S. Layton who died in 1921.[15] It was, however, before this that, on the instigation of Professor Sir German Sims Woodhead, the Hospital obtained its Biochemist and the Laboratory was divided into two departments. The Clinical Pathologist, with his attendant, was on the upper floor and the Honorary Biochemist, Dr Wolf, with his attendant, was on the lower floor.[16]

After Dr Layton died the staff proposed that the post-mortem and pathological work should be amalgamated and placed under the honorary directorship of Dr Gaskell and that under his supervision an appointment of Clinical Pathologist should be made after advertisement. Dr Gaskell was made Honorary Clinical Pathologist[17] and Mr H.W.C. Vines M.A., M.B., of Christ's College, was appointed Clinical Pathologist at £300 p.a.[18]

In September 1921, Dr J.F. Prideaux, Medical Officer in Charge of the Psychological Department, left the hospital after two years' service, having received an appointment with the Ministry of Pensions.[19] After his resignation the appointment did not seem to be popular. There was only one application for the position and that candidate, Dr James P. Lowson, was appointed. He was the University Demonstrator in Experimental

Psychology at Cambridge and had been neurologist to the Third Army Psycho-neurological Centre in the War and then in charge of a military hospital at East Preston, Sussex, until demobilisation.[20] He resigned a few months after taking the Addenbrooke's position to work in Brisbane[21] and the vacancy was taken by Dr Archdale of the Cambridgeshire Mental Hospital. He resigned shortly afterwards too as he was leaving Cambridge[22] and the position was taken by Dr P.C. Cloake, M.B., of 27 Owlstone Road, Newnham, who was again the only applicant. He was to resign also after a year.

In December 1921, Professor Sir G. Sims Woodhead died. He was Honorary Consulting Pathologist to the Hospital and a member of the John Bonnett Memorial Laboratory Committee. He was succeeded in 1923 in both positions by the new University Professor of Pathology, Dr H.R. Dean.[23] The Clinical Pathologist, Mr H.W.C. Vines, retired after two years' service and Mr C.H. Whittle, M.B. B.Ch. (Cantab) was appointed.

Dr Cloake, who was in charge of the Psychological Department resigned in 1923 because of other engagements and Dr A.F. Reardon, Medical Superintendent of the Cambridgeshire Mental Hospital, was appointed.[24]

In April 1924, the subject of the Biochemical Department of the John Bonnett Clinical Laboratory came up for review. Because of the increasing importance of biochemistry in the diagnosis of disease and the treatment of patients the staff felt that the demands on the time and finances of Dr Wolf, the Honorary Biochemist, had become too great and should be shared to a greater extent by the Hospital.[16] The work had soared – from 70 examinations in the year previous to the appointment of Dr Wolf to over 1000 in the past year – and Dr Wolf bore all the expenses of his department, which were about £300 p.a., except for £100 contributed by the Hospital. He also worked without a qualified assistant.

Dr Gaskell was currently Honorary Pathologist, Dr Whittle was Clinical Pathologist at a salary of £300 a year from the Endowment Fund, and he had an attendant who received £2 a week. Dr Wolf carried on his department at his own expense, apart from the £100 from the Hospital, had bought his own equipment at a cost of about £1,000, and paid his attendant £3.15s. a week. However, the previous year the Hospital had also paid £112.8s.2d. to balance the Laboratory Account.

The Clinical Pathologist was allowed to take private practice but had to hand over 25% of his fees to the Hospital. The Biochemist divided his time between his own research work and hospital work. The staff wanted the Hospital to pay all Dr Wolf's expenses and also provide him with a qualified assistant.

After the Finance Committee had considered the matter it was decided[25] that the allowance made to Dr Wolf be increased from £100 to £250 p.a. but there was to be no qualified assistant as the Finance Committee said the Hospital could not afford it.

Biochemistry was not the only department in the Hospital to feel the strain of additional work. A Clinical Assistant had to be appointed to the E.N.T. Department to help Mr Bowen[26] and a third Honorary Dentist was appointed, Mr H. Curtis, L.D.S. A new post of Surgical Registrar to have charge of patients' records[27] was approved and Mr V. Pennell, M.B., B.Ch., F.R.C.S. (England) was appointed and to commence his duties at the end of June.[28] The next year Dr F. Roberts of The Gables, Histon, was appointed Clinical Assistant in the X-Ray Department 'where the work is very heavy'.[29]

The following February, 1925, the Regius Professor of Physic, Sir Thomas Clifford Allbutt, K.C.B., F.R.S., died. He had still been regularly attending to teach the medical students. He was Senior Physician of the Hospital but, apart from a period during the war when the majority of the staff were mobilised on Active Service, he had never taken beds.[30]

The General Committee resolved that Lady Allbutt be told his 'advice and skill so freely and generously given have been of the utmost value to the Hospital during the period of 33 years for which he has held the post of Regius Professor of Physic in the University and whose eminence both as a Physician and as a writer has conferred lustre upon the hospital . . .' Now (1991) his portrait hangs in the Clinical School library between the busts of Paget and Humphry.

The next Regius Professor of Physic was Sir Humphry Davy Rolleston, President of the Royal College of Physicians. He was elected to be a Physician of the Hospital in 1925.[31]

In November 1925, Dr Reardon, the Honorary Medical Officer in charge of the Psychological Department, had died and his position was filled by Dr H. Travers Jones, Medical Superintendent of the Fulbourn Mental Hospital.[32]

For a number of years past there had been suggestions that the Hospital should admit fee-paying patients out of those who, while not able to pay the full charges of a Nursing Home, could still pay a modified fee. In 1926 the General Committee decided to take these suggestions further and bye-laws to carry it out were drafted and submitted to the staff for consideration. The staff, however, 'informed the General Committee that they do not consider the scheme of taking in paying patients is workable under the existing conditions of the hospital . . .' so the idea was dropped again for the time being.[32]

Dr Shillington Scales was to retire from the post of Honorary Physician in charge of the X-Ray and Electrical Department at the end of 1926. Over the years the value of the work had grown and by 1926 it had become 'of very great importance in the treatment of patients'. Two applications were received for his appointment, one withdrew and Dr Ffrangcon Roberts, his Clinical Assistant, was recommended for the post by the Selection and Advisory Committee. The General Committee did not agree. It was decided to advertise the post afresh and Dr Scales was asked to stay on for another three months.[33] However, on 28 February Dr Scales died and Dr Ffrangcon Roberts, M.A., B.Ch. (Camb), M.R.C.P. (Lond), D.M.R.E. (Camb), was appointed.[34] This was a controversial appointment (see next chapter).

Mr Bowen, the Surgeon in charge of the E.N.T. Department, was given an Honorary Clinical Assistant in 1926, Mr A.S.H. Walford. It was said: 'The work in this Department had increased greatly during the last few years, and it was essential that the surgeon in charge should have assistance to enable him to deal efficiently with the number of patients.'[35] It is not clear if this was a second assistant to the one appointed in 1924 but it seems more likely to be a replacement. Mr Bowen resigned his position on 30 September 1927, although continuing as a general surgeon to the Hospital, and Mr Walford M.A., M.B., B.Ch. (Cantab), F.R.C.S. (Eng), M.R.C.S. (Eng), L.R.C.P. (Lond), was appointed to be Honorary Assistant Surgeon in charge of the E.N.T. Department.

At the end of 1927 Dr Lloyd Jones, Honorary Physician, retired and became a member of the honorary consulting staff. He had given 28 years' service to the Hospital, having been elected Honorary Assistant Physician to the Out-patient Department in 1899. In 1919 when Professor Bradbury retired, Dr Lloyd Jones had become Physician to in-patients with charge of beds, and on the death of Dr Laurence Humphry in 1920 he became Senior Physician.

On Dr Lloyd Jones' retirement Dr Aldren Wright became Senior Physician, and Dr Haynes, one of the Honorary Assistant Physicians, became a Physician to in-patients with charge of beds. Dr Leslie B. Cole of 13 Trumpington Street, Cambridge, filled the vacancy of Honorary Assistant Physician.[36]

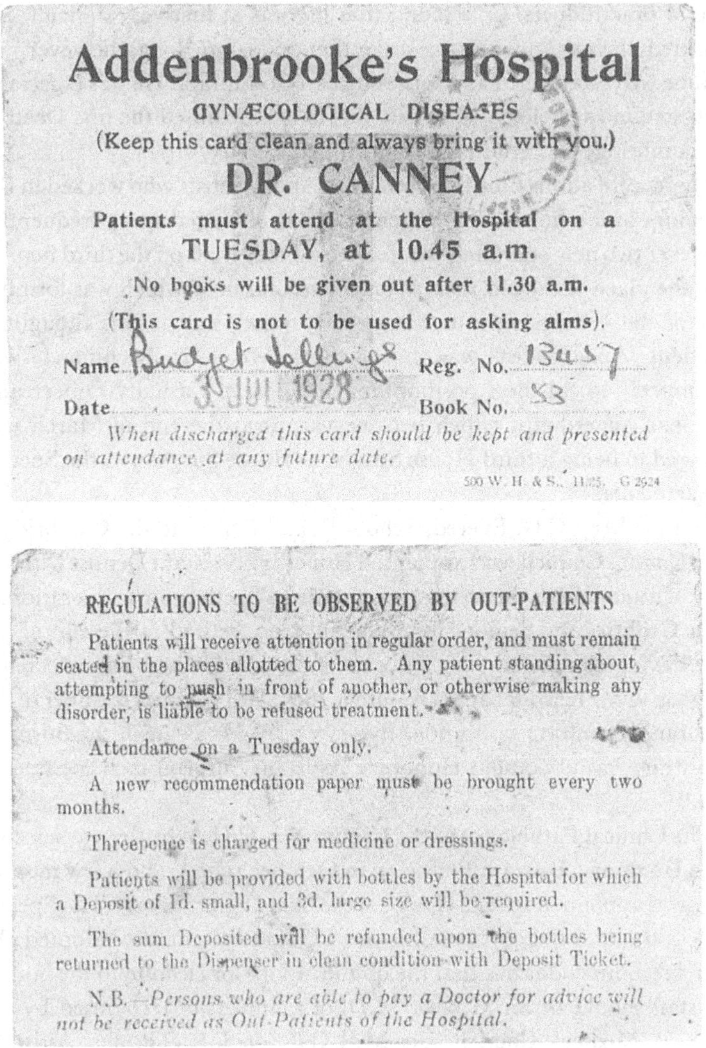

Addenbrooke's Hospital
GYNÆCOLOGICAL DISEASES
(Keep this card clean and always bring it with you.)
DR. CANNEY
Patients must attend at the Hospital on a
TUESDAY, at 10.45 a.m.
No books will be given out after 11.30 a.m.

(This card is not to be used for asking alms).

Name .... Reg. No. 13457
Date 30 JUL 1928 Book No. 53
When discharged this card should be kept and presented on attendance at any future date.
500 W. H. & S., 11.25. G 2924

REGULATIONS TO BE OBSERVED BY OUT-PATIENTS

Patients will receive attention in regular order, and must remain seated in the places allotted to them. Any patient standing about, attempting to push in front of another, or otherwise making any disorder, is liable to be refused treatment.

Attendance on a Tuesday only.

A new recommendation paper must be brought every two months.

Threepence is charged for medicine or dressings.

Patients will be provided with bottles by the Hospital for which a Deposit of 1d. small, and 3d. large size will be required.

The sum Deposited will be refunded upon the bottles being returned to the Dispenser in clean condition—with Deposit Ticket.

N.B.—*Persons who are able to pay a Doctor for advice will not be received as Out-Patients of the Hospital.*

Fig. 49. Both sides of a gynaecological out-patient's card, 1928.

Leslie Cole (1898–1983) had served in the Royal Field Artillery 1916–1918 in India and Mesopotamia before going up to King's College, Cambridge, and St Thomas' Hospital. After graduating M.B., B.Chir., 1923, he went on to become Resident Assistant Physician at St Thomas', the most senior of the junior appointments. He was determined not to do general practice and to be a true Consultant and this was how he came to Cambridge in 1927. Almost all the Consultants up to that time were really general practitioners. Cole found that life was at first very difficult. He admitted having given some anaesthetics; before long, however, he became well established and successful as a Consultant. He was especially interested in cardiology. (Later he was to be appointed the first Dean of the Cambridge Postgraduate Medical School, 1957–1965.)

There were at this time five Honorary Anaesthetists who worked in the mornings and who seemed in general to be changed quite frequently. However two new operating theatres were being built on the third floor to take the place of the old theatre on the second floor which was forming part of the conversion into a maternity ward, and it was thought a Resident Anaesthetist was necessary.[37] Mr J.H. Richmond was appointed[38] to this new position and the post of Casualty Officer and Resident Anaesthetist which became vacant at the end of March was changed to being a third House Surgeon, 'House Surgeon to the Special Departments'.

In 1928 Mr J.C.G. Evered, School Dental Officer to the Cambridge-shire County Council, was appointed Honorary Assistant Dentist with the duty of attending to the treatment of patients' teeth prior to operation.[39]

Dr Griffiths, the Senior Honorary Surgeon, retired at the end of the year having completed over 33 years of service. He had been elected a Surgeon to the Hospital at Midsummer 1895. He became a member of the honorary consulting staff under Bye-law 17.[40] Mr Pennell, the Surgical Registrar, was appointed Honorary Assistant Surgeon in succession to him.[41]

The Clinical Pathologist to the Laboratory, C.H. Whittle, was selected to be Honorary Assistant Physician in October 1929,[42] and a few months later was appointed to take charge of the Skin Department.[43] The Special Selection and Advisory Committee of October 1929 also adopted the staff's recommendations that the qualifications for election to the honor-ary staff should be an M.B. or M.D. of a university recognised by the General Medical Council, an M.R.C.P. or F.R.C.P. for Assistant Physicians, and an F.R.C.S. for Assistant Surgeons.

Candidates for the post of Assistant Physician to the Radiological Department must hold a Diploma in Radiology as well as an M.B. or M.D., and the qualification for Assistant Surgeons was also to apply to the surgical Special Departments, namely Ophthalmic, Aural, Orthopaedic, and Gynaecological.

The Senior Physician to the Hospital, Dr Aldren Wright, retired according to the bye-laws at the end of 1929 and Dr G.S. Haynes became

Senior Honorary Physician. After Dr Wright's retirement he planned to leave Cambridge[44] but apparently remained an Honorary Consulting Physician until his death in 1942. When he wrote resigning from the various committees of the Hospital he said 'After so long a connection – beginning in 1891, when I joined the Hospital as a Student – it is difficult now to realise my severance . . .'

In April 1930, the General Committee accepted the staff's recommendations to amend Bye-law 53[45] in order to allow Physicians and Surgeons to follow up their cases and to obtain better facilities for teaching.[46] It was now to be allowed for Physicians and Surgeons to take out-patients provided they took them on a day other than that on which an Assistant Physician or Surgeon was taking them and that a certain number of beds was given up to the Assistant Physician or Surgeon.[47] 'The necessity for this is recognised in progressive hospitals, and we consider it will add to the efficiency of the Hospital,' said the staff. The bye-law in question was already obsolete as out-patients were now seen on all days except Sunday, rather than the Mondays, Wednesdays and Saturdays specified.[48]

More changes to the bye-laws were approved in mid 1930. In February the staff had proposed a temporary provision under which Dr Budd, the Senior Honorary Anaesthetist, and Dr Wolf, the Honorary Biochemist, should be made members of the honorary staff.[49] A temporary provision was not thought possible, however an alteration in the bye-laws was approved[50] and the staff were asked whether the Honorary Pathologist should not also be a member, and the Dental Surgeons, and the remaining Honorary Anaesthetists. The staff[51] considered that it might not in every instance be desirable to make the Senior Honorary Anaesthetist and the Honorary Biochemist full members of the staff. They suggested amending Bye-law 20 and adding a new Bye-law 20a so that officers in charge of Special Departments could become members of the staff 'in recognition of loyal and distinguished service to the Hospital' as well as the Honorary Consulting Physicians and Surgeons, the Physicians and Surgeons, and the Assistant Physicians and Assistant Surgeons.

The General Committee then asked the staff to consider whether there was any longer a useful purpose served in distinguishing Assistant Physicians and Surgeons from Physicians and Surgeons since all now took out-patients, and the staff agreed there was not.[52] They also requested that the retiring age be restored from 60 to 65 since if the senior men continued in 'active and vigorous practice' after retirement the junior men might be compelled as in the past to take general practice 'with its many and irregular calls on time and energy.' It was to the advantage of the Hospital that 'the number of Consultants should not be in excess of the needs of the district'. This was agreed.[53]

The amended bye-laws[54] defined the honorary medical and surgical staff as

> the Honorary Consulting Physicians and Surgeons, the Physicians, the Surgeons, and the Physicians or Surgeons in charge of Special Departments as defined in Bye-law 13. The Anaesthetists and the Dental Surgeons shall be summoned to Meetings of the Staff only when matters concerning their respective Departments are under consideration.
>
> The General Committee, after consultation with the Staff, may appoint to membership of the Staff the Pathologist, the Senior Anaesthetist, the Biochemist, the Senior Dental Surgeons, or any other officer in charge of a Special Department, in recognition of loyal and devoted service to the Hospital.

Bye-law 13 defined the Special Departments as Ophthalmic, Ear and Throat, Gynaecological, Orthopaedic, Skin, X-Ray and Electrical. The Psychology Department was excluded as the staff wished[55] this.

In September the General Committee took advantage of the new bye-laws and agreed to make Dr Budd and Dr Wolf members of the staff.[56]

In 1932 Dr W. Langdon-Brown, the Regius Professor of Physic, was elected as Physician under the agreement between the University and Addenbrooke's. Also the staff requested, and it was agreed, that they should be allowed white coats on request.[57]

The following year Mr R.W. Butler, M.A., M.B., M.Ch. (Cantab), F.R.C.S., was elected Honorary Surgeon; and Mr E.G. Recordon, M.A., M.B., B.Ch. (Cantab) was elected Honorary Surgeon in charge of the Ophthalmic Department.

In December Dr Travers Jones resigned as Medical Officer in charge of the Psychological Department, a post he had held for the past eight years. He agreed to carry on until other arrangements were made. It had been decided that the Department was to be reorganised and in future the session would be divided into two parts, one for cases of nervous disorders such as attended the present clinic, and the other for a child guidance clinic. The following October (1934), charge of the Psychological Department and Child Guidance Clinic was taken over by Dr R.A. Noble.[58] He was assisted by Mrs Crosthwaite as Social Worker. The work of the Department increased and within a few months the General Committee had agreed to the appointment of Honorary Clinical Assistants, of a Psychologist to assist Dr Noble and also of a trained Social Worker since

Mrs Crosthwaite resigned. Dr Noble was also elected to be an Honorary Physician instead of Honorary Medical Officer in charge of the Department.[59]

It had already been decided that the Psychological Department should be designated a Special Department, along with the Ophthalmic, Ear Nose and Throat, Gynaecological, Orthopaedic, Skin, Radiological, and Urological Departments,[60] and the name had soon been changed to the Psychiatric Department.[61] Cambridge Town Council decided that year to make a grant of £75 p.a. towards the expenses of the Child Guidance Clinic, subject to the approval of the Ministry of Health.[62]

In 1935 the Regius Professor of Physic Sir Walter Langdon Brown retired and his successor Dr John A. Ryle was elected a Physician in his place.[62]

Although, by the terms of the Hospital's Scheme of Management a limited number of the honorary staff were allowed to attend General Committee meetings as advisers, they were not members as such. In 1909 they had tried and failed to get the right to vote. In 1937 they asked that, in order to secure closer co-operation between the General Committee and the honorary staff, they should be allowed to nominate annually three of their members as ex-officio members. The General Committee and the Charity Commissioners agreed to this request.[63]

Also in 1937 the General Committee heard from the B.M.A. and the honorary staff on the subject of the payment of medical and surgical staffs of Voluntary Hospitals out of Contributory Scheme funds.[64] The staff felt the principle should be applied but said they would not press for its application at present. Their attitude would depend on keeping the numbers of the honorary staff to an economical level and the strict application of income limits to those joining the Contributory Scheme.

The General Committee thanked the staff and said they would bear these two points in mind. As Dr Haynes was to retire at the end of the year advertisements were to be inserted for an Honorary Physician.

Dr Wolf was also to retire at the end of 1937 from the post of Honorary Biochemist[65] and it was decided to advertise for a salaried Biochemist with a medical qualification. It was hoped the successful candidate would be associated with the Biochemical Department of the University. The Regius Professor of Physic, who either just had, or was just about to, issued the first of his two Memoranda on the future of Addenbrooke's with special reference to the interrelationships between it and the University, gave his views on policy and they were supported by the Professors of

Biochemistry and Pathology. It was considered that it would not be possible to obtain the services of an Honorary Biochemist and it was decided to recommend that the post of Clinical Biochemist be abolished. Dr Wolf was to be elected Honorary Consulting Biochemist. On his retirement at the end of the year he presented the apparatus, chemicals, books and furniture which he used in the Biochemical Laboratory, to the Hospital.[66]

Mr N.R. Lawrie, Dr Wolf's salaried assistant who had earlier been a Beit Fellow and Honorary Clinical Assistant[62] for three years was appointed Biochemist.[67]

In October of 1937 the staff recommended the appointment of a non-resident whole-time radiologist at a salary of £500 p.a. They decided against having an Honorary Radiologist as that would go against the spirit of their letter to the General Committee on the subject of payment of the honorary staff and would tend to raise their numbers to an uneconomic level. They also recommended the passing of certain bye-laws which would give the University Department of Medicine a definite footing in the Hospital and give power to the Assistant Director of the Department to act as an Assistant Honorary Physician of the Hospital.[68]

Dr Haynes retired at the end of 1937 and F.B. Parsons, who had been an Honorary Anaesthetist 1931–1936,[69] was appointed Honorary Physician in his place.[70] It was recommended he should be informed he would be wise to retain the position of Police Surgeon 'for a time if he considers it fit to do so'.

Dr A. Maxwell Evans was appointed Assistant Radiologist for a year from 15 February 1938, but he resigned shortly afterwards to go to Canada[71] and Dr L. Werbeloff was appointed.

Later in the year arrangements were made for the Regius Professor of Physic's Research Assistants to undertake work in some of the Special Departments and to act as part-time Assistants to the Heads there[72] and the General Committee of 25 October 1938 received a letter from the Regius Professor of Physic: 'It looks now as if the emergency has passed', however the whole of his department had offered to put their services at the disposal of the Hospital in the event of war 'until such times as they were individually called to other forms of service'.

In the Annual Report for the year ended 30 September 1938 it was announced among the changes in the medical staff that Dr R.A. McCance, M.A., F.R.C.P., who was later to become the University Professor of Experimental Medicine, had become an Honorary Assistant Physician.

In April 1939,[73] 29-year-old P.H.R. Ghey, the Resident Surgical Officer, was selected for the appointment of Honorary Surgeon from 1 January 1940, to fill the vacancy that would be created by the retirement of Dr H.B. Roderick at the end of 1939. However the War was to intervene and affect these plans.

The General Purposes Committee received a letter from the B.M.A. in July[74] with regard to the position of Consultants and Specialists on the visiting staffs of Voluntary Hospitals who in the event of an emergency would be employed on whole-time Government service. They made several recommendations. No new appointments were to be made on a permanent basis during the war or for twelve months after it, and temporary appointments should be terminable within twelve months of the conclusion of hostilities. Also it was desirable that the period of war service of an absentee practitioner should be added to the retirement age of his hospital appointment, and that hospital appointments of absentee practitioners which would normally be terminated due to the age limit should be continued, the period of war service being added to the age limit. The Committee agreed to recommend that the B.M.A. be informed that these matters would be borne in mind.

At the end of November it was clear that Ghey would not be able to take up his appointment because of absence on military service and it was decided to ask Roderick to act as his deputy instead of retiring.[75] Ghey joined the R.A.M.C.,[76] but it was agreed that his appointment at Addenbrooke's should be kept open for him.

A number of deputies were organised for the staff in the forces:[77]

Staff in Forces	Deputy
Mr R.W. Butler	Mr S. Riddiough
Dr L.B. Cole	The Regius Professor of Physic and Dr L.C. Martin (Out-patient Department)
Dr P.H.R. Ghey	Dr H.B. Roderick
Mr E.G. Recordon	Miss M. Perrers Taylor
Dr Ff. Roberts	Dr F.R. Berridge, Dr J.S. Mitchell
Mr A.S.H. Walford	Mr C. Hamblen Thomas

In July a letter came from the Regius Professor, J.A. Ryle,[78] to say he had taken a new job, an Emergency Medical Service appointment as physician to a sector attached to Guy's School. The teaching and clinical research activities of his department in Cambridge had greatly diminished and the new appointment would give him much wider scope to exercise his functions as a physician and also, while conditions allowed, as a clinical teacher. Dr McCance and Dr Martin were prepared to deputise for him and he named others who would be ready and willing to assist in Addenbrooke's if needed.

Addenbrooke's must have found itself short staffed at this time since a drive was instituted for the return of members of the honorary staff on military service.[79] Requests for the return of Ghey, Butler and Cole had been forwarded to the War Office but it was said they could not be spared as they were holding important military posts. Nevertheless the Secretary-Superintendent had written a further letter to the Ministry pressing for Dr Cole's return. In October[80] the Central Medical War Committee agreed to take up the question of Cole's release. However Mitchell was now in danger of being called up. His name had apparently been put on the list of medical men who could possibly be spared from the area and the local Medical War Committee wanted to know if Addenbrooke's wanted to reserve him for work at the Hospital. It was agreed that, subject to the approval of the honorary staff, an official application should be submitted for his reservation for work in the X-Ray Department.

The next month Ghey was released from the army and was able to take up his work as an Honorary Surgeon. He was to take over Dr Roderick's beds and also to attend the Out-patient Department on two days a week but Roderick was to continue in charge of the clinic both at Addenbrooke's and in the area. Ghey had additional work as a surgeon under the Emergency Medical Service but this would not interfere with his work at the Hospital.

In December the General Committee heard[81] that the Central Medical War Committee (C.M.W.C.) had refused to return Major R.W. Butler or Lt/Col L.B. Cole. They had been asked again however.

All these efforts began to bear fruit. In January[82] the General Committee heard that the C.M.W.C. had approved the release of Cole. A telegram had been received from him to say he would be sailing the same night. The next month[83] they heard that Mr A.S.H. Walford had been released from the R.A.M.C. and had returned to duty at the Hospital.

In a further development, the Ministry of Health decided that Addenbrooke's was a suitable place in which to establish a Fracture Department. About 100 beds at the Leys were earmarked for it and Mr R.W. Butler was released from Military Service in June to undertake the necessary surgical work.[84]

In November[85] the staff asked, and it was agreed, that Butler be appointed Honorary Surgeon and Honorary Surgeon in charge of the

Orthopaedic Department at Addenbrooke's. Roderick was to be Honorary Consulting Surgeon to the Orthopaedic Department but to continue his present work of assisting in out-patient clinics of the Orthopaedic Department and in running and organising Orthopaedic Clinics in outlying towns. Mr Butler was anxious he should continue to do this until the work of the Hospital returned to peace-time conditions. Roderick was to have beds only at the Leys; his allocation of beds at Addenbrooke's was to cease.

The staff also reiterated their earlier statement about reserving the right to claim for payment 'should circumstances demand'. They had considered the Government's scheme for regionalisation of the hospitals in the Cambridge area and while approving of it in principle they felt it was going to affect their economical position.

They said that with the establishment of a Maintenance Fund the Hospital had largely ceased to be a charitable institution and had become 'the instrument of a sickness benefit society. On this account a system whereby members of the Maintenance Fund received free of charge the services of the Staff at the expense of private patients was anomalous.'

They had in the past suggested that the weekly Maintenance Fund payment should be increased from 2d. to 3d. to cover payment of the staff but they had been told this would lead to a diminution of membership and had been refused. The weekly payment had since been raised to 3d. notwithstanding.

The regionalisation scheme and the altered conditions to be expected after the war lent added weight to their arguments. When hospital facilities were increased patients with higher incomes would be drawn in and also there would be a more equal distribution of incomes and 'the small number of paying patients will no longer be able to support the payment of specialist services for the increased number making use of the hospital'. The staff said they felt 'bound to protect themselves and their successors' and felt it necessary to remind the General Committee of their previous resolution 'that the Honorary Staff reserve the right to re-open the claim for payment should circumstances demand'.

The Hospital was having to deal with yet more work and with it came the need for increasing the number of paid medical staff. A salaried full-time Gynaecological Assistant to Dr Canney was agreed in the first quarter of 1942 and Dr F. Schmelz, M.D. (Prague), M.R.C.S., L.R.C.P. (Eng), was appointed.[86] In the second quarter a salaried full-time Assistant Clinical Pathologist was agreed and Dr B. Traub was appointed.[87] He resigned at the end of January 1943,[88] and Dr F. Gunz was appointed.[89]

In April 1943, there was some discussion at the General Purposes Committee meeting[90] about the wartime assistance being rendered by various medical personnel and some changes in the bye-laws recommended by the Honorary staff in this connection. It was decided to ask for the General Committee to have the power to deviate from three of the bye-laws (nos 21, 22 and 23) in order to secure an adequate medical and surgical staff for the war emergency period, and this was done.[91] As a result, Dr J.F. Gaskell and Mr W.H. Bowen, who were due to retire under the age limit, were re-elected Honorary Physician and Honorary Surgeon respectively for a further year.

It was also recommended that the following temporary Honorary Surgical appointments be made for the period ended 31 December 1943:

Miss M. Perrers Taylor, Temp. Hon. Asst Surgeon to the Ophthalmic Department;

Mr S. Riddiough, Temp. Hon. Asst Surgeon;

Mr C. Hamblen Thomas, Temp. Hon. Asst Surgeon to the ENT Department;

Mr Oswald Lloyd, Temp. Hon. Asst Surgeon to the Gynaecological Department;

Mr W.G. Watson, Chief Assistant to the Ophthalmic Department.

As Dr Watson was ill the General Purposes Committee had written to the Authorities asking for Major E.G. Recordon's release from Army Service. This was obtained and he was to take up his duties in the Ophthalmic Department from 6 September 1943.[92]

The war had brought increased rates of pay and improved conditions of employment to nursing and other hospital personnel but they had to be paid for. In the General Committee's report for the last quarter of 1943[93] when it was announced that the Hetherington report on the wages and hours of duty for domestic workers in Institutions was to be implemented at Addenbrooke's at an additional annual expenditure of £3,100, a note of warning was sounded. 'Addenbrooke's is anxious to be in the van of progress regarding reforms but a note of warning must be uttered about the Hospital's financial state' '. . . unless the general income is augmented in the near future the year of 1944 will result in a heavy deficit, mainly owing to the increases of salaries and wages which are estimated to amount to over £11,800 in the full year'.

As a result the rate of contributions to the Maintenance Fund was increased from 3d. to 4d. per week per member[94] the next year.

In June 1944, an Out-patient's Appointment Scheme was introduced to reduce patients' waiting time. It involved making group appointments throughout the period of the clinics.

The following year it was decided to advertise the posts of Dr Gaskell and Mr Bowen who were still working although beyond retirement age; the new appointments were to commence on 1 October 1946, when all wartime Honorary Assistant appointments were to be terminated.[95] Two additional posts were to be created: a second Honorary Surgeon to the Gynaecological and Obstetric Department, and an Honorary Radiologist.[96] It was also decided that there should be a physician devoting himself entirely to dermatology in charge of the Department of Dermatology once more beds were available for the work and there should also be a new E.N.T. Honorary Surgeon when the demand for more beds had been satisfied.

In February 1946, the Examination Halls annexe closed and the bed complement of the Hospital was reduced to 358 from its full wartime complement of 811. The flow of the freshly wounded must have stopped but there would have been many disabled soldiers in the wards, and attending out-patients in addition to the normal complement of patients. In the report of the General Committee to the Quarterly Court for the quarter ended 31 March 1946, it said: 'This reduction (in beds) is having the effect of swelling the number of patients on the waiting list and the position is regarded as a serious one.' It was known that the Hospital would have to be enlarged and the Joint Advisory Committee of representatives of the Hospital and of the University had been asked to prepare a plan.

In the same report it was announced that because the General Committee had accepted the recent recommendations of the Rushcliffe Committee and the Joint Industrial Council relating to the wages of nursing, domestic and portering staffs, the Hospital would be involved in an additional expenditure of approximately £5,490 in 1946 and £6,350 in 1947.

Professor J.S. Mitchell was to be accorded the title of Director of the Radiotherapeutic Centre and he was to be granted an honorarium for the work he undertook for the Hospital. A second Ophthalmic Surgeon was to be appointed to the staff.

This was certainly a time of expansion. The General Committee of

27 August 1946 received the draft report of the General Board of the University on the arrangement with Addenbrooke's, the establishment of certain additional University offices in this connection, and the constitution of a School of Clinical Research and Post-graduate Teaching.

Arrangements between Addenbrooke's and the University with regard to the development of a School of Clinical Research and Postgraduate Teaching were in the process of being finalised and the University took over responsibility for the pathological and biochemical services of the Hospital from 1 October 1946, on the understanding that the Hospital would provide its share of the cost.[97]

Mr Brian Donnelly, M.R.C.S., L.R.C.P., D.M.R., was appointed full-time Assistant Radiologist to the Douty X-Ray Clinic and the appointment of a second Honorary Surgeon to the Ear, Nose and Throat Department was to go ahead. Mr K. Wilsdon, M.B., B.Ch. (Oxon), M.A. (Oxon), F.R.C.S. (Edin), was selected for this position, to take up his duties from 1 January 1947.[98] The position of Chief Assistant Surgeon to the E.N.T. Department was to terminate at the end of 1946 and the present holder Mr Robert Williamson was thanked[99] for his services.

A number of new appointments were to take effect from 1 October 1946. Laurence Martin, M.A., M.D. (Cantab), M.R.C.P. had been selected as Honorary Physician[100] out of five applicants; Mr B.M. Truscott, M.B.E., M.B., B.S. (Lond), F.R.C.S. (Eng) as Honorary Surgeon out of 22 applicants;[101] Dr G.F. Wright, M.A., M.B., B.Chir., M.R.C.S., L.R.C.P., D.O.M.S., to be Honorary Ophthalmic Surgeon out of five applicants;[102] S/L Brian Donnelly to be Assistant Radiologist;[102] Mr F.R. Berridge, M.A., M.B. (Camb), D.M.R. (Lond), B.Ch. (Camb), M.R.C.S., L.R.C.P., to be Honorary Radiologist out of three applicants;[102] Mr T.W. Harrison L.D.S., R.C.S. (Eng), and Mr C.D. Farris, M.R.C.S. (Eng), L.R.C.P. (Lond), L.D.S. (Eng), to be Honorary Dental Surgeons out of three applicants; Mr Oswald Lloyd, M.D., B.S. (Lond), F.R.C.S. (Eng), L.R.C.P. (Lond), M.R.C.O.G., to be Honorary Surgeon to the Obstetrics and Gynaecology Department out of six applicants;[100] Mr R.S. Quick, B.Sc., to be Senior Physicist;[100] and Miss J.L. Findlay, B.A. (Hons), to be Junior Assistant Physicist.[102]

The Radiologist Dr Berridge was to receive an honorarium of £500 for the first three years of his appointment unless the State Medical Service came into operation before the expiration of that time.

Recommendations received from the Rushcliffe Committee on the subject of increases in salaries for senior nursing personnel and student

nurses were accepted by the General Committee, to take effect retrospec-
tively from 1 January 1946. It was estimated they would cost the Hospital
an additional £3,515 for that first year.[97]

An agreement was arrived at between the University and the Hospital
and under these arrangements certain university officers were given
positions on the staff of the Hospital.[103] Professor R.A. McCance,
Professor J.S. Mitchell and Professor H.A. Harris, the Head of the
Department of Anatomy, were made Honorary Physicians, and Drs M.
Haynes, R.I.N. Greaves, and Raymond Williamson, who were the
Readers in Medicine, Bacteriology, and Morbid Histology respectively,
became Assistant Honorary Physicians.

In addition, the Chairman and Vice Chairman of the General Com-
mittee, the Chairman of the Finance Committee, and the Chairman of the
Building Committee were all appointed to serve on the Council of the
Medical School.

The E.N.T. Department was designated the Department of Otolaryn-
gology, and it was agreed it should be given the use of the converted
maternity wards after the transfer of the abnormal maternity work to the
County Hospital, Mill Road.

Prior to the take-over of the National Health Service the assets and
liabilities of the Private Wards Insurance Scheme were, as from 1 April
1947, to be transferred to the new British United Provident Association
Ltd, which had been inaugurated by the Nuffield Provident Guarantee
Fund. Members would be able to obtain current benefits until 31 March
1948, when they would be eligible to join the new association.[104]

Two more new appointments were planned in August 1947.[105] For one,
that of Honorary Paediatrician, an application was to be made to the
Ministry of Health and it was thought to pay him an honorarium of
£1,000. It was expected that the Local Authorities would also wish to
make use of his services and they would pay the Hospital accordingly.

The second appointment was that of thoracic surgeon. Papworth Hall
and White Lodge Hospital (Newmarket) were about to lose the services of
their visiting London Thoracic Surgeon and it was felt that the time was
opportune for Addenbrooke's to make such an appointment. White
Lodge and Papworth might also be able to use him and contribute. Their
payment would obviate the need to subsidise the appointment and a
further advantage was that Addenbrooke's might not need to provide
beds since there was a complete thoracic unit at Papworth.

Mr G. Kent Harrison, M.D. (Toronto), F.R.C.S. (Eng), aged 40, was selected as Honorary Thoracic Surgeon[106] to take up his duties on 1 December 1947. Dr D. Gairdner M.B., B.Ch., M.R.C.P., D.M., was to be selected as Honorary Paediatrician.[107]

Dr Canney was due to retire at the end of 1948[108] and in May of that year Miss Janet Bottomely M.B., B.S. (Lon), F.R.C.S. (Eng), M.D. (Lond), M.R.C.O.G., was selected out of fourteen applicants to be Honorary Surgeon to the Gynaecological and Obstetrical Department from 1 January 1949.[109]

Meanwhile the honorary staff had finally requested payment for their services. The subject had been brought up again in August 1947,[110] when a circular letter was received from the British Hospitals Association jointly with the British Medical Association on the subject of the payment of part-time visiting medical staff. There was to be a meeting of the Association of Voluntary Teaching Hospitals to discuss the matter and the staff were to appoint a sub-committee to look into the subject and then discuss it with the General Purposes Committee.

At the meeting between the General Purposes Committee and the staff the Hospital was asked to pay £750 p.a. to all full members of the staff excluding those in general practice and those holding full-time academic or university appointments. Also £250 p.a. was to be paid to each Honorary Anaesthetist.[111] The Ministry of Health was asked to approve that a global sum be paid to the Honorary staff fund for distribution, to cover honoraria from 1 October 1947 until the appointed day.

The following payments were to be made:

1. At the rate of £750 p.a.

   Honorary Physicians (Drs Cole, Parsons and Martin)
   Honorary Surgeons (Messrs Pennell, Butler, Ghey and Truscott)
   Honorary Ophthalmologists (Messrs Recordon and Wright)
   Honorary Gynaecologists (Dr Canney and Mr Lloyd)
   Honorary Laryngologists (Messrs Walford and Wilsdon)
   Honorary Radiologists (Drs Roberts and Berridge) – the present
      honorarium of £500 paid to Dr Berridge to cease
   Honorary Dermatologist (Dr Whittle)
   Honorary Psychiatrist (Dr Noble)
   Honorary Thoracic Surgeon (Mr Kent Harrison) – appointed as
      from 1 December 1947.

2. At the rate of £1,000 p.a.

   Honorary Paediatrician (Assuming appointment commences on 1
      February 1948).

3. At the rate of £250 p.a.

   Honorary Anaesthetists (Drs Budd, Richards, Youngman, Cooper, Simpson, Windsor Lewis and Keates)

4. At the rate of £125 p.a.

   Honorary Dental Surgeons (Messrs Curtis, Smith, Freeman, Harrison and Farris)

5. At the rate of £100 p.a.

   Honorary Chief Assistant to the Ophthalmic Department (Miss Perrers Taylor).

6. At the rate of £50 p.a.

   Honorary Clinical Assistants (Drs Roscoe, Kodicek, Wade, Riddiough, Elliott, Silberstein, Gilbert, Lawson, Hedgcock, Roughton).

The estimated total global sum to be paid to the honorary staff between 1 October 1947 and 5 July 1948 was £13,713. This included 10% to cover deputies, but excluded the Director of the Radiotherapeutic Centre (Professor J.S. Mitchell) who should continue to be paid his existing honorarium of £500 p.a. The payments also excluded the work done by the honorary staff in connection with the treatment of school children, maternity and child welfare patients, surgical tuberculosis and Ministry of Pensions and Emergency Medical Service (E.M.S.) work. Confirmation was given to the payment of these honoraria at the Quarterly Court of 24 February 1948.

~ 37 ~

A controversial appointment

Conrad William Röntgen discovered 'X-rays' in November 1895. No medical discovery before it had been so widely and so rapidly publicised. By the beginning of February 1896, the B.M.A. had commissioned an investigation into the clinical uses of X-rays and before the end of that year the first British monograph on radiography had been published, and many hospitals had acquired X-ray machines.

Addenbrooke's itself was not among the pioneers, which was perhaps fortunate for patients and staff as the hazards of X-rays were at first unsuspected. However, X-rays were taken of Addenbrooke's patients as early as 1896 by Mr W.H. Hayles, a member of the staff of the Cavendish Laboratory, together with Mr Everett. Mr Hayles was said to be probably the first man in England to take an X-ray.[1]

It was in December 1902 that the possibility of obtaining an X-ray machine at Addenbrooke's was discussed. 'Röntgen photographs which in many surgical cases are necessary' were taken privately and were costing the Hospital about £20 a year. Money was collected by various Friends of the Hospital and, in October 1903, an X-ray apparatus was obtained from the Cambridge Instrument Company for £60.17s.4d. How successfully it was used is not recorded but there were evidently many technical difficulties.

In February 1905, the Surgeons were made responsible for taking their own X-rays, 'to be developed by a photographer in the town'. Only a month later it was agreed that the House Surgeon should take the X-rays, 'except in special cases'. About a year later the medical staff reported that this procedure was unsatisfactory. The Committee approved their recommendation that Mr Field, the Dispenser, should undertake the X-ray work and be paid 2s. for 'taking and developing each skiagram'.

In July Mr Field was authorised to visit London 'for the purpose of obtaining all the information he possibly can in connection with radiography and the X-ray apparatus'. In January 1907, Mr Field duly visited London and spent one day with Dr Hugh Walsham who was in charge of the X-ray apparatus at St Bartholomew's Hospital. Mr Field continued to combine the duties of Dispenser and Radiographer and when, in 1909, Dr Shillington Scales was appointed Honorary Medical Officer in charge of the X-Ray Department, he acted as his assistant.

The next important expansion of the facilities for diagnostic radiology came in 1914 when new X-ray rooms were taken over and an appeal was launched for £250 for a new apparatus to make 'instantaneous skia-graphs'. This appeal emphasises the value of a machine with which it would be possible to take skiagraphs of children without anaesthetic and reminds us of the very long exposure required with the early machines.

Radiotherapy at Addenbrooke's began in 1909. The Hospital was, as usual, desperately short of money. It was epidemic scalp ringworm which made it possible to acquire new apparatus, partly at the expense of Cambridgeshire County Council. Scalp ringworm was a serious public health problem among school children. Before the introduction of the antibiotic griseofulvin it was often necessary to keep infected children away from school for as long as a year, unless temporary hair loss could be induced by X-rays. In 1909 the Cambridgeshire County Council asked the Hospital to undertake this treatment and offered to pay half the cost of the necessary apparatus. It was decided that a new Siemens apparatus would be suitable for the ringworm cases and the general purposes of the Hospital. It was purchased at the end of 1909 and was in use by the early months of 1910, under the supervision of Dr Shillington Scales, assisted, of course, by Mr Field who was voted an extra £15 per annum for this work.

Although the Hospital lagged behind many others in making use of X-rays in diagnosis and treatment, it was unusually fortunate in finding in Dr Shillington Scales a man exceptionally well qualified to take charge of these potentially dangerous machines.

He was born in London in 1867 and qualified as an engineer. He was interested in the application of the physical sciences to medicine and published books on microscopy and electro-cardiography. He did not come up to Cambridge as a student until 1902. He took the Natural Sciences Tripos in 1905, and it was to qualify for the appointment to the Hospital that he took the M.B. examination in 1909. He remained a practical engineer, making much of the equipment for his department. He later gained a great reputation as a teacher of radiology and electrology. In the early days he must have been one of the relatively few medical men who fully understood the scientific basis of the work he was doing, for it would not be unjust to describe many of the early radiologists as enthusiastic amateur photographers.

~ 333 ~

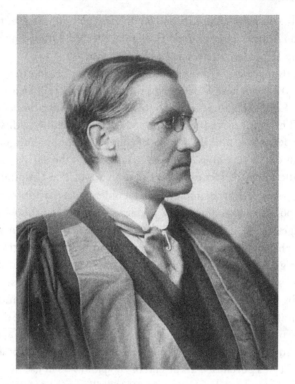

Fig. 50. Francis Shillington Scales, 1867–1927

It proved difficult to find accommodation for the new department. It was finally decided to adapt the sitting room used by the laundry maids but it was not until November 1912 that the Medical Committee drew attention to the dangers of working under such cramped conditions.

The work of the X-Ray Department had been steadily increasing and it was presumably to attempt to reduce the volume that it was agreed that recommendations for X-ray be signed by one of the senior medical staff, or in their absence by a House Surgeon in the case of emergency.[2]

When the first war-wounded reached the Hospital in December 1914, the House Sub-Committee agreed to charge the army 2s. per skiagraph; this would cover the cost of the plates and make it possible to compensate Mr Field for his extra work in developing them.

After 1915 a similar amount was charged to the County for the chest X-rays for the tuberculosis patients.

In August 1919, the impending departure of the Sister of the X-Ray Department prompted Scales to propose a review of the staffing of this department. He had four sisters in ten years and it took six months to train them and even then some of the work was too arduous for a woman. He suggested a trained male assistant should be appointed in the place of the Sister at a salary of £200 per annum; he would pay £50 out of his own pocket and in return would get some help with his private work. The assistant would take X-rays, give treatment and do repairs.

Meanwhile, numerous reports of X-ray damage had appeared in the medical journals and at its meeting on 28 May the General Committee approved the following X-ray certificate: 'I herebye consent to . . . undergoing X-ray treatment and I herebye hold the Hospital and the person who administers the treatment exempt from liability should any permanent loss of hair ensue.'

Scales insisted that the electrotherapy work should be carried out by a trained nurse under his guidance and he did not need a Sister. The only objection to this scheme was that it involved 'a male assistant and masseuse working together'. After much discussion it was agreed that a part-time assistant should be employed at £120 per annum. He would work in the Hospital from 9 a.m. to 3.30 p.m. six days a week. Ernest Mann of Soham was engaged as the assistant.

In 1922[3] it was pointed out that the X-Ray Department had from the beginning been hampered by the fact that the current from the town mains was alternating and that rectification to direct current had to be carried out with a dynamo. The dynamo originally installed was quite inadequate and the electric lift disturbed the use of the apparatus. The University, finding direct current essential, had installed its own power station from the Downing Street site; it was near enough to the Hospital to allow this source of supply to be used. Electricity from this source would not cost more than was now paid to the Cambridge Electricity Supply Company. A cable was, therefore, laid from the University to the Hospital. This arrangement proved to be satisfactory and the X-Ray Department functioned well enough but after 3.30 p.m. each day only emergencies could be accepted.

In December 1924,[4] a request was received for X-ray facilities for Huntingdon patients. The X-Ray Department were prepared to be helpful but thought it advisable to transfer such cases to Addenbrooke's Hospital because of the 'difficulty which would arise in making a diagnosis unless the X-ray Department is in touch with a clinician'. In 1925[5] the appointment of a clinical assistant to the X-Ray Department was approved for one year. The only applicant was Dr F. Roberts, who was appointed.

In the following year Dr Scales informed the Committee that he was due to retire at the end of December. There was some debate about the choice of his successor and eventually it was decided the post should be readvertised and that Dr Scales be asked to continue for an extra three months.

Dr Shillington Scales died on 28 February. There had been two applicants for his post, Ffrangcon Roberts and K.J. Yeo. There were further discussions and Committee meetings and, although it was eventually agreed to appoint Dr Roberts, it is clear that his arrival was as controversial as his departure proved to be.

Ffrangcon Roberts was born in 1888 in Bethesda, Carmarthenshire, where his father was a general practitioner. He won a scholarship to Clare College, Cambridge, and after gaining first class honours in both parts of his Tripos he went to St Thomas' Hospital in London for his clinical training and graduated in 1913. He returned to Cambridge as a lecturer in physiology and he was on the staff of the First Eastern General Hospital where he was in charge of nerve injuries. He was then sent to Salonika as a radiologist. At the time of his appointment he had never even seen an X-ray tube but he bought a book on the subject and studied it on the voyage out.

At the end of the war when he had taken the M.R.C.P. he returned to Cambridge and to physiology. In 1925 he took the recently established diploma in radiology and was elected to the staff of Addenbrooke's. In 1939 he joined the R.A.M.C. from which he was later invalided out.

He was very active in medical politics and in 1952 he published a book entitled *The Cost of Health* in which he predicted with remarkable precision the financial difficulties which the Health Service was later to experience. He died on 3 August 1974, at the age of 85.[6]

The University had established in June 1919 a Diploma in Medical Radiology and Electrology, which was the first of its kind in Britain. The University ran a special course; it was highly successful and in the year 1920–1 there had been 69 entries. The co-operation between the Hospital and the University appears to have been unsatisfactory, however, and in 1927[7] Dr Roberts expressed doubts about the practicality of complying with a request of the Faculty Board of Medicine that teaching facilities be given to the University lecturer. Under the circumstances it was not surprising that a University Committee for Medical Radiology gave notice of their intention to remove from the Hospital the X-ray apparatus that belonged to the University.[8] The Committee later agreed to allow the apparatus to remain in the Hospital until the next September. The

Hospital was obliged to spend £582.5s. to replace the University's apparatus.

On a number of occasions the possibility of the Hospital acquiring a supply of radium had been brought up. The Chairman attempted to raise by special appeal the £1,500 it was estimated would be required. By January 1927, the Radium Fund had reached £1,166.18s.od. and the Secretary[9] was authorised to order radium and equipment to the value of £1,405, with the Hospital providing the balance.

The relationship between Dr Roberts and the Governors was no better than that with the University. In July 1928,[10] the Governors had refused to allow Dr Roberts the use of the lecture room for special classes during the long vacation term, on the grounds that it was 'practically in constant use'. The following March they received a report that they had requested on the cost of the X-Ray Department since his appointment. The report showed that a total of £2,427.9s.5d. had been spent including £1,872.12s.od. for new apparatus. It should, however, be said that some of this expense was probably due to improved accommodation for the Department and the replacement of equipment which Dr Roberts considered was out of date and dangerous, the medical staff having supported him in this.

In 1931 a donor, at first anonymous,[11] but later revealed to be Mrs Douty, the widow of the former Surgeon to the Hospital, gave the funds for the construction of the Douty X-Ray Clinic. It was opened on 25 November 1932. The formal opening was performed by Sir Humphry Rolleston, first President of the British Institute of Radiology and a friend of Dr Douty. It was said that the new clinic was the brainchild of Dr Roberts and the architect Mr William Keay, who had visited French, German and Austrian clinics over a period of three years and coupled this experience with their own ideas in its design.[12]

The commemorative programme included a description of the department and a chart showing the increase in the number of X-ray examinations from 483 in 1917 to 3270 in 1931.

By 1937, however, the inadequacy of the accommodation provided by the Douty Clinic was becoming obvious.[13] The honorary staff requested that a whole-time paid assistant to the radiologist should be appointed. The Governors suggested that a second Honorary Radiologist should be appointed as they were concerned about the out-patient delays and the lack of cover during the holidays.

Mrs Rees-Mogg presented £1,000 and after much discussion Dr A.

Maxwell-Evans was appointed as Assistant Radiologist.[14] He stayed only about four months[15] and Roberts was authorised to engage temporary help since Professor Ryle said he could provide a research worker in the department on 1 October next.

In October 1939,[16] the General Committee agreed in principle to a request from Roberts that the Research Assistants[17] Drs J.S. Mitchell and F.R. Berridge should be allowed to carry on his practice at the Hospital during his absence on active service, and a financial arrangement was suggested. This was similar to an arrangement likely to be made in London, whereby the Hospital was to receive one third of the receipts and the remaining two thirds was to be shared between the owner of the practice and his locums. (The next month it was agreed that the salary of Dr Roberts' lay assistant, K. Titterington, was to be first charge on the gross receipts.)[18]

Mitchell and Berridge were also appointed to deputise for Roberts on the therapeutic and diagnostic sides respectively. They had been appointed to the department because the work was too much for Roberts alone.[19]

But less than a year later, trouble had brewed in the X-Ray Department and a Special Meeting of the General Committee was called[19] to consider 'a very difficult matter . . .'

Roberts had returned from military service and resumed control of the X-Ray Department, and now Professor Ryle, Dr Berridge (who was a full-time member of the Emergency Medical Service and available for work at the County Infirmary, Mill Road, and Newmarket as well as Addenbrooke's) and Dr Mitchell were all threatening to resign unless he could be persuaded to retire. Ryle thought that 'Dr Roberts' return to the X-Ray Department so jeopardises efficient running and so interferes with and upsets the work of others that the position was impossible.'

The General Purposes Committee had had a one-and-a-half hour discussion. They thought it essential that the services of one or both of the present Medical Assistants should be retained and they resolved that Roberts should be invited to resign. Berridge and Mitchell must stay as heavy demand would probably be made on the department if there were air raid casualties.

There had apparently been difficulties between Roberts, Ryle and the research doctors on a previous occasion over a year ago but this had been overcome after a good deal of effort.

Roberts had been interviewed but had not offered to resign, in fact the

Chairman thought he would challenge the decision and a letter had indeed been received from his solicitors.

The General Committee resolved unanimously to take legal advice as to the steps required to remove Dr Roberts from his post but agreed that Roberts should have the opportunity to express his point of view.

Messrs Hempsons of Henrietta Street, London, solicitors, were consulted.[20]

Roberts approached both the B.M.A. and the London and Counties Medical Protection Society and, in August 1940,[21] members of the General Purposes Committee had a meeting with Dr Hill, deputy Secretary of the B.M.A. Dr Hill suggested, on behalf of both societies that the case should be referred to an independent committee. The General Purposes Committee made certain counter-proposals; briefly, these were that the case should go before a single lawyer arbitrator and that Roberts should meanwhile take sick leave.

The arbitration was decided upon[22] and in the interim the Chairman of the General Committee was to write to members of the honorary staff on active service and approach those at home, together with members of the General Committee, in order to collect evidence.

The statements gathered were sent to Counsel[23] who advised a compromise, saying that he thought the Hospital's case would be proved but much would be made of Roberts being deprived of his position after returning from the Forces and that efforts would be made to prove the trouble had arisen out of a personal quarrel with Ryle.

The compromise arrived at took the form of an undertaking[24] by Roberts not to interfere with the work of Berridge and Mitchell or anyone appointed in their place but to 'consult with and co-operate with' them; to 'treat all patients with consideration and refrain from personally questioning any patients as to their eligibility to receive treatment in the hospital'; and that if the General Committee were to appoint another physician to share the charge of the X-Ray Department or work in it, that 'I will loyally support the Committee in giving effect to such decision.' A Special Committee was to organise the Department.

Roberts returned to duty on 7 April.[25]

When the Radiotherapeutic Centre became an independent department at the Leys School in March 1943, Dr J.S. Mitchell was made director.[26] He went to Canada for a year on a research project at the request of the Government[27] recommencing at Addenbrooke's in December 1945,[28] then he took up the new chair of Radiotherapeutics.

When the Leys School was closed down as an annexe of Addenbrooke's after the war, the radiotherapy machines were temporarily stored.[26] One was used briefly on the ground floor of the Cavendish Laboratory until the prefabricated hut promised by the Government was put up on the Hospital site and opened in October 1946.

~ 38 ~

Efforts to improve the nurses' pay and training

The commitment of so many members of the Hospital medical staff to the Army at the outbreak of the First World War left the Hospital danger-ously understaffed and was paralleled in the nursing arrangements.

Miss Constance Crookenden (Fig. 51), Matron of Cray Valley Hospital since 1908, was, in August 1913,[1] appointed to succeed Miss M.G. Montgomery as Matron of Addenbrooke's and succeeded her also as Matron of the First Eastern General Hospital. Miss Crookenden had trained at St Thomas' Hospital 1899–1902 and became State Registered in 1921. She was State Registered Nurse No. 81. She took up her duties in October 1913.

The General Committee had over the years given its support to the Queen Alexandra's Imperial Military Nursing Service, guaranteeing to supply six nurses in time of war or national emergency. These were requisitioned in the early days of the war, two going to work in France, and Miss Till, Sister of Bowtell Ward, volunteered for service with Queen Alexandra's Naval Nursing Service. The Matron, Assistant Matron, Out-patients' Sister, Sister of the X-Ray and Electrical Department, Night Sister, and Sister of Griffith Ward were all mobilised for duty at the First Eastern General Hospital.[2]

The general shortage of nurses was so great that the General Com-mittee felt obliged[3] to ignore Matron's protest at the presence of Volun-tary Aid Detachments (V.A.D.s) gaining experience in the wards. The 'Voluntary Aid Detachments' had been organised in 1909 by a joint Committee of the British Red Cross Society and the Order of St John of Jerusalem. V.A.D.s, who were often virtually untrained but considered themselves socially superior to the regular nurses, were to be for many years a root cause of jealousy and ill feeling.

There had been demands for the State Registration of nurses since at least the 1880s although Florence Nightingale disapproved. Mrs Bedford Fenwick, the vigorous ambitious former Matron of St Bartholomew's

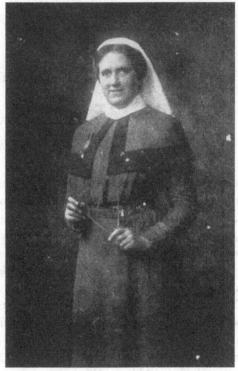

Fig. 51. Miss Constance Crookenden, Matron of Addenbrooke's,
1913–1921.

Hospital, to which post she had been appointed in 1882 at the age of 25,
founded the British Nurses Association in 1887 which worked for State
Registration and from 1891 maintained its own register. The College of
Nursing, established in 1916, had an eye to registration too and the Nurses
Registration Act became law in 1919.

The proposed Register was a subject of controversy for years. Viscount
Knutsford of the London Hospital wrote to Addenbrooke's Governors in
June 1914,[4] asking them to support opposition to the Bill for the State
Registration of Nurses then before Parliament. The Governors pledged
their support.

So serious had the nursing shortage become by 1915 that the House
Sub-Committee[5] decided to increase the salaries of probationers from £5
to £8 for the first year, from £10 to £12 for the second, while the third
year remained at £20, and a few months later increased the salaries of
Sisters to £40 p.a.[6] Sisters at the Eastern General Hospital were paid £50
p.a.

In January, 1916, the question of the registration of nurses was raised again by a letter from Mr Arthur Stanley, Chairman of the Joint War Committee, British Red Cross Society and Order of St John, who said: 'There is no unanimous feeling either amongst those responsible for the training of Nurses or amongst Nurses themselves in favour of any system of State Registration. Nevertheless I am convinced that something should be done at once to co-ordinate the various interests involved . . .' He suggested founding a College of Nursing.[7]

This time the Governors, at least those attending the House Sub-Committee[8] were in favour of registration and also of a College of Nursing 'on the lines of the Royal College of Physicians and Surgeons'.

Many nurses joined the Nursing Service of the army and navy as soon as they had completed their years of training. A return made at the request of the War Office in November 1916[9] showed that only three nurses in the Hospital held a certificate of three years' training, and only ten more were due to be certified in the next year. There were 32 probationers of whom 11 would finish training in 1918 and 21 in 1919.

In May 1917,[10] the Hospital received an appeal from Lord Derby, Secretary of State for War, for nurses with a three-year certificate of general training to join military service. He had not picked a good time; several nurses had been off duty unwell, and one had contracted diphtheria and was being looked after by two special nurses who had had to be engaged for the purpose. Matron told the House Sub-Committee that one nurse, Nurse Lane, had joined the Military Nursing Service, and another, Nurse Jennings, had promised to do so but beyond this she held out no hope of further assistance in the matter. The Matron's salary was increased, perhaps because of the difficulties of the time, from £100 p.a. to £120 p.a. with the usual allowance of £5 p.a. for uniform and board, etc.

At the beginning of the next year[11] it was resolved to increase the salaries of the rest of the nursing staff as from 1 January and for the duration of the war. The Assistant Matron was to get £60 for the first year, £65 for the second, and £70 for the third year, the Night Sister £45 for the first year and £50 for the second, Ward Sisters £40 for the first year, £45 for the second, and £50 for the third, the X-ray Sister £45 for the first year, £50 for the second, and £55 for the third, and probationers' salaries were to go up from £8 to £12 for the first year, from £12 to £16 for the second, from £20 to £24 for the third, and from £25 to £30 for the fourth. It was only a year and a half however before more rises had to be implemented.

In February 1918,[12] the Matron's salary was increased again, this time to £150 p.a. with £5 p.a. for uniform. In the September of that year[13] the House Sub-Committee agreed that owing to the rationing of gas the nurses should be allowed only candles in their bedrooms and they should not have more than four baths each per week. Things did not improve; there was an influenza epidemic in the town at the end of that year and 'very few members of the staff escaped'.[14]

In 1919 some landlords and landladies required back the rooms hitherto occupied by nurses[15] in order to let them out to members of the University returning from the war. This was in spite of an allowance apparently made in the rent of Hospital properties in which nurses stayed[16] and resulted in an acute shortage of accommodation.[17] More nurses were also required, both to take some of the heavy load off those already engaged and to meet 'modern requirements' and this made the situation even more serious.[18] The Hospital authorities hoped that money from the War Memorial Committee's appeal might help here as for some other of the Hospital's needs and, although they did not get as much as they hoped for,[19] a new Nurses' Home was completed in 1924.

Salaries went up again in 1919.[20] The Assistant Matron was entitled to £70 p.a. rising by annual increments of £5 to a maximum of £90, but the present holder, Miss Leach, who had only recently been demobilised[21] and held the Royal Red Cross, first class,[22] was to receive £80 p.a. rising annually towards the maximum. The X-ray Sister was to receive £60 p.a. rising by annual increments of £5 to a maximum of £80. The Night Sister was to receive £5 p.a. more than the Ward Sisters under similar conditions. The Ward Sisters were to receive £50 p.a. rising by annual increments to a maximum of £70 p.a., and the probationers' salaries were to go up from £12 to £16 p.a. for the first year, from £16 to £20 for the second year, from £24 to £28 for the third year, and from £30 to £35 for the fourth year.

The Matron's principal problems immediately after the war were, as has already been shown, a shortage of probationers and a shortage of accommodation for nurses and masseuses.

A shortage of probationers was the experience of hospitals throughout the country. During the war, girls had successfully held down well-paid jobs, previously the province of men. They were reluctant to accept the rigid discipline and poor pay of hospital nurses. An advertisement in the *Nursing Mirror* brought only four applications, all from unsuitable candidates;[23] it was agreed to advertise after Christmas in the *Nursing Post*, *The Church Times* and *The Times*, but to no avail. Eight nurses were leaving in

August[24] and there were no probationers coming. The Matron was authorised to engage Staff Nurses at £45 p.a., rising to £50 after six months, and Humphry Ward was temporarily closed.

Various attempts to make the conditions of service of probation more attractive did not go far enough. These changes included the introduction of a 56-hour week[25] although this would require the engagement of additional probationers. Since these probationers were not obtainable six additional Staff Nurses were authorised[26] to make possible the introduction of the shorter week, but six months later[27] the shortage of nurses still made it impossible to implement the 56-hour week although three wards were closed.

It is not surprising that Miss Crookenden, the Matron, decided to resign.[28] She did so after eight years in her post, in June 1921, to become proprietress of a nursing home. Later, in 1924, she was to found the Addenbrooke's Missionary Guild which made a link with St Stephen's Hospital, Delhi.

There were 31 applicants for her post[29] at Addenbrooke's and Miss Annie Common Bell was appointed and began work in October. She had trained at St Thomas' Hospital 1910–1914, had been Assistant Matron at Northampton General Hospital 1918–1920 and was Matron at Herefordshire General Hospital. She became State Registered in 1922 and was No. 4950.

The new Matron's duties, apart from taking measures to overcome the shortage of nurses, included the introduction of the new curriculum which the General Nursing Council (G.N.C.) had introduced and which the Nursing Committee had agreed to arrange.[30] In July 1922 the Matron attended a conference called by the G.N.C. at which the syllabus was finally agreed. The first compulsory State Examination would be held in 1925 but a voluntary examination would be held in 1924 as some hospitals had introduced the training syllabus in 1921.[31]

A badge was designed[32] which would be presented, on payment of 5s., to each nurse on the completion of her training, together with her certificate of training. It showed the University, County, and Borough arms together with a view of the front of the Hospital.

In October 1922, the Hospital was notified by the G.N.C. that it had been approved by the General Nursing Council for England and Wales as a training school for nurses.[33] The provision of a Sister Tutor presented problems. Eventually[34] it was agreed to share a Sister Tutor with the West Suffolk General Hospital; she would spend three days each week in each hospital. Miss J.E. Whittam was appointed at £120 p.a. with board, lodging, washing, indoor uniform, plus travelling expenses. She was to start on 19 February.

The Building Committee was asked to consider the provision of more accommodation for nurses, but finding the nurses to occupy it remained a problem. In February 1922, advertisements for Staff Nurses brought no applicants. The salary was raised from £45 to £50, and to £55 for those who had their midwifery certificate.[35] Only one suitable applicant answered the next advertisement.[36] A partial solution to the nursing shortage was provided by entering into agreements with other hospitals to help with the training of their probationers.

Miss Bell evidently did not find her work congenial. As early as June 1923,[37] she asked for a testimonial as she was applying for another appointment. She made a further unsuccessful attempt to leave in April 1925,[38] and the following month was appointed Matron of the General Infirmary at Salisbury.[39] Gertrude Moggach was chosen from a large field to succeed her.

Miss Moggach[40] trained at the Bradford Royal Infirmary 1912–1915 to which she returned as Sister and Night Superintendent after spending a year in the army. She then became Sister at the West London Hospital, Night Sister and Assistant Matron at the Royal Hospital for Sick Children, Aberdeen, Assistant Matron at the Preston Royal Infirmary and finally, in March 1924, Matron at the General Infirmary, Bury. She had become State Registered in 1922.

The shortage of nurses continued. Miss Moggach appointed a Home Sister for the first time[41] in 1925. Her duties were, among other things, to take charge of the Maids' Annexe, preside at the servants' meals, assist with the care of the linen, and act as required for relief duty of the Assistant Matron and the Night Sister.

In April 1926,[42] Lord Knutsford wrote with some suggestions and mentioned that the wages of Sisters and nurses appeared to be rather low. It is not clear whether his advice had been sought. The Secretary-Superintendent was asked to make enquiries of other similarly sized hospitals for particulars of salaries paid and uniforms provided. He approached nine hospitals and as a result the salaries of probationers and Staff Nurses were raised[43] and more uniform provided for the probationers. Sisters' salaries had been raised when Lord Knutsford's letter was received.[44]

Some of Miss Moggach's reforms were not kindly received by the

Sisters. It had long been the custom that Sisters' rooms off the wards should be used as their private sitting rooms; until the 1880s many Sisters had also used the room as a bedroom. A proposal from the House Committee that Sisters' rooms should no longer be used as private sitting rooms (since a general Sisters' sitting room had been provided in the Peckover Home) was referred to the General Committee. It was also thought that Sisters should not appear in the wards except in uniform, and when off duty should separate themselves from the wards.[45]

Enquiries at six other hospitals showed they were agreed on the new policy of Sisters having a general sitting room and the House Committee was equally divided on the problem. The General Committee confirmed the original decision but only by seven votes to six.[46]

Later, however, the General Committee rescinded their resolve[47] and referred the matter back to the House Committee. In March three Sisters submitted their resignations – 'under the present regime they find it impossible to continue their work'. The proposed loss of their private sitting room was not their only grievance; they also objected to the Matron's rule that Sisters of wards on the same floor should not go off duty together. The Matron replied that other hospitals had the same rule.[48] A compromise solution to the problem of the Sisters' rooms was eventually approved. The Sisters' rooms were only to be available for the Sisters' use whilst in uniform and on no occasion after 10.30 p.m.; they might, however, keep their personal effects in their rooms and take tea there.[49]

This decision seems to have satisfied the Sisters for, in September 1927,[50] the following letter was read to the General Committee: 'The Sisters wish to thank the Committee for providing such a prettily furnished general sitting room for their use when off duty. It is a most comfortable little room and is much appreciated.'

Nurses in training were still being received from other hospitals but there cannot have been a shortage at Addenbrooke's any longer for, in October 1927, the Nursing Committee reviewed the situation and recommended changes in the Affiliation agreements.[51]

There were at that time fourteen probationers from other hospitals – four from the Brompton Hospital, one from the Saffron Walden Hospital, and nine from the Wisbech Hospital – compared with 34 from Addenbrooke's itself. The Matron thought that the proportion of outside probationers to those belonging to the hospital was unduly large 'and that as the training at Wisbech was not equal to that at Addenbrooke's, the probationers coming from Wisbech had an unsettling effect upon those belonging to the hospital and that this was accentuated by the outside probationers being sometimes senior in standing to the home probationers.' Some minor adjustments were made.

In January 1928,[52] the Matron reported the resignation (after six years) of the Assistant Matron, Miss McLean, who was seriously ill and had been advised to give up work immediately. She was sent a letter of sympathy and paid her salary until the end of March, then the end of June,[53] then the end of September,[54] then until the end of December[55] since as late as October she was said to be still seriously ill. Mrs Lamplugh was recommended for her position[56] but only stayed a year.[57] She had trained at Addenbrooke's, then was Sister of the Out-patient Department, and before her appointment had been Assistant Matron and Sister Tutor at the Guest Hospital, Dudley.

The Matron herself was ill in June 1928. The Secretary-Superintendent reported to the House Committee[58] that she was off duty through illness and that on 7 June she had undergone a severe operation by Mr Arthur Cooke. She was off again in April 1930, when she was given sick leave to go to Droitwich for a month as she was suffering from rheumatism;[59] it seems with hindsight that the work at the top of the nursing hierarchy was proving rather much for its incumbents.

During the Matron's absence Mrs Lamplugh, the Assistant Matron, acted for her, and the former Sister Tutor, Miss Whittam, was engaged for three months to act as Deputy Assistant Matron.[60] The Matron was back at work by August, however, when she is found reporting to the House Committee.[61]

At the beginning of 1929 it was decided that the Sister Tutor should be allowed to spend more time at Addenbrooke's since, owing to the larger number of nurses now being employed there, she said she was unable to give sufficient time to them on the current basis of spending two days away each week. The agreements with the Huntingdon and Wisbech Hospitals whereby each had one day of the Sister Tutor's time were reconsidered and that with Huntingdon was terminated, the Nursing Committee considering the one extra day allowed to be sufficient[62] for their purposes.

The Matron seems then to have turned her attention to the off-duty time and holidays of the nursing staff and decided it was more than adequate. First she obtained permission for the holidays of the Sisters who worked 50 hours per week to be altered from five weeks per year to four weeks plus a long weekend, and for the off-duty time for nurses to be reduced to two hours on each of three days a week, and three hours on two days, instead of three hours on each weekday as it had been. They retained four hours off duty on Sundays and one day off in each week. She is said to have thought this would be acceptable to the nurses as it might have the effect of reducing the period of training to three years instead of it having to be extended to three and a half years to pass the State Examinations.[63]

She then suggested that nurses in training should have three weeks' holiday a year instead of four because, she explained, the present system by which they took their holiday in two parts, a week after six months and three weeks after a year, led to the difficulty of arranging for two breaks in the first year when it was necessary for them to have special teaching to be able to sit for the Preliminary State Examinations. It also led to problems for nurses who lived at a distance from Cambridge and were unable to meet the expense of taking two holidays a year.

The Nursing Committee recommended the reduction,[64] and so did the House Committee, but the General Committee[65] asked them to think again. The reason for this was probably the fact that it had caused a minor rebellion amongst the nurses. Details are not given in the Minutes[66] but the nurses apparently wanted their holidays to remain unaltered and came to some sort of agreement between themselves, no doubt with the idea of persuading the Committee members to change their minds. They also seem to have made other complaints, including one about their hours: the average number of hours worked was shown to be 60 approximately. As a result of this the Matron was asked to draw up an amended timetable which adhered to the 56-hour week.

Two months later the desired timetable was produced but as the off-duty times for the Night Nurses were thought inadequate 'the Secretary-Superintendent was instructed to ascertain from the Matron, on her return from her holidays, if the return is correct in this respect, or if it needs amendment . . .'[67] In view of the complaint by 35 of the nurses in their letter to the Nursing Committee Chairman 'that Nurses are frequently on night duty for five months at a time working an 84 hour week with only one night off in a month' it was agreed the Matron should be told 'that the Nursing Committee do not consider that any Nurse should be on night duty for a longer period than three months at a time.' A new timetable was subsequently approved (see Table 9).

Meanwhile the enlargement of the Peckover Nurses' Home was proceeding which meant that some nurses were temporarily accommodated in Bowtell Ward which had been closed to patients,[68] and as advertisements had failed to produce any applications it was agreed to

Table 9. Nurses' timetable, 1929

Timetable for nurses on day duty

Breakfast	Wards	Lunch	Dinner	Wards	Tea	Off duty	Supper	Bedroom	Lights out
6.40a.m. or 10a.m.	7a.m.	10a.m. to 10.45a.m.	1.15p.m. or 2p.m.	1.45p.m. or 2.30p.m.	4.30p.m. or 5p.m.	8.30p.m.	7.30p.m. or 8.30p.m.	10p.m.	10.30p.m.

Off duty time: One whole day each week. Three hours daily on two days a week, two hours on three days a week, and four hours on Sunday.

Timetable for nurses on night duty

Breakfast	Wards	Midnight meal	Dinner	Off duty	Bed
8.10p.m.	8.30p.m.	Nurses are relieved for this meal	8.15a.m.	8.15a.m. to noon	12.30p.m. (12.45p.m. Sundays)

Two nights off are given monthly.

offer higher rates of pay for new Staff Nurses. The rate for a State Registered Nurse with the C.M.B. certificate was raised from £60 p.a. to £65 and that for State Registered Nurses from £50 p.a. to £60 p.a. which was what other hospitals were offering.[69] A month later it was realised the post of Assistant Matron could not be filled at the salary offered either, namely £100 rising by £5 to £120 p.a., and the Nursing Committee agreed that it should be readvertised at £120 rising by £5 p.a. to a maximum of £140 p.a.[70] which did result in a number of applications. At the same time consideration was given to the Matron's request for an increase to her salary which had commenced in September 1925 at £180 p.a. and had been increased a year later to £200 p.a. Comparisons were made with the salaries paid in five other hospitals, all of which paid their Matrons more, and then the Chairman intimated he would propose a rise of £50 p.a. although apparently no recommendation was decided.[71] The House Committee resolved not to recommend the increase either but the General Committee disagreed and Matron received her rise.[72]

A timetable for the nursing staff was then approved as outlined in Table 9.[73]

The question of offering a gold medal for the best all round nurse in training had been under consideration for two years,[74] the matron being in favour. In October 1929, it was decided to accept an offer from Mr Bowen (probably Mr W.H. Bowen, Honorary Surgeon in charge of the Ear, Nose and Throat Department) for £100 for the endowment of a gold medal in perpetuity but the regulations for its award were not approved for another year.

The General Committee had been considering at intervals the possibility of joining the Federated Superannuation Scheme for Nurses and Hospital Officers that had been prepared by the King Edward's Hospital Fund for London and which had by this time been adopted by 103 London hospitals associated with the Fund and by 111 provincial hospitals. The details had been gone into and it was found that 30 members of the administrative and nursing staffs would be eligible and the cost to the Hospital if it joined the scheme would be £483 p.a.[75] Only recently a favoured applicant for the post of Theatre Sister[76] had said she would not accept the post unless arrangements were made for the continuance of her membership of the Pension Scheme. She did not get the job but it was an indication of the times and there must have been some pressure on the Governors to fall into line.

It was agreed to adopt the scheme and, in March 1930, various regulations were made out. The scheme was to be compulsory for all eligible employees joining the Hospital after 1 April 1930. Officers whose salary was over £100 p.a. and nurses who were State Registered were eligible. Two members of the Dispensary staff, one member of the X-Ray Department, two masseuses, three office staff, fifteen nurses and the Matron joined.[77]

There was more evidence of low pay at Addenbrooke's when the Matron reported she had failed to obtain a Staff Midwife at £65 p.a. as other hospitals offered not less than £70 p.a., and she also asked for a higher rate of pay for nurses trained at Addenbrooke's who remained on as Staff Nurses after passing the State Examination, who were still apparently only receiving £50 p.a. These matters were referred to the Nursing Committee[78] who appear to have written to the College of Nursing.

The Nursing Committee was also requested by the House Committee to interview in future all candidates recommended for appointment as Sisters. It was decided to ascertain the procedure adopted at the Norwich, Ipswich, Reading, Oxford, Guy's and St Bartholomew's Hospitals[79] but after doing so and finding that their Nursing Committees, like Addenbrooke's, accepted the Matron's appointments, and being told that the Matron when appointing a Sister consulted the medical staff, they decided to retain the present practice.[80]

The regulations for the award of the Catherine Bowen Medal were approved in November 1930.[80] The medal was to be of gold and inscribed on one side with the name of the Hospital and of the medal, the name of the recipient and the year of the award, and on the other 'In aeturnum misericordia aedificabitur'. It was to be given to the nurse who obtained the highest number of marks during the three years of her training, these being awarded for a number of virtues such as general conduct, neatness and academic work. It was not to be given if the marks obtained were not at least 80% of the total maximum available, and if the nurse with the highest number of marks had at some time committed an act which was detrimental to the honour of the award then the gold medal was to go to the nurse with the second highest number of marks.

Quotations of £6.10s. had been received for the special dies and £4 for the medal itself if it was in 15-carat gold, and £5 if it was in 18-carat gold. The chairman of the Nursing Committee promised to give a replica medal in silver as a second prize.

At the same meeting it was agreed to accede to the request of Canon

Crookham, Chairman of the North Cambridgeshire Hospital, and issue a training badge to their nurses who were at present without one. It was suggested that the badge should bear on its face 'North Cambridgeshire Hospital, Wisbech, affiliated to Addenbrooke's Hospital, Cambridge'.

The Wisbech Hospital had recently had the services of the Sister Tutor, which had been shared with Addenbrooke's, withdrawn because of the larger number of nurses now at Cambridge.[81]

A discussion on nursing salaries now followed. The College of Nursing had produced a report on what it considered should be the minimum salaries of members of nursing staffs from the Matron downwards.[80] Addenbrooke's made some enquiries as to the rates of pay at other hospitals, found they did not come off too badly out of the comparisons, and made some recommendations. The Matron, for example, who was currently receiving £250 p.a. was to have her salary increased by annual increments of £10 to a maximum of £300 p.a. and State Registered Staff Nurses, who appear to have been getting £50 p.a. were to have their salaries raised to £60 p.a. The Assistant Night Sister was to get the same as Ward Sisters, namely £75 p.a. rising by annual increments of £5 to £90 p.a.,[82] although what she was receiving before is not stated. Later,[83] the Out-patient Sister, who had been receiving £70 p.a. rising by annual increments of £5 to £85 p.a. was awarded the same salary as Ward Sisters, and the Theatre Sister had a rise to £85 p.a. increasing by annual increments of £5 to £100 p.a. instead of £80 increasing by increments of £5 to £90 p.a.

The first Catherine Bowen Medal (for 1930) was awarded to Nurse A. Woolerton (probably the same person who in 1947 became Assistant Matron),[84] and the silver replica medal to Miss J.C.M. Hawthornthwaite.[85] They were presented at the General Committee meeting on 28 April 1931 by the Chairman, the Revd C.A.E. Pollock, and a month later 'It was agreed to accept with grateful thanks the offer made by Mr Bowen to provide for the endowment of the Nurses Silver Medal.' For the next presentation, however, a special meeting was arranged in which the giving of the medals and other prizes was combined with a reunion of past and present members of the nursing staff.[86] This annual prize giving and nurses' reunion continued[87] until 1937 when it appears to have been replaced by a smaller event.

Nurse Woolerton was appointed Sister of Musgrave Ward about a year after she finished her training[88] and a Miss Hawthornthwaite was to become Sister of Griffith Ward.[89]

The salaries of the Out-patient Department Sister and the Theatre Sister had not been considered in the recent review and so in February[90] the House Committee recommended bringing them into line by putting the Out-patient Department Sister on to the same level as Ward Sisters, and the Theatre Sister was to receive £85 rising by annual increments of £5 to £100 p.a. instead of £80 rising by annual increments of £5 to £90 p.a.

Hospital patients were generally woken early: in January 1930 in Addenbrooke's they were having their breakfast at 6 a.m.[91] There was a move made towards later breakfast at this time and it was suggested that the breakfast time should be changed to 7 a.m. Matron was against this,[92] 'in addition to the rearrangement of all the work it would mean that the Doctor's visiting hours to the wards would have to be altered and also the times of the operating hours'. However, she agreed to a change to 8 a.m.[93] shortly before the Hospital received a request from the Isle of Ely Federation of Women's Institutes (W.I.s), said to represent some 2,000 women, who in support of a resolution passed by their National Federation, wished the Hospital to adopt the routine successfully carried out by the Middlesex Hospital where no patient was disturbed except for urgent reasons before 7 a.m.[94] The W.I. thought the present system of early waking of hospital patients for washing, etc. was 'a cause of justifiable complaint, and against the best interest of the recovery of the patient . . .'.

The Committee was able to reply with the new breakfast time and say that now patients were not called until 6 a.m., 7 a.m. was inconvenient, they said, since owing to the peculiar circumstances pertaining in provincial hospitals it would be impossible to have the wards ready for the visiting staff at 10 a.m. or to have the patients ready for the operating theatre at 9 a.m. Also, it should be borne in mind that lights were put out at night at 8 o'clock.

In 1932 with new wards being completed, the Nursing Committee examined the staff situation and the accommodation they had available for them. In 1926 the Hospital had had 190 beds with 169 on average being occupied daily; there were 73 nurses on the staff at that time. In 1931 there were 200 beds of which 194 were on average occupied, and there were 103 nurses. In 1932 there were 200 beds and 105 staff including three masseuses, one X-ray assistant and Matron.[95]

It was estimated that fifteen more staff would be required for the private wards, ten for the children's wards, five for the eye wards, and sixteen for the proposed new septic wards. Also an administrative Sister, a Sister for the X-Ray Department, and nurses for the Orthopaedic Clinic would be needed. At present there were 108 beds in the Nurses' Homes and 99 assigned.

After some adjustments to the figures it was decided that nine additional rooms had to be provided for the nursing staff and it was agreed that accommodation near the Hospital should be sought. Enquiries were to be made as to the availability of 25 and 26 Trumpington Street and the architect was to be consulted on their conversion and as to whether Nurses' Home No. 2 could be enlarged by adding on another storey (the third storey was actually added in 1933).

In November that year it was agreed to found a Preliminary Training School (P.T.S.) and it was suggested that 25 Trumpington Street should be used.[96] The P.T.S. actually opened in March 1935, in nos 25 and 26 Trumpington Street.[97]

In 1935 it was agreed to increase the Matron's salary in two annual increments of £12.10s., from £300 to £325, the first increment to be backdated to 1 October 1934.[98] Miss Moggach had apparently done much for the Hospital during her time there and probably well deserved this rise which was granted in spite of the staff's comment that on medical grounds they considered the Matron's present salary adequate.[99]

The next year[100] the Matron applied for the appointment of a Junior Administrative Sister but after collecting information on the number of members of their administrative staff from other hospitals of comparable size the appointment was considered unnecessary.[101]

An enquiry was made into the nursing administration and a report submitted to the General Committee in which it was said that there was too much overlap of work by the Matron and staff and too little delegation by Matron. 'The Committee realise that during the last few years the Matron has carried out her work in the Hospital during a time of rapid expansion and change with complete disregard for herself. She has endeavoured to carry on her own shoulders a task which is too great for any single individual. This can only be remedied by a system of delegation such as the Committee recommend.'

They suggested that the Matron be given three months leave on full pay and maintenance allowance, and that before her return the duties would be reorganised to relieve her of undue strain. A Sub-Committee had been appointed to consult with her to this end before she went on leave.

The Matron appears to have gone on leave as recommended,[102] however in September a Sub-Committee of Dr Gaskell, Mrs Peart, and Mr Butler reported that they felt a Junior Administrative Sister *was* necessary 'as the present staff is insufficient to carry out the duties and in consequence the Administrative Sisters are unable to take their off-duty times'. The Junior Administrative Sister was to be appointed at £80 p.a.

Up until the Nurses Registration Act of 1919 no basic standard of education had been required from nurses. After it the General Nursing Council still wanted to raise the standard of the profession and in 1932 passed a resolution that a test educational examination should be instituted. When no objections were received a rule was drawn up in 1935 and submitted for the Minister's approval.

A conference of interested parties was held in November 1936, at the Ministry of Health and later the British Hospitals Association (B.H.A.) sent Addenbrooke's a summary[103] of the proceedings.

It was said that the reasons for the proposed test were: the lack of general education of many candidates for the Preliminary State Examination caused a lower standard to be adopted by the General Nursing Council than was desirable; after one year's training many girls took up nursing despite a failure in the Preliminary State Examination; the lack of a preliminary test created a barrier in the minds of educated girls who might otherwise enter the profession, and their parents; and, finally, it was economically disadvantageous to train for a year girls who could never be expected to pass the professional nursing examinations.

The British Hospitals Association had consulted the views of Boards of Management and Matrons of hospitals with training schools and replied that the test might deter girls from entering the profession and would not, in view of the preliminary trial period now adopted, raise the standard of education of probationer nurses. They were assured that the test would be really simple. No girl of a reasonable standard of education could fail to pass or should be afraid of the examination.

As a result of this conference the B.H.A. was advising hospitals to support the G.N.C. in their proposed rule. Addenbrooke's wanted some points raised.

In July 1937,[104] there was a communication from the Minister of Health on the subject. The test examination for training school entrants was to begin 1 January 1938.

In May 1937,[105] a report on the accommodation available to nursing staff was made with reference to a suggestion that no. 27 Trumpington Street should be taken over to provide additional rooms. Now in the

Peckover Home, Nurses' Home No. 2, and the Maids' Home Extension there were a total of 144 bedrooms occupied by nurses and there were 155 nursing staff in this accommodation. It was recommended that no. 27 Trumpington Street should be made over to the nurses until the whole question of further accommodation had been settled.

The General Committee received a letter from the College of Nursing in October[106] appealing for the Hospital Board to establish a maximum 96-hour working fortnight. The Chairman reported that this matter had been considered by the Eastern Regional Committee (presumably of the British Hospitals Association) when the recommendation had been accepted in principle, 'and we shall endeavour gradually to introduce this schedule'. The question was referred to the House Committee 'with a view to the possible reduction of the working hours of the nursing staff'.

In November the Matron asked to be released from work in connection with housekeeping.[107] The request was referred to the Nursing Committee, but it was agreed that her living accommodation in the Nurses' Home was unsatisfactory and she was to have the ground floor and first floor in 27 Trumpington Street.

Two months later she resigned on health grounds,[108] her resignation to take effect from August. She had given thirteen years' service. The Chairman said she had done much reorganisation work to improve the efficiency of the Hospital and it was at her instigation that the Preliminary Training School was inaugurated. Although she would not be entitled to a pension for another five years a pension had been in principle agreed and she was to leave at the end of July as she had her holiday owing.

When the terms of appointment of the new Matron were considered[109] it was recommended that the housekeeping be separate from the Matron's duties and when a Housekeeper was appointed she must be responsible to a Sub-Committee of the House Committee and not be under the control of the Matron. The Matron had control of nursing and massage staff and was responsible for domestic staff; she was also responsible for nursing the patients, for seeing that food was satisfactorily served to the patients, the nurses and servants, and for organising the training of nurses. Her salary was to be £300 p.a. with annual increments of £12.10s. to £375, and her retiring age was to be 55.

The next month, March 1938,[110] the Matron asked to be released at the end of the month on account of her health. The House Committee agreed without waiting for the confirmation of the General Committee and she was given leave of absence on full pay.

Shortly afterwards[111] the General Committee decided to separate the Hospital catering from Matron's duties and place it in the hands of dieticians. They were proceeding to appoint a Dietician-Housekeeper and Assistant Dietician-Housekeeper at an early date to supercede the Nursing Housekeeper and Dietician. No. 27 Trumpington Street was to be converted for the Matron and two Dietician-Housekeepers.

Thirty-three applications were received for the Matron's position and five candidates interviewed;[112] Miss C.H. Alexander, Senior Tutor at the London Hospital was recommended and to commence duties early August.

In spite of the appeal in 1937 from the Royal College of Nursing for a 96-hour working fortnight it had still not been implemented a year later for, in September 1938,[113] the General Committee are found considering their future policy bearing in mind the facts that improvements were needed in the Maids' Home and the main kitchen and there had been a rise in the patients' waiting list over the past twelve months. The House Committee were asked to prepare a report showing the additional number of nurses and/or maids required to put the 96-hour fortnight for the nursing staff into practice, the additional staff needed should a new unit of 30 beds be built, and also the additional accommodation that would be required for staff in both these cases.

It was estimated that the nursing staff would have to be increased from 159 to 179 in order to institute the 96-hour fortnight and the increased cost of all the staff involved would be £2,670 p.a. If the maids too were to get a 96-hour fortnight, eight additional maids would be required. To staff an additional 30-bed unit, one Sister, one Staff Nurse and ten nurses in training would be required plus maids and kitchen personnel.[114] The report, together with particulars of the additional accommodation that would be needed, was referred to the Building Committee,[115] but the war appears to have supervened.

Meanwhile changes were made in the nursing curriculum in order to accept completely the General Nursing Council's regulations for training. The results of the alterations were to be that nurses on the Supplementary part of the Register (i.e. Registered Fever, Children's or Mental Nurses, or those who had passed the Preliminary State Examination) be accepted on the same standard as second-year nurses with the option of staying for a third year as a Staff Nurse if suitable; the Hospital examinations, medals and prizes were to be eliminated and more frequent tests set and corrected by the Matron and Sister Tutor; and the Hospital certificate and badge were not to be issued until the nurse had passed the State Final Examinations.[116] The sums resulting from the endowment fund for the Catherine Bowen Gold Medal were, with Mr Bowen's permission, to be spent on books for the nurses' reference library.

Now that there was a shortage of nursing staff again it must have been with a sense of relief that the House Committee greeted a request for affiliation from the Matron of St Nicholas and St Martin's Orthopaedic Hospital, Pyrford. After two years training at Pyrford, nurses would be received at Addenbrooke's as second-year nurses with corresponding pay, and stay for a further two years' training. The scheme was approved in principle and the details were to be settled later.[117]

A week later it was also agreed, after a request from the College of Nursing, that retired trained nurses should undergo a three-week post-graduate course at the Hospital to bring them up to date with nursing methods so that they would be available in the event of a national emergency.[118]

Just prior to the outbreak of war Mrs John Chivers (who was connected with the neighbouring Chivers jam firm) offered her house at Histon to the Hospital. It was found to be suitable to house the Preliminary Training School, and the transfer would free premises for housing additional nurses so the offer was gratefully accepted.[119] The Preliminary Training School was not to be moved, however, until the present accommodation was actually required.

The equipment from the Preliminary Training School was moved to Homefield, Histon, some time before[120] the end of July 1940, and training there was planned to commence on 8 August. This was considered an opportune time to begin training nursing auxiliaries, as recruits could be housed in the old Preliminary Training School. They were to have one week's training in theory and one week in practical work in the wards. Immobile and part-time auxiliaries paid a fee of 1 guinea weekly during training for board and lodgings and the Government refunded £2.9s. towards the cost of the board, lodging and laundry during training of those recruits who enrolled for full-time mobile service.

The Leys School was taken over as an annexe to Addenbrooke's and it was decided it should be established as a hospital capable of dealing with all types of case, but that it should primarily be used for the treatment of Service cases and E.M.S. patients. Miss E.M.C. Cawthorne, Matron of the Central London Throat Hospital, was appointed to the Leys and designated Sister-in-Charge.[121]

A plan was formed for trebling the capacity of the Preliminary Training School so that it held 30 probationers in order to augment the staff at the Leys. There was a general shortage of trained nurses and the Preliminary Training School had a waiting list;[122] the General Purposes Committee felt that in view of the general good some risks ought to be taken. However the plan was abandonned as 'the Ministry of Health were not prepared to accept any post-war liability, either financial, or by way of accommodation for patients and the scheme had been dependent upon such accommodation being available at the Ley's School'.[123] If there were insufficient patients available after the closing of the Leys annexe the nurses would not be able to obtain an adequate training.

For the additional work she had undertaken, the Matron, Miss C.H. Alexander, was awarded £50 for the period 1 August 1939 to 1 August 1940, and the same again for 1940–1941;[124] however she resigned[123] in the latter year to take up the post of Matron of the London Hospital. Her resignation was to take effect from 1 October.

There were 36 applications[125] for the Matron's post and Miss E.A. White, Matron at the Swansea General and Eye Hospital, was selected. She was to receive a commencing salary of £325 p.a. plus £100 p.a. during the time that the additional beds at the Leys and Examination Halls were in use. Her previous posts had included Assistant Matron at the Royal Northern Hospital, London, Assistant Matron at the Metropolitan Hospital, London, and Sister Tutor at the Prince of Wales General Hospital, and she had trained at the Leicester Royal Infirmary. She took up her duties on 21 November 1941.[126]

The shortage of nurses in some hospitals had caused the Minister of Health to pay increased rates to trained nurses in the Civil Nursing Reserve, and also to arrange for the recruitment and training of probationers and to pay them higher salaries than were in general operation. This produced certain anomalies and the Government agreed to subsidise temporarily increases that would bring the pay of all nursing staff to certain minimum levels. First-year student nurses were now to get £30 p.a., those in their second year £35 p.a., those in their third year £40 p.a., and those in their fourth year £50 p.a. until State Registered, £70 p.a. when State Registered. Staff Nurses were to get £90 p.a. Senior nurses' salaries were also to be reviewed. The General Committee[127] agreed to pay these increases as from 1 August 1941. The amount involved with regards to the 137 student nurses would be an additional expenditure on the part of the Hospital of £670 p.a. plus a Ministry grant of £670 p.a., and with regard to the seven Staff Nurses the Hospital would have to pay an extra £115.10 while the Ministry would pay £670.

In 1943 it was decided to appoint a second (Assistant) Sister Tutor.[128] The present Sister Tutor was training approximately 180 nurses instead of the maximum of 60 recommended by the Royal College of Nursing. The new appointment would cost the Hospital £300–350 p.a. It was also resolved to establish a Bursary of £100 for the purpose of enabling an Addenbrooke's trained nurse to take the Sister Tutor's course.[129] Applications were to be invited from nurses who had completed their training and left the Hospital, as well as from residents. Candidates should have had varied Hospital experience including that of holding a post as Ward Sister. The money was to come from the general funds of the Hospital and to be provided for two years; after that the matter was to be reviewed.

The Matron and Sister Tutor wanted to re-institute the Hospital examinations and no objection to this was raised.

The Matron, Miss E.A. White, resigned in 1944 as she was getting married. Her resignation was to take effect on or about 20 May.[130] Thirty-four applications were received for her post[131] and Miss L.J. Ottley, who had been Matron of the Royal Gwent Hospital, Newport, for six years, was selected.[132] She was 42 years old, had trained at the Radcliffe Infirmary, Oxford, had been one year as Charge Nurse and Holiday Sister at the Radcliffe, had done one year's private nursing, had been for three years Ward Sister and Night Superintendent at the Royal Sussex County Hospital, Brighton, for one year Sister Tutor and Home Sister at the Buchanan Hospital, St Leonards, and for two years Assistant Matron, Croydon General Hospital.[131] She took up her duties on 1 July 1944.

In September Messrs Chivers & Sons Ltd wrote asking for the premises at Histon presently being used for the Preliminary Training School to be vacated as they wanted to use them for expansion.[133] They were to be answered that the Hospital had recently bought a house in Cambridge and that, as soon as this was available for members of the nursing staff, arrangements would be made for the Preliminary Training School to leave Histon. In 1945 it moved back to Hospital premises and soon afterwards into the property known as Owlstone Croft which was to be renamed Addenbrooke's Training School, Owlstone Road.[134]

In July 1945,[135] with the Civil Nursing Reserve staff, who formed the majority of the staff in the annexes, rapidly decreasing in numbers and few candidates coming forward to take their places, the Matron reported that the nursing staff of all wards was now below the margin of safety and could not be further decreased. She suggested that School House Ward should now be closed and this was done.[136] McArthur Ward was also to be closed[137] and Holloway Ward too if the staffing position deteriorated. At the same time permission was given to the senior staff to become non-resident if they wished and the hospital was to pay £70 p.a. to landladies.

The Leys was handed back to the school authorities on 8 November 1945,[138] and the Examination Halls to the University on 28 February 1946. When the Leys closed there was an acute shortage of accommodation available for the nursing staff. Owlstone Croft, which was to be purchased for the Preliminary Training School the next year, was requisitioned by the Ministry of Health and occupied 3 November 1945. In 1946 the 'New Nurses' Home' was renamed the Nightingale Home.[139]

During the First World War, nurses had given anaesthetics.[140] In some centres the practice had been continued, although in Addenbrooke's in 1930,[141] following the death of an out-patient under an anaesthetic given by the Out-patient Sister, certain regulations had been adopted. These were to the effect that the nursing staff were not to give general anaesthetics, except rectal anaesthetics, and also that Resident Medical Officers were not to perform operations involving general anaesthesia unless a second Medical Officer was present to give the anaesthetic.

During the Second World War, owing to the shortage of skilled anaesthetists, two Sisters were trained at Addenbrooke's in the speciality. This gave rise to a controversy in the medical press,[140,142,143,144] particularly because of a finding of the Canadian High Court that the use of a nurse–anaesthetist constituted negligence on the part of the surgeon.[145] Despite this, one of the Sister–anaesthetists, Sister P.N. Kemp, continued in the job from 1940 until six months after the end of hostilities.[146]

In 1946 and 1947 the Sisters, Staff Nurses and Civil Nursing Reserve received pay rises. These were still subsidised by the Ministry of Health.[147]

In 1947 an arrangement was made with Huntingdon County Hospital whereby their student nurses were allowed to enter the Preliminary Training School before beginning training.[148] A similar arrangement had been made with the North Cambridgeshire Hospital, Wisbech, five years previously[149] when affiliation with the Royal Westminster Ophthalmic Hospital for general nursing training had also been agreed.[150] Plans were going ahead for the building of the new Hospital and meanwhile temporary buildings were to go up on the existing Hospital site in order to increase the bed complement as quickly as possible; further temporary buildings were to be provided at Owlstone Croft for the accommodation of additional nursing staff.[151]

~ 39 ~

The Training School for Nurses

Nursing before Florence Nightingale was not the honourable profession it is today; it was indeed as Florence herself said[1] '*preferred* that the nurses should be women who had lost their characters, i.e. should have had one child'. The surgeons regarded sex on demand with the nurses to be one of their perks and the packed hospital wards in which the nurses often slept, sometimes in with the male patients, were filthy, stank, and infections were rife.

When Florence returned from the Crimea she opened the Nightingale Training School for Nurses at St Thomas' in 1860. There was medical opposition as well as some support but among her allies was Sir James Paget, enior surgeon at St Bartholomew's and brother of the Cambridge physician. It may have been through his influence that Addenbrooke's opened a Training School for Nurses in 1877 under Miss Alice Fisher, who was one of the Nightingale trainees.

Miss Fisher 'was undoubtedly one of the outstanding personalities in nursing in the nineteenth century'.[2] She was born in 1839, the daughter of a distinguished astronomer and mathematician, and had published four novels by 1875. She had spent 1874–1875 at the Nightingale Training School.

In her relatively short life Miss Fisher is said to have reformed nursing in Cambridge, in Oxford, in Birmingham, and finally in one of the largest hospitals in the United States, the Blockley Hospital in Philadelphia, where she died in 1888.

Nursing at the end of the nineteenth century cannot have been much different from the way it is today from the point of view of the struggling nurse, judging by a poem published anonymously in the first, and possibly the only, edition of *The Hospital Inkstand*, November 1888, and filed away under Addenbrooke's Hospital at the local library.

THE NURSE
Who follows on with folded hands,
And listens to the Staff's demands?
Who never sits, but always stands?
The Nurse.

Who labours on with watchful eye?
Who listens to the patient's cry?
For help and comfort always by?
                    The Nurse.

Who measures out the gruesome dose?
And ope's the window when it close?
And huddles on the patient's hose?
                    The Nurse.

Who's 'jumped on' when the things go wrong,
Or when she breaks out into song,
While she's at work the hours long?
                    The Nurse.

Who's haunted by the busy broom
And duster, imps of musky gloom,
That flaps around her sleeping room?
                    The Nurse.

Who's never free from care or toil,
And turpentine and mats and oil?
Whose life's a never ending moil?
                    The Nurse.

Whose brains are tried to comprehend
The 'hows' and 'whys' the 'mar or mend'?
Who puzzles to the bitter end?
                    The Nurse.

Who glides about with stealthy tred
Silent and noiseless round each bed?
Or 'dumps' enough to wake the dead?
                    The Nurse.

Who breaks the china, burns the mat,
Misplaces this and loses that?
Bears blame borne elsewhere by the cat?
                    The Nurse.

In 1888, the year this poem was written, 30 probationers were under
training and 433 had been trained as nurses since the school began. The

Matron was M.N. Cureton, and Dr Laurence Humphry M.B. was 'Lecturer to the Nurses'.[3] The training involved 'classes of preparation' given by a Miss Young, head nurse of Griffith Ward, instruction in massage from a certificated lady masseuse residing in the Hospital, and courses of lectures given by the medical staff which were each followed by an examination. If the practical work and technical knowledge were satisfactory, certificates were awarded at the end of a year.

The next year it was decided to build a special ward for sick probationers, funded partly by the Governors, partly by the proceeds of a bazaar, and partly by friends of Miss Alice Fisher to perpetuate her memory.[4] It was completed in 1890.

By 1891 a total of 511 probationers had been trained and permission was being given to those who wished to stay on for a second year. Former students included one Lady Superintendent of a Home for Nurses, two Matrons, two Assistant Matrons, two Sisters in London Hospitals, one Sister in a Provincial Hospital and one Staff Nurse. Miss Young, who had been giving her special classes in nursing for nine years now had another appointment in Cambridge but was continuing to instruct the probationers, and a Miss Kelly had started teaching bandaging. Dr Laurence Humphry was now M.A., M.D. There were still 30 probationers being trained per year, and the Alice Fisher Ward for Sick Probationers had been 'a great comfort especially during the last Influenza epidemic'.[5] It was to so continue the next year.

In 1892 Mr Frederick Deighton became Lecturer to the Probationers. In 1893 there was no mention of Miss Young and the probationers now needed two years for a certificate. This was related to the decision during the past few years of a Lords' Committee that nurses should have at least three years' training. The Matron and Staff Nurses had all had three years in a recognised school and were members of the Royal British Nurses Association which had held its first provincial meeting in Cambridge in 1889.[6]

In 1894 Frederick Deighton was still Lecturer to the Probationers and that year he succeeded Sir G.M. Humphry as Honorary Surgeon. There was urgent need for an improvement in the probationers' sleeping accommodation because 'In the cubicles they occupy there is neither privacy nor quiet, as the Day and Night nurses share the same rooms and the sleep of the latter is frequently and unavoidably disturbed', and 'The Probationers often break down from inability to get sufficient sleep.' Accommodation for more probationers was required too, 'the supply being insufficient for the demand. During the past year £40 was expended on extra nurses.[7] Some of the Governors had suggested that the place of the charwomen be taken by ward maids and a separate building built for them and the hospital servants. Since the beginning of the school the fees paid by probationers amounted to £11,452.

The Peckover Home was begun in 1895 with extra accommodation in it and space for each nurse to 'have a room to herself and every necessary comfort'.[8] It was completed in the summer of 1896 at a cost of £4,184, £2,000 of which was given by the Lord Lieutenant, Mr A Peckover. It contained 38 bedrooms and 6 bathrooms. A covered way to the main building was built in 1897[9] and the cost met by a Mrs Adams and her friends; it was said to be 'quite an ornament to the gardens'. The architect, Mr W.M. Fawcett, gave his services gratuitously. The main part of the Cubicles Building was made over to the ward maids as sleeping accommodation.[10] Occupation of the new home was followed by a 'marked improvement in the general health of the nurses'. However three of the Staff Nurses still had to sleep in their sitting rooms off the wards.

Probationers now had to have three years' training for a certificate as a duly qualified nurse, and as a result no longer had to seek admission to other schools for the remainder of their training; Staff Nurses when off duty could leave the wards in the hands of the senior probationers. The Training School had a good reputation and was booked up for the next two years.

In addition to the usual lectures and classes, Mr Byles the House Surgeon was giving two courses of lectures on elementary anatomy and physiology.

In 1897 in his report Mr Deighton said that since the commencement of the School £15,822.7s.6d. had been received from the probationers and £5,703.3s.7d. paid out in nurses salaries. 'Addenbrooke's Hospital is unique both in the smallness of the sum paid in salaries, and in the largeness of the amount paid in fees.' He also said 'Addenbrooke's continues to keep up its good name . . . Matron has received 220 applications for 12 vacancies . . . she is constantly being asked for Addenbrooke's Nurses to fill posts in other Hospitals.'[9]

The next year the school did away with its system of having two grades of probationers, the one paying the higher fees doing the lighter work and having different privileges. Before 1896 much of the work now delegated to the ward maids had been done by the probationers paying the lower fees. Fees were set at an intermediate level between the two grades, at £10 per quarter for the first year, £5 per quarter for the second year, and the third year was free. In this third year a suitable probationer might be made a Staff Nurse and deputise for Sister. Now there were generally about 40 nurses and probationers in residence, together with eight ward maids, ten female servants and porters; 248 applications had been received for the twelve probationer vacancies.[10]

In 1898 Dr Lloyd-Jones, who had been appointed Assistant Physician, became Lecturer to the Probationers. He too was proud of the fact that 'This is the only Training School where so much is received in fees from Probationers, and where so little is paid in salaries.' The third-year probationers were still acting as Staff Nurses, and 'Several Addenbrooke's Nurses have gone out to nurse the sick and wounded in South Africa . . .'[11]

By 1901 the fees had halved and by 1903 a slight increase in nursing staff had been made to give members a day off fortnightly 'in addition to her two hours off daily'. By 1 January 1906, owing to the 'constantly growing difficulty experienced in obtaining the requisite number of probationers', fees had been abolished altogether, salaries were to be paid and the probationers also supplied with material for indoor uniforms. This change was estimated at costing the Hospital £400 per year and was said to be bound to result in an increase in salaries; however, it had resulted in 366 applications and 'rendered unnecessary the hiring of Special Nurses'.[12] Addenbrooke's was one of the latest, perhaps the last, hospital to take this course.

The next report of interest on the Training School appears during the First World War when Miss Constance C. Crookenden was Matron. Owing to the great demand for highly trained and experienced nurses to look after hospital wards, the salaries of the Sisters had been increased, and the nurses' salaries had followed suit.[13] In the following year salaries continued to rise.

Miss Crookenden's successor was Annie Bell, formerly Matron of Herefordshire General Hospital, who had trained at St Thomas'. She secured a 56-hour week for the nursing staff. This concession involved the hospital in considerable expense as additional nurses had to be engaged and then, as the Nurses' Home was not large enough, some nurses had to be lodged away from the Hospital. With a view to providing further accommodation for them, nos 12, 13, and 14 Fitzwilliam Street were purchased from St Peter's College (Peterhouse) out of the Geldart Bequest in 1921.[14] It does not sound as if the Training School had enlarged significantly, however, as in the next year only eleven nurses were awarded Certificates of Training.[15]

The State Registration of Nurses was to become compulsory in 1925, and to provide the training necessary for the State Examination, a Sister Tutor was engaged in 1923 to be shared between Addenbrooke's and the West Suffolk General Hospital at Bury St Edmunds. She was Miss J.E. Whittam, Sister Tutor of Lord Mayor Treloar Cripples' Home.[16] Addenbrooke's also had an agreement with the Brompton Hospital whereby some of their nurses received part of their training in Cambridge.

Nurses' Home No. 2 (Nightingale) was occupied in December 1924. It had 49 bedrooms and other rooms including a class room and offices. Its Memorial Tablet read

TO THE HONOURED MEMORY
OF THOSE FROM THIS COUNTY, BOROUGH AND
UNIVERSITY
WHO SERVED IN THE GREAT WAR,
AND ESPECIALLY OF THOSE WHO CARED FOR
THE SICK AND WOUNDED
THIS NURSES' HOSTEL WAS ERECTED
1924

By 1926 there were still only twelve candidates accepted for the Training School although another nine entered from the affiliated hospitals. There were a total of 48 probationers among the 73 nursing staff, the remainder consisting of one Matron, one Assistant Matron, one Home Sister, one Sister Tutor, one Night Sister, six Ward Sisters, one Theatre Sister, one Out-patient Sister, one X-ray Sister, three Masseuses and eight Staff Nurses.[17] Twelve nurses completed their three years' training and passed out of the school, five staying on as Staff Nurses.

The probationers were now paid £20 for their first year, £25 for the second, and £30 for the third, and still received help with their uniforms. The Training School was said to be 'Approved by the General Nursing Council for England and Wales'.

The number of applications received for training, the numbers accepted, and the size of the nursing staff rose steadily. By 1932 there were 126 nursing staff of whom 88 were probationers; there had been 400 applications for places in the school and 38 had been accepted. Twenty-two nurses completed their three years' training, thirteen of them remaining on for a fourth year as Staff Nurses. There were 35 candidates for the State Examinations, and the School awarded its students prizes; one of these was a gold medal that had been founded in perpetuity, to go each year to the best all-round nurse throughout her training.

At the end of 1932 Dr Haynes suggested establishing a Preliminary

Training School for candidates who wished to join the nursing staff, and the Nursing Committee provisionally agreed.[18] It was suggested that the new school should be in no. 25 Trumpington Street which would become available when the resident medical staff moved into new quarters in a year's time. It was to teach a compulsory course which would last eight weeks. There would be five groups each of eight candidates in a year.

Matron attended a special meeting of the House Committee the next year.[19] It was said that when the extension to the Hospital was built it would be necessary to admit 35 probationers a year; eight at a time should enter the Preliminary Training School. The architect Mr Keay was to be asked if the required accommodation could be provided at 25 and 26 Trumpington Street and to submit a sketch plan.

In December[20] the cost of the conversion was estimated at £1,000 but five months later[21] another £600 was said to be needed. The Preliminary Training School actually cost about £2,500 including furniture and equipment and opened in March 1935[22] to the first group of eight nurses. Only candidates with previous training and who had passed the Preliminary State Examination were exempt.

The course at the Preliminary Training School cost £5 for instruction, board, residence and laundry.[23] Probationers had then to be aged 18–30, of average height, and with a satisfactory medical certificate. At the Preliminary Training School they learned anatomy, physiology, hygiene and sanitation, dietetics, sick-room cookery, first-aid, and theoretical and practical nursing, including bandaging and practical housewifery. If satisfactory and if they passed their examinations in the Preliminary Training School, candidates entered the wards for another two months at a salary of £20 per year. They then spent the next two years ten months (making three years on the wards) as probationers. Each probationer was expected to enter for the Preliminary and Final State Examinations held by the General Nursing Council. Certificates were awarded at the end of the third year if the probationers passed the examinations after each course of lectures. There were gold and silver medals, and prizes for proficiency in the Training School.

Meanwhile another storey had been added to Nurses' Home No. 2,[24] and teaching in midwifery, public health, tropical diseases and district training was available to students.[25] There was also a sports club and a Missionary Guild.

By 1939 the total nursing staff had grown to 160 of which 113 were student nurses and probationers. Thirty-seven entered the Preliminary

Training School that year and 27 nurses completed their training.[26] A change on 1 January abolished the Hospital examinations and concentrated the course on passing the Final State Examination without which now no certificate or badge was awarded. This meant complete acceptance by Addenbrooke's of the regulations for training laid down by the General Nursing Council for England and Wales.

Also in 1939 many former Addenbrooke's nurses were called up for the Queen Alexandra's Imperial Military Nursing Service Reserve or the Territorial Army Nursing Service, and members of the British Red Cross Society, St John's Ambulance Corps, Women's Voluntary Service and A.R.P. First Aid Workers gained experience in the Hospital in order to join the Civil Nursing Reserve or the staff for a First Aid Post.

Affiliation schemes agreed in 1939 and 1942 with the Hospital of St Nicholas and St Martin, Pyrford, the Royal Westminster Ophthalmic Hospital, London, and the North Cambridgeshire Hospital, Wisbech, brought more nurses from other hospitals for training.[27]

Since the commencement of the war, the Preliminary Training School had been accommodated at 'Homefields', Histon. In 1945 it returned to the Hospital premises.[28] The same year a property known as Owlstone Croft, at Newnham, was requisitioned for nurses' quarters since there was an acute shortage following the closing down of the Leys School Annexe. In 1946 Owlstone Croft was purchased for the Preliminary Training School at a cost of £12,500[29] and the course was extended from two months to three.

～40～

The special departments

The term 'special department' is sometimes applied as a euphemism for the department of venereal diseases. In the history of the Hospital, however, and here, it is applied to departments admitting primarily patients with diseases affecting a particular organ or requiring a particular form of treatment.

Midwifery and gynaecology

According to the Rules and Orders of the Hospital, 1766, no woman big with child should be admitted. This rule was enforced but exceptions were made when other diseases complicated the pregnancy.

In the seventeenth century most midwifery was carried out by women without training and usually of poor levels of education.

Towards the end of the eighteenth century a new class of midwife developed; these were women of better education and character who had received some training and whose work became recognised. A Chair of Midwifery had been established in Edinburgh in the 1720s for the training of midwives.

In many areas most of the midwifery practice was in the midwives' own hands but the introduction of midwifery forceps, which were not used by midwives, increased the practice of midwifery by doctors. Midwifery was, however, not yet a subject for compulsory training and until the Medical Act of 1858 there was no obligation for the future general practitioner to have received any training or experience in midwifery.

In the nineteenth century general practitioner midwifery reached its peak and some general practitioners built up very large practices, for example, Dr W.J. Young of Harston, Cambridgeshire (1869–1948), acquired a high reputation. He was responsible for over 2,000 deliveries without a maternal death.[1]

The records of the Cambridge Medical Society, founded in 1880, show that obstetrics and gynaecology was the subject of 40 papers compared with 83 on general surgical topics and 34 in general medicine during the period 1890–1913.

Gynaecology evolved late as a specialty for it was dependent on both anaesthesia and the development of bacteriology. The first operation to be carried out was the removal of a massive ovarian cyst. Tapping such cysts often led to death from infection. Ovariotomy by abdominal section was successfully carried out in 1809 and again in 1813 and 1816 by Ephraim McDowell (1771–1830) in the U.S.A.[2] Among early British ovariotomists was George Murray Humphry (See Chapter 16).

A hazard of hospital obstetrics was puerperal fever, the risk of which was far greater among hospital patients than in those delivered at home.

As the range and variety of gynaecological operations increased, the speciality of gynaecology developed. The first gynaecologist at Addenbrooke's was Edward Douty and he was succeeded by Frederick Deighton in 1897. Deighton was also in charge of the Ear, Nose and Throat Department.

Women in the late stages of pregnancy had always been regarded as ineligible for admission by the Hospital but a few were admitted on account of the co-existence of other medical and surgical problems. In October 1917, the Cambridgeshire County Council asked the Hospital to admit necessitous women 'where special difficulties may occur in connection with the confinement'. It was estimated that there would not be more than twelve such cases each year. The General Committee of 22 October referred the matter to the honorary medical staff.

The next month[3] the staff reported that hitherto it had been the custom for cases of difficult labour to be admitted and that some had come in every year. An increase in numbers would be impossible in the present accommodation. It was recommended that such women be admitted, as before, so far as Mary Ward would allow, upon payment by the Council of 6s. per patient per day. The staff did not require any payment.

The Council then requested that they be allowed to subscribe 5 guineas per annum to obtain a supply of recommendations to enable them to refer cases to the Out-patient Department for examination.[4] This was agreed.

On 11 February 1918, the House Sub-Committee agreed that cases of difficult labour should be admitted from the Borough on the same terms as from the County.

On 12 May 1919, the General Committee referred to the medical staff a letter from Dr Laird asking, on behalf of the Borough Council, if the Hospital would consider establishing an ante-natal clinic. A fortnight later[5] the General Committee likewise referred to the staff a letter from

Frank Robinson, the County Medical Officer of Health, asking for terms for Maternity and Child Welfare services, including the admission of children with non-infectious illnesses from 'prejudicial' home conditions.

A month later[6] the General Committee received a report from the medical staff in favour of both proposals and the House Committee later decided[7] that ante-natal consultations could be provided at 10s.6d. for the first visit and report, and 2s.6d. for each subsequent visit. They also agreed that cases of normal confinement might be received, when the home conditions were prejudicial, for 7s. maintenance per day. The confinement fee of the Ministry of Health should be paid direct to the surgeon in attendance on the case. Children under five with non-infectious ailments could be admitted for 5s. per day. The maintenance fee for abnormal confinements admitted under the 1917 (County) and 1918 (Town) agreements should be increased to 7s. per day.

Similar arrangements were to be made with the Isle of Ely County Council and the Diocesan Maternity Home.

The Dental Department

In the early days of the Hospital, tooth extractions were the responsibility of the Apothecary, and later of the House Surgeon. Outside, extractions formed part of the routine work of surgeons but were also performed by tooth drawers, some of them itinerants who worked in the open air at fairs and markets. Others, by apprenticeship, achieved considerable skill.[8]

By the middle of the nineteenth century few general hospitals in London had yet appointed a dentist so it is interesting that as early as 1855 George Paget proposed that a Dental Department be established. He was, however, overruled by his colleagues and the question did not arise again until 1883[9] when the proposal came in a letter from the Secretary of the Eastern Counties Dental Association (E.C.D.A.). In the interim, dentists in Britain had become an organised profession with a recognised diploma and steadily increased status.

The letter from the E.C.D.A. was to inform the Governors that 'this Association is of opinion that in the interests of the public and for the efficiency of medical charitable institutions it is expected that a qualified dental surgeon should be attached to the medical staff of all general hospitals and dispensaries . . .'. The matter was referred to the medical staff.

On 3 November 1886, the Weekly Meeting agreed to recommend the establishment of a dental department. It was later decided it was to be for two years in the first instance and there should be two Honorary Dentists, registered under the Dental Act (of 1878). Each should attend the Hospital for one hour once a week.

At a poll held on 7 February 1887, Mr Alfred Jones, Jr, and Mr W.A. Rhodes were elected.

Between 7 March and 30 September 1887, 723 operations in the Dental Department were recorded. In December the next year the Board recommended that the Dental Department should be definitely established and on 31 December Rhodes and Jones were elected for a period of six years.

W.A. Rhodes (1856–1918) was a Yorkshire man who came to Cambridge in 1878. In 1879 he registered under the Dental Act and in 1881 he took the L.D.S. (Ireland). He ran a very successful practice, first in Trumpington Street and then in Silver Street. He was president of the Eastern Counties Branch of, and in 1913 President of, the British Dental Association.[10]

Alfred Jones (d. 1927) had succeeded his uncle in practice at Cambridge and was himself succeeded by his son. When the British Dental Association met in Cambridge in 1885 it was under his presidency, and he was among the first dentists to use prolonged nitrous oxide anaesthesia with a nasal inhaler.

In 1894 the appointments of both Dentists were renewed for a further period of six years,[11] and in 1900 Mr Rhodes decided not to seek re-election. He was elected Consulting Dentist to the Hospital instead.

Mr Jones' application for re-election was approved; however, in his letter he suggested that Honorary Dentists should be made full members of the surgical staff. The medical staff replied[12] that 'they were unanimously of the opinion that it was impossible to comply with Mr Jones' request . . . The qualifications they are required to possess are not such as would justify the Governors in permitting them or expecting them to share the serious responsibilities of the surgical staff.'

Staffing the Dental Department became a perennial problem after Mr Rhodes' resignation. It was inevitably increased by the needs of the armed forces during the First World War, but, after 1921, as a consequence of the new Dentists' Act, the supply of dentists improved.

Ophthalmology

The development of the specialties at Addenbrooke's depended on a variable combination of factors.

In ophthalmology the work of the itinerant operators during the eighteenth and the early nineteenth centuries provided treatment for cataracts. Chevalier Taylor was a surgeon in Norwich who from 1734 made repeated tours about Britain and Europe operating and lecturing. Most general surgeons undertook some procedures in the eye and discouraged the appointment of specialist ophthalmic surgeons.

On 7 February 1878, a committee set up on the instigation of Professor Humphry did not agree to the appointment of an ophthalmic surgeon. Instead they approved a proposal by the surgeons 'to place the ophthalmic cases under the care of one or other of their number'. This was to be George Wherry.

A steady increase in the number of patients referred to the Eye Department led to repeated complaints of overcrowding. On 13 November 1905, Mr J.C.W. Graham was appointed Clinical Assistant in the Ophthalmic Department and two years later he was joined by Dr Ponder who was succeeded in November 1909 by Dr Davies of Histon.

In 1911[13] Wherry complained of overcrowding which he blamed on children sent after school inspections. One Saturday morning he had found over 100 people waiting.

The overcrowding problem continued. The General Committee of 14 October 1912 claimed that the Department was being abused and that the services of an Almoner were required.

On 28 May 1917, the General Committee ordered a notice to be sent to all medical practitioners informing them that because of increasing difficulties in the Eye Department cases for refraction could no longer be seen. There was general agreement that no senior appointment of an eye surgeon should be made until the end of the war.

Mr Arthur Cooke, who had succeeded Mr Wherry in charge of the eye wards on the latter's resignation, took them over again when he returned from France in 1919 after the First World War.[14]

Dermatology

Dermatology developed as a specialty during the nineteenth century. At first the rashes of the acute fevers were of interest to the Physician, whilst syphillis and the other venereal diseases were considered to be surgical problems.

Gradually the Department developed in the charge of a physician with a special interest in the subject. At Cambridge this was Aldren Wright who was a general practitioner.

The most widespread and chronic condition which the Skin Department was called upon to treat was ringworm of the scalp caused by a fungus, microsporum audouini. This infection, which spread rapidly from child to child, caused bald patches with broken hairs and fine scaling. From the Middle Ages onwards there are references to the infection usually under the popular name of 'scald head'. Most commonly the condition persisted from its onset in early childhood until it cleared spontaneously at puberty. There was no effective treatment and the application of powerful irritants could cause much discomfort and leave permanent scars.

After the discovery of X-rays the possibility of clearing scalp ringworm within a reasonable period of three months or so by this form of epilation was an attractive one. It was the willingness of the Local Authority to pay for the treatment of school children with ringworm that prompted the opening of the skin clinic.

On 5 December 1908, the Town Clerk wrote to ask if the Hospital would undertake the treatment of ringworm with X-rays. The next year[15] the purchase of suitable apparatus for £120 was authorised. A private donor gave £50[16] and the Education Authority also agreed to contribute £50.[17]

In 1920[18] Wright's request that he be allowed to continue to see outpatients who attended for diseases of the skin was approved and it was agreed that 'The Special Department of Diseases of the Skin' be placed under his care.

On 4 April 1922, the Medical Officer of Health for Hertfordshire asked for terms for treating patients with the form of tuberculosis of the skin known as lupus. This was referred to Dr Shillington Scales. The next year[19] the Hospital was asked by Dr Bullough, County Medical Officer of Health for Essex, on what terms they would treat scalp ringworm in children. He negotiated a fee of 2 guineas per case.[20] In this way two large groups of patients were added to the many others treated at public expense.

Another group similarly covered were those with venereal diseases.

In 1930 Dr C.H. Whittle, the Clinical Pathologist, succeeded Wright in charge of the Skin Department[21] and Dr L.B. Cole took over Venereal Diseases.[22]

Ear, Nose and Throat Department

The first mention of an Ear, Nose and Throat Department is on 23 March 1892, when Mr Deighton was allowed up to £24 to purchase instruments for the 'throat and ear department'. Eighteen years later[23] the General Committee approved the medical staff's recommendation that an Honorary Clinical Assistant to the Department be appointed. Mr W.H. Bowen was elected.[24]

Surgery of the ear, nose and throat received a strong incentive to develop when tonsillectomy became a very common operation for the treatment of children who were the financial responsibility of the Local Authority. The House Committee of 12 June 1922 received a letter from the Education Secretary of the Isle of Ely County Council asking for terms for the removal of tonsils and adenoids. An arrangement of 25s. per case was agreed, maintenance being extra.[25]

During the Second World War[26] it was agreed to use the Leys School sanatorium for all E.N.T. cases. Private patients were also admitted.[27]

Orthopaedics

The development of the Orthopaedic Department at the Hospital is of particular interest since in some parts of the country it was held up by the general surgeons who strongly resented the loss of patients always regarded as coming within the province of surgery. This was not the case at Addenbrooke's. An Orthopaedic Department was already in existence by 1915 (see Chapter 36). It was under the care of Griffiths.

At a meeting of the General Committee on 16 December 1918, a letter was received from the Ministry of Pensions concerning the establishment of an Orthopaedic Centre in Cambridge. The letter was referred to the staff and two weeks later[28] their 'hearty approval' of a clinic for the orthopaedic treatment of discharged soldiers was obtained.

The Ministry wished to establish 26 Orthopaedic In-patient Centres in the U.K.[29] and it was hoped that one of these would be at Addenbrooke's. It was to be linked to established clinics at Ely, March, Wisbech, Peterborough, Bedford and Huntingdon where out-patients would be treated. By 20 October 1919,[30] the General Committee were able to tell the Ministry that such a centre had been established.

Demand for orthopaedic services must have fallen off in the years after the war, however, for the General Committee of 13 January 1925, accepted the recommendation of the staff 'that the work of the Orthopaedic Department having lapsed' it should be re-started under Dr Roderick.

~ 41 ~

Addenbrooke's and the University, 1900 to 1948

In his essay 'Cambridge Medicine and the Medical School in the Twentieth Century', Leslie Cole[1] says that after the death of Paget and Humphry there appears to have been for the next 50 years a swing away from clinical medicine in the University. A number of University clinical appointments were suppressed:

> Downing Professor of Medicine, discontinued 1930 on the death of Professor Bradbury.
>
> Professor of Surgery (1883–1915), suppressed on the death of Professor Howard Marsh.
>
> University lectureships in Medicine (1883–1911), Surgery (1883–1912), Midwifery and Obstetrics (1883–1909), and Medical Jurisprudence (1883–1916), were all suppressed or vacated.
>
> Readership in Surgery (1898–1903), suppressed.
>
> Demonstrator of Surgery (1901–1926), suppressed.

And four special diplomas which had been established were also discontinued:

> Diploma of Public Health (1875–1932)
>
> Diploma of Tropical Medicine and Hygiene (1904–1932)
>
> Diploma of Psychological Medicine (1912–1927)
>
> Diploma of Medical Radiology and Electrology (1919–1936)

He describes the beginning of the century: 'It appears that clinical work was casual and much of the syllabus repeated later at a London Hospital. After 1900, when both Humphry and Paget were dead, with the rise of the pre-clinical school and the increase in importance of the tripos, clinical teaching was gradually pushed more and more into the background and had decreased considerably by the outbreak of war in 1914.'

In 1913[2] a scheme was suggested to bring the laboratory and hospital work of the students closer together. There were then about 20 students attending the Hospital, each term and long vacation, usually while also working in the laboratories for their second M.B. Part II (Pathology, Bacteriology and Pharmacology). It was proposed that the present honorary staff should hold University appointments with the title University Teacher, and that the student's fees be collected by the University and supplemented by a grant from the Board of Education and used to pay each University Teacher £50. A further £100 p.a. (in addition to the £300 already paid to the Hospital by the University) should be paid from the Board of Education grant into a fund towards the teaching of students, and the Special Board for Medicine should be responsible for teaching arrangements. Further action was deferred until the University moved in the matter.

In June 1914,[3] an agreement was reached. The Special Board for Medicine had applied to the Board of Education for a grant to the Medical Departments and the Board of Education had suggested the staff of the Hospital should be brought into closer touch with the University, changes being made to enable the Vice Chancellor of the University to accept responsibility for the expenditure of the money granted by the Board of Education.

The Board of Education's Visitors were to view the Hospital when viewing the various Departments of the Medical School in order to report on the facilities for teaching. The Honorary Physicians, Surgeons, Assistant Physicians, Assistant Surgeons and Pathologist were, with the exception of those holding professorial rank, to become 'University Teachers'. The Special Board for Medicine became responsible for the teaching of the students working in the Hospital, and an extra £50 p.a. was to be paid to the Hospital. In addition £100 p.a. was to be allowed for apparatus required by the staff for special methods of treatment or in the teaching of students, and any other apparatus required for teaching was to be the responsibility of the University. In agreeing to the proposition the General Committee thought it should be intimated to the Special Board for Medicine that £100 per year to the General Fund would be appreciated.

In 1916 the Mistress of Girton and the Principal of Newnham applied to the Vice Chancellor for admission of their students to the first and second M.B. examinations and this was approved in a Grace of 18 November 1916.[4] The first woman medical student at Addenbrooke's appears to have been admitted in 1918. There is an apology in the

Minutes[5] from a Miss E.K. Saunders of Newnham College for one of their students having begun attendance on the course at Addenbrooke's under the impression that it had been opened to women students. It was referred to the medical staff who reported[6] that they approved of the principle of women medical students attending the Hospital.

A Grace was passed on 20 October 1921, to confer degrees by diploma on duly qualified women but a diploma for an M.B. was not presented to a woman until May 1925.[4]

In 1918 the General Committee received draft suggestions relating to Clinical Medicine from Sir Clifford Allbutt.[7]

He described how before the war the relations of Addenbrooke's Hospital with the University had been gradually improved, for example, 'the co-operation of the Regius Professor of Physic, the Professor of Surgery and the Professor of Pathology with the Hospital Staff had been arranged and defined'.

He said that during the war progress had been arrested and there were altered conditions of general medical service such as health insurance organisation, the enlargement of public health legislation, and special provisions for tuberculosis and V.D. But now that agreement had been reached to reconstruct all services, he believed that closer co-operation with the University in research, and with local medical practitioners, should be considered. He suggested there should be a new officer in the Clinical Laboratory to carry out additional observations in the wards, and that the Hospital should inform medical practitioners of their patients' admission, discharge and treatment, and also make records available.

The proposals were received with sympathy,[7] but detailed consideration was postponed until the medical and surgical staff 'can find time to give their advice thereon'.

Leslie Cole (Fig. 52) was elected Assistant Physician to Addenbrooke's Hospital in 1928, coming from a senior appointment at St Thomas'. He says:[1] 'In general, at Addenbrooke's, sickness appeared in a more florid form against a background of dirt, deformity, under-nutrition and anaemia, and extreme examples of disease and neglect came from the Fens. Nursing, diet, investigation and treatment were well below the standards of a London teaching hospital which were much lower than today.' Under the voluntary system the prosperity of a hospital and its area were linked and as Cambridgeshire was poor 'a first class service could hardly have been possible'.

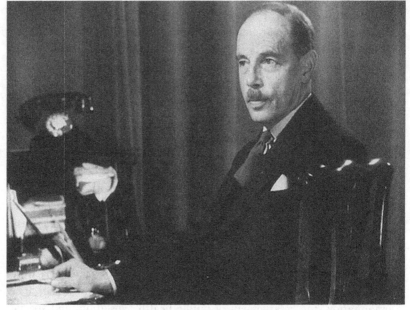

Fig. 52. Leslie Cole, 1898–1983. Physician to Addenbrooke's for
nearly 40 years and first Dean of Cambridge School of Clinical
Research and Postgraduate Medical Teaching.

In 1931[1] a syndicate was appointed to consider the medical courses and
examinations in connection with those for the B.A. Until 1934 it was not
compulsory for medical students taking the M.B. to take a Tripos, and
increasing numbers of them did not; for example, between 1906 and 1911,
77% took it, and between 1920 and 1926 only 44% did. One of the aims of
the syndicate was to set up a Medical Sciences Tripos under a single
Faculty Board instead of the Natural Sciences Tripos under several
Boards controlling medicals and non-medicals alike. Some changes were
made but the proposal for a single Faculty Board to control medical
examinations was rejected. Another proposal, that the teaching of applied
anatomy, physiology, and pathology should be undertaken by members
of the staff at Addenbrooke's, resulted in two liaison officers, a physician
and a surgeon, being appointed, but little time for it was allotted to the
students. A Medical Sciences Tripos was finally introduced in 1966.

In December 1934,[8] a Sub-Committee was appointed to change the
bye-laws of the Hospital as required by the contemplated change in
University regulations for medical degrees.

The new bye-laws, as well as allowing the Regius Professor of Physic to be a Physician and hold beds in the Hospital, and lecture there, allowed the Professors of Anatomy, Physiology, Biochemistry and Pathology, and the Reader in Pharmacology, and officers of their departments to demonstrate on out-patients. The Professor of Pathology was permitted to conduct post-mortem examinations. Material such as blood or urine was to be provided for teaching purposes and facilities given for conducting the University examinations.[9]

In 1935 a new Regius Professor of Physic, John Ryle, was appointed and set up a Department of Medicine with laboratories for research in the Pathology Department. Cole says: 'The benefit conferred on the hospital was immense.'

In July 1937,[10] the General Committee received the first of two memoranda from Ryle.

He said: 'With the establishment in October 1936 of an active Department of Medicine in the University, and the generous welcome . . . it has become possible to visualise and plan developments for the future of far-reaching importance alike to the Hospital and the University. There is now, in fact, no reason why Addenbrooke's should not become one of the most important medical centres in this country . . .'

Dr Cole and Mr Butler were the liaison officers with the University in connection with 'work for the examinations, provision of teaching materials and a certain amount of undergraduate teaching.

'The primary functions of the Department include clinical research and training for clinical research, correlative experimental work in the university laboratories, and some undergraduate teaching.'

He made some suggestions for a closer liaison between Hospital and University, such as sharing the work of essential laboratory services, and said that routine and research in clinical medicine were inseparable in that especially elaborate investigations on a case might be research but the results benefit the patient. The Department of Medicine would be responsible for some of this work but the number of investigations carried out in the Hospital laboratories was bound to increase and the Hospital would have to bear this.

He said that Addenbrooke's was currently receiving from the Department of Medicine in return for facilities and friendly co-operation, 'the services of five or more highly qualified and well-trained young men, a follow-up department for certain types of case, a vastly improved system of records and the services of a whole-time secretary'.

This memorandum was referred by the General Committee to the honorary staff and to the General Purposes Committee; however, in November[11] the Regius Professor of Physic wrote again withdrawing his previous memorandum and introducing a new one. He was proposing a full statement on future developments for consideration by the Faculty Board and later presumably by the General Board of the University. He suggested that eventually a Committee representing the University, the Faculty Board, the Department of Medicine and the Hospital Governors might be appointed to review the whole matter. The new memorandum would be circulated for consideration by the General Committee and other bodies concerned.

The new memorandum[12] described the existing department of medicine quite clearly.

Its functions were as follows.

1 The prosecution of clinical and correlative research.
2 The training for clinical research of selected workers.
3 The provision of opportunity and material for workers in other departments having close relationships with medicine.
4 The encouragement of collaborative experimental work in the University laboratories and the establishment of a closer liaison between the Departments of Pathology, Physiology, Pharmacology, Psychology, Biochemistry and Anatomy on the one hand and Addenbrooke's on the other.
5 The provision in association with the honorary staff of illustrative clinical teaching.

The staff consisted of the Regius Professor of Physic, the Assistant Director of Research (Dr J.F. Brock), five Elmore research students, two other research students, a German woman doctor with an endowment from the Handson Bequest, two secretaries, a laboratory technician, and two laboratory boys. Accommodation for the unit was in the Pathology Department, and the Regius Professor had eight beds allocated to him for research purposes.

The Department of Medicine was obviously working in quite close contact with the Hospital, for the departmental programme for the week consisted of: a joint staff round on Monday mornings at which cases of difficulty or special interest were presented and discussed; a departmental conference on Monday evenings; ward visits by the Regius Professor and Assistant Director of Research on Tuesday and Saturday mornings; a departmental staff round with the Regius Professor on Thursday afternoons; a follow-up session on Friday afternoons; and a fortnightly clinical conference or symposium held on Thursday evenings in term time.

The Department was in Addenbrooke's at that time by friendly arrangement but the Governors were planning to make it an Associate Department of the Hospital. Also the honorary staff had recommended that the Assistant Director of Research should be accorded the status of Honorary Assistant Physician. Meanwhile the research students accompanied the Honorary Physicians on their ward rounds once a week and, being engaged on various problems of their own as well as having routine duties in the Hospital, they split their time equally between ward work and the laboratory.

Part of the plan for development of the Department involved including its personnel in the clinical services of the Hospital and in the special services concerned with medical diagnosis and investigation. To this end, further research assistantships were to be created in specialities such as pathology and psychiatry, funded by the Rockefeller Foundation who were giving £1,600 annually for five years.

So far, said the memorandum, the Department had made no heavy demands upon the University or the Hospital owing to the provisions of the Elmore Bequest (this provided for scholarships for medical research at the University and for assisting medical education there).[13] It had been helping the Hospital in administrative work, medical records – a new filing system had been introduced – investigation and follow-up studies (the importance of follow-up had only latterly received recognition in England).

The Department needed offices and laboratories of its own and two ten- or twelve-bed research wards. It was thought that a quarter of a million pounds would provide both for the building of this research wing and its endowment.

'Patients would not as a rule be specifically admitted for research upon their particular diseases, but would be transferred as occasion demanded from other wards or the out-patient department to the research-wards for special investigations and specially controlled treatment.' Their expenses would be shared by Hospital and Department.

'Either building or endowment or both, or alternatively a part of both, might well be considered a very appropriate object for a larger private benefaction or for a special appeal.'

Representatives of the Hospital and the University met to discuss the Regius Professor's letter[14] and, in May 1938, the Hospital's Building

Committee reported[15] that space for the research block could be found on Hospital ground. However the war seems to have supervened.

During the Second World War the Twentieth General Hospital was the successor to the First Eastern General Hospital of 1914. It was commanded by Charles Budd who had been Senior Anaesthetist at Addenbrooke's.[1] Cambridge and East Anglia took in many evacuees and the Leys school, which had been evacuated to Pitlochry, was opened up as an annexe of Addenbrooke's. Cole[1] says: 'There was no run-down of the pre-clinical school as in the 1914–18 war, most medical students continued a shortened course, with a depleted staff, and pre-clinical and clinical examinations continued at Cambridge as usual.'

During the war the Department of Medicine seems to have become sadly depleted. In 1939 there were eleven doctors working as research assistants in the Hospital[16] but in 1945[17] there was only one medically qualified person on the staff, the Reader in Medicine, Dr R.A. McCance, who was working with four ladies, two of whom had Ph.D.s, plus four laboratory assistants and a secretary.

Meanwhile, however, in 1942, an Interdepartmental Committee on medical schools had been appointed by the Minister of Health and in 1943 the Hospital held discussions on the desirability of Addenbrooke's becoming a full teaching centre.[18] It was expected that Government post-war policy would be to divide the country into areas each one centred on a university teaching hospital, and the General Committee and staff were in favour of having an active clinical teaching school 'so that this Hospital in association with the University may assist to the fullest extent in the health services of the country'. It was decided to make approaches to the University[19] in order to receive their support.

In October that year[20] it was agreed to send a 'Memorandum on the Future Developments as Between the Hospital and the University of Cambridge, with special reference to Clinical Teaching and Research', to the Interdepartmental Committee on Medical Schools and also to the University Registry for submission to the Council of Senate. It had been drawn up by representatives of the Hospital after meeting with representatives of the University.

It allowed that 'Regular clinical teaching prior to qualification, of undergraduates and graduates of the university and other students has never been extensive, and in recent years has been very limited, since for various reasons it has been customary for the vast majority of Cambridge medical students to go to one of the London Hospitals for their clinical training.' However, all Cambridge medical students attended Addenbrooke's for their final clinical examinations and there was a strong tradition of teaching in the Hospital. For example: the honorary staff participated in short courses of elementary undergraduate clinical teaching each year; a few students (although only one to four per year during the last ten years) elected to do the greater part of their clinical courses at Addenbrooke's; the University Department of Medicine, which undertook some clinical teaching although being primarily occupied in research, was an Associate Department of the Hospital; and up to the war regular refresher courses of post-graduate teaching for practitioners had been given several times a year under a Ministry of Health scheme.

The University representatives had indicated that the University would be glad of a closer liaison with the Hospital in that the Council of Senate would welcome the establishment in Cambridge of the central hospital of the Eastern area, and also a post-graduate school of clinical research. If the latter were to be set up the Council would be prepared to consider the possibility of a pre-graduate school of clinical medicine.

The Hospital, however, did not agree that a pre-graduate school should be left as a mere possibility, and several arguments were put forward in favour of establishing one in Cambridge, the main one, from the Hospital's point of view, seeming to be that it would raise the standard of medical work done at the Hospital more than a post-graduate school, since, for example, workers of distinction would be recruited to fill the senior posts.

But: 'Bearing in mind that the Department of Medicine is already an Associate Department of the Hospital, the General Committee are willing to co-operate in the further elaboration of a Post-graduate School of Clinical Research . . .' and that if either type of Teaching School be established then it was reasonable that the Charity Commissioners be approached to alter the scheme of management of the Hospital to give the Council of Senate direct representation on the General Committee.

In February 1944,[21] the Chairman of the General Committee reported that a Committee of the Faculty Board of Medicine had also issued a report in connection with the establishment of a School of Clinical Research at Cambridge. It had been received, and was to go in addition to the Council of the Senate with a request that it be sent to the Interdepartmental Committee. More discussions were to be held.

In March the Interdepartmental Committee published its report. It agreed with the University.[1]

A Joint Advisory Committee was set up to consider and advise on all matters of common interest to the Hospital and the University. It was to consist of the Regius Professor of Physic, six members nominated by the Council of Senate, six by the General Committee (these were the Chairmen of the General Maintenance Fund, and House Committees, and Mr R.W. Butler, Dr L.B. Cole, and Mr A.S.H. Walford as honorary staff representitives), and the Secretary-Superintendent was to be Joint Secretary.[22] The Committee approved the development of a School of Clinical Research and Post-graduate Teaching and made proposals that were to link Addenbrooke's and the University more closely than ever before in their history, particularly the provision by the University departments of all the pathological and biochemical services of the Hospital[23] although being reimbursed for the costs of routine work. The other undertakings included provision for the honorary staff to be represented on the council of the Medical School, for the School departmental heads to be members of the honorary staff and further members of University Departments to have status in the Hospital, for School departments to be Associated Departments of the Hospital, and for financial arrangements between the Hospital and the University. The Hospital also provided beds for the Professors of Experimental Medicine and Radiotherapeutics as well as for the Regius Professor of Physic, and the honorary staff became recognised teachers in the University.[24]

The new school, constituted 1 October 1946,[24] comprised four professorial departments: Haematology under the new Regius Professor Sir Lionel Whitby, Experimental Medicine (1945) under Professor McCance, Radiotherapy (1946) under Professor Joseph Mitchell, and Human Ecology (1948) under Professor Banks.[1]

In August 1947, the General Purposes Committee received a report of the visit to Addenbrooke's of Dr Clarke of the Ministry of Health with regard to its designation as a teaching hospital, and also correspondence in which the University informed the Ministry it would welcome such a designation.[25] Plans were in progress for a new larger Addenbrooke's 2 miles away, and 5 acres on the selected 40-acre site had been reserved for University buildings.[1] The future of the Hospital under the National Health Service seemed assured.

Modern times

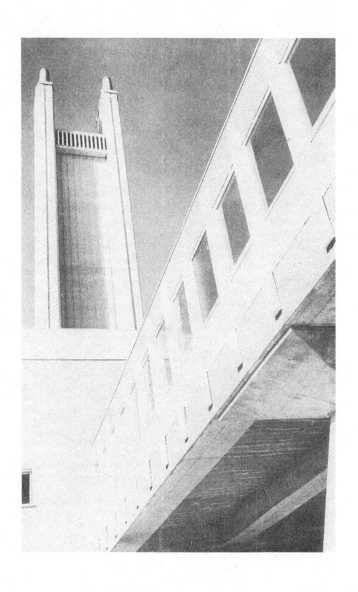

~ 42 ~

The early work of the Board of Governors

The final meeting of the Quarterly Court of Addenbrooke's Hospital took place on 23 May 1948, and that of the General Committee of the Hospital on 22 June 1948, that is some weeks after the administration of the Hospital had become the responsibility of the National Health Service (N.H.S.). The N.H.S. Act which had become law in November 1946, took effect from 5 July 1948 and from that date the administration of Addenbrooke's Hospital was the responsibility of a Board of Governors appointed by and accountable to, the Minister of Health. This structure lasted until 1974 when the first of several reorganisations of the N.H.S. was made, and it is with this period of nearly 26 years that this epilogue to the history of Addenbrooke's Hospital is concerned. Let us first look back to the final months of the old administration and examine the issues which were then dominant.

On 26 August 1947 the General Committee reported to the Quarterly Court that the finances of the Hospital were in 'a less than satisfactory state'. The Committee recommended that the bank borrowing limit be raised to £60,000 and, bearing in mind that the N.H.S. Act had received the Royal Assent in November 1946, the Ministry of Health be asked to give financial assistance until July 1948. At the same meeting the Committee recommended that the well-known firm of London architects, Messrs Easton and Robertson, be appointed as architects of a new Hospital to be built on a site in Trumpington which it was hoped would shortly be acquired. And at a later meeting on 27 April 1948 the same Committee agreed to place on record their desire '. . . that the new Board of Governors of the Teaching Hospital should perpetuate the name of Addenbrooke's in association with this (new) Hospital'.

More mundane matters were also engaging the General Committee, and much of the meeting held on 23 December 1947 was devoted to the question of transferring the superannuation contributions of employees and to safeguarding their pension rights when the State through the

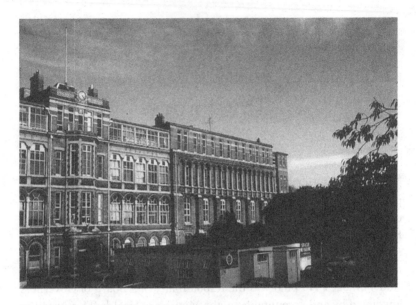

Fig. 53. Addenbrooke's Hospital, Trumpington Street, as it was
between 1960 and 1984 when the last patient moved from the
original site to the new Hospital at Hills Road. (Photo by O.G.
source W.G.C.)

Board of Governors became the employing authority in the following
July. When the final meeting was held there was no account of any
recognition of the historic nature of the occasion, and indeed the
Committee continued with its routine business until the end. However,
the three topics of finance, the new Hospital, and staff concerns, provide a
foretaste of things to come and a sense of continuity with the past (Fig. 53).

It would be wrong to suggest that either the general public or the staff of
the Hospital were greatly concerned about, or indeed aware of, the
changes that were taking place. This is not perhaps surprising when one
considers the nature of those changes: administrative in the grouping of
hospitals, financial as far as the source of funds was concerned, and above
all political. Out-patient clinics continued to be held, the shortage of beds
in all specialities remained bringing with it the high occupancy rates
which has always been a characteristic in Cambridge; and to all intents
and purposes, the general practitioner service remained unchanged.

What then were the main changes over which the politicians had
battled for so long and which between 1946 and 1948 had divided the
medical profession? What was new was that a 'Hospital Service' had been

created and groups of hospitals created into more-or-less single administrative entities. As far as Addenbrooke's was concerned, it had been designated under the Act as a Teaching Hospital for medical students. This differentiated it from non-teaching hospitals which, although similarly grouped, were administered by Hospital Management Committees who were accountable to Regional Hospital Boards, who in turn were responsible to the Ministry of Health. Boards of Governors accounted direct to Whitehall and the Addenbrooke's Board, entitled 'The Board of Governors of the United Cambridge Hospitals' had responsibility for Addenbrooke's as well as for:

The Maternity Hospital, Mill Road;
Brookfields Hospital, Mill Road;
Chesterton Hospital, Union Lane;
The Home of Recovery, Hunstanton.

Fulbourn Hospital, as a psychiatric hospital, was not part of the United Cambridge Hospitals and was administered by its own Hospital Management Committee (although, from the outset, psychiatric out-patients were seen at Addenbrooke's). One of the continuing subjects which was to occupy members and officers was the organisation of joint services where the responsibility to provide clinical services was shared between the Regional Hospital Board and the Board of Governors.

The organisation of joint services was one of the issues which engaged the Board of Governors and its committees – joint that is with both the Regional Hospital Board, and the University. Earlier reservations about a national service, held mainly by some doctors, were soon forgotten and attention was directed at what was described as 'the abnormal rise in the Waiting List'. In June 1948 this stood at 1842, and by March 1950 it had risen to 2912. The shortage of beds, and of space especially at Trumpington Street, were continually under discussion and here the medical voice was predominant. Lay members of the Board contributed mainly to the debates on ways to overcome the shortage of finance that was available to do what was seen as needed.

Although the shortage of nurses, particularly of skilled ones, was often mentioned, there is little indication that the Matrons and other senior nurses were directly involved in decision taking. Their influence was brought to bear through the Secretary-Superintendent, a state of affairs which was common in most hospitals and was increasingly resented by the nursing profession. Doctors for their part recognised the crucial role of nurses, especially of Ward Sisters, but were little involved in the problems of nurse management. The routine medical business was largely devoted to the identification of members of the medical staff, and to determining whether or not they were to be accorded consultant status. This was clearly a difficult task with so many doctors practising privately, as general practitioners, and for the University; a few worked for the City and County Councils.

The appointment of Messrs Easton and Robertson as architects to the new Hospital was soon followed by detailed discussions about the plans. The site that had been earmarked was defined in the minutes of the General Committee of 28 January 1947 as follows '. . . of 60 acres on the Pemberton Estate, bounded on the east side by Trumpington Road, on the south by Trumpington Hall, on the west by land scheduled for a municipal golf course, and on the north by land scheduled for playing fields.' A joint University and Hospital planning committee was established and at an early meeting Mr Murray Easton said that 'to provide what may be required, the buildings would have to be high, that the site would be fully covered, and that the Hospital authorities should keep in mind the need to secure a larger area than the 60 acres to allow for any eventual developments.' We shall return to the history of the planning of the new Hospital and note now only the early recognition of the need to plan for expansion as medical science developed, an issue which has remained unchanged in its intractibility throughout.

Mr T. Knox-Shaw, M.C., M.A., Master of Sidney Sussex College, had been appointed Chairman of the Board by the Minister but thereafter the new authorities were left to make their own arrangements for the organisation of the services for which they were responsible. The early meetings of the Board were largely devoted to routine matters and at the first meeting on 25 June 1948, as the first item of business, Mr R.H. Parker, M.C., D.L., M.A., was elected Vice Chairman. The Board then proceeded to make its two senior appointments: that of J.A. Beardsall, O.B.E., F.H.A., and of P.A. Hollings, A.S.A.A., A.H.A., as Secretary to the Board and Finance Officer respectively. The former had been Secretary-Superintendent and the latter Accountant, to Addenbrooke's Hospital.

Under the N.H.S. Act all authorities were required to set up at least two standing committees: a Finance Committee and a Medical Committee. In Cambridge a General Purposes and Finance Committee was established, in addition to the Medical Committee, Chair of the former being taken by the Chairman of the Board. This signified the importance of financial issues, and indeed virtually no matter which was discussed at any of the committees did not at some stage pass before the eyes of the members of the General Purposes and Finance Committee.

The Medical Committee was made up of eleven consultants, elected by themselves to serve in a general capacity – that is they did not represent their own specialities; the Chairman and the Vice Chairman of the Board were *ex officio* members of the committee. This generalist characteristic of the Medical Committee was a source of strength throughout its history and the time-consuming and onerous task of serving on it for not less than three years at a time was shared out over the years amongst a large number of the senior staff; the task of Chairman was even more demanding and of course the Chairman had to be a member of the Board of Governors. The first Chairman of the Medical Committee was the Regius Professor of Physic, Sir Lionel Whitby, C.V.O., M.C., Master of Downing College.

Other committees set up in 1948 were the House Committee which was concerned with the domestic and local issues of the several hospitals, the Building Committee which had responsibility for the maintenance of the 'estate' for which the Board was accountable to the Minister and the Planning Committee. This last which was also chaired by Mr Knox-Shaw was to assume considerable significance as policies to build a new hospital were developed. Its membership was small and included as well as the Vice Chairman of the Board, the Chairman of the Medical Committee, one other representative of the consultant staff, the Chairman of the House Committee (Mrs Parsons who was to become Chairman of the Board in 1966) and two representatives of the University of Cambridge, one of whom was Dr H.M. Taylor, the Secretary General of the Faculties. Finally, and as an interesting comment on the priority given to the important subject, the Board appointed a Medical Records Committee.

The Board was required to submit its estimates of future financial need to the Minister by October 1948, and for the period to the end of March 1950 these were estimated to be £427,634 (net) for the cost of running the hospitals, and £145,198 as the capital that was needed. Agreement with the University had been reached over the continuation of the sharing arrangements for running the Pathology and Biochemistry Laboratories, but there were difficulties with the County Council over the details of the transfer of staff from the Council to the Board, and particularly over the payment of their salaries. An 'Endowment Fund' was created which was separate from the finances provided by the Government and which could be used for purposes related to the running of the hospitals not provided for by the State; never large, this Fund throughout the years was able to finance most valuable research projects as well as provide amenities for patients and opportunities for staff, not otherwise attainable.

~ 43 ~

Planning a new hospital

In 1948 the time was not ripe for the development of clinical specialities. These had to wait for the burgeoning years of the 1960s and onwards. Indeed the Hospital was still very conscious of the less than complimentary comments about it which had appeared in the Goodenough Report published in 1944 and in fact the Medical School was not equipped to undertake the clinical training of students, at least not on any large scale. The battles to establish such training were still to come.

Powerful people were, however, in positions of influence. The Master of Sidney Sussex, as we have seen, was Chairman of the Board of Governors. The Regius Professor of Physic was Sir Lionel Whitby, C.V.O., M.C., F.R.C.P., and from the outset he took a leading part in the administration of the Hospital. As Chairman of the Medical Committee he attended its monthly meetings as well as those of the General Purposes and Finance Committee and of the Board itself. He was also a member of the Planning Committee, set up originally as a joint committee with the University but later to assume greater significance as the plans for a new Hospital developed (Figs. 54–57).

Far-reaching matters of future policy did not, however, come before the Medical Committee during the early years. In September 1948 an outbreak of Sonne dysentery occurred which threatened the already stretched hospital facilities as beds and operating facilities were reduced. A highly critical report on the toilet facilities in the residencies and kitchens was considered by the Committee and forwarded to the Board with a strong recommendation that remedial action be instituted forthwith. In October of the same year a report was received from the Nuffield Hospitals Provincial Trust which recommended a total revision of the medical records system in operation in the Hospital, and later in the same year a report, which was even more before its time, was received from the Regius Professor of Physic (R.P.P.). This was on the need to establish a Home Care Nursing Service – a service which was staffed and organised from the Hospital and which had as its objects an improved service to

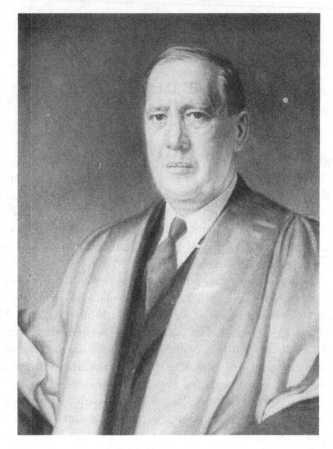

Fig. 54. Sir Lionel Whitby, C.V.O., M.C., M.D., F.R.C.P., Hon.
D.Sc. (Toronto), D.P.H., Regius Professor of Physic, 1945–1956.

patients, a better use of scarce hospital beds, and a reduction in the rising waiting lists.

1949 saw a similar mixture of medical administrative topics but during this year the Medical Committee spent some time discussing what were clearly difficult medical staffing matters. First came the need properly to identify the medical staff of the Hospital and then to establish the appropriate status and grade of each one. This called for two special meetings, in March and May, in addition to the routine monthly meetings. These were followed in July by the decision to ballot every member of the consultant staff asking each to place themselves on one of three 'merit' grades and also to name three senior colleagues who would

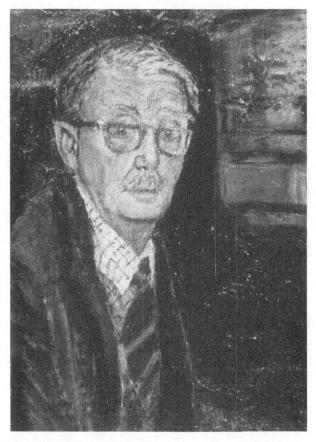

Fig. 55. Professor J.S. Mitchell, C.B.E., M.A., Ph.D (Cantab),
F.R.C.P., F.F.R., F.R.S., Regius Professor of Physic, 1957–1975.

act as adjudicators for the award of 'merit' gradings; this ballot was to be
carried out anonymously.

The case for a premature baby unit (March); the installation of a call
system for doctors (April); a procedure, worked out jointly with the
Regional Hospital Board, for the reception and treatment of patients
suffering from poliomyelitis (July); and the perennial issue of the extent to
which general practitioners working in Cambridge should have direct
access to hospital facilities such as pathology, X-ray and physiotherapy
(October), were also considered. A further outbreak of Sonne dysentery in
November 1949 brought to light the fact that the earlier strictures of the
two physicians (Dr L.C. Martin and Dr M.H. Gleeson-White) had not

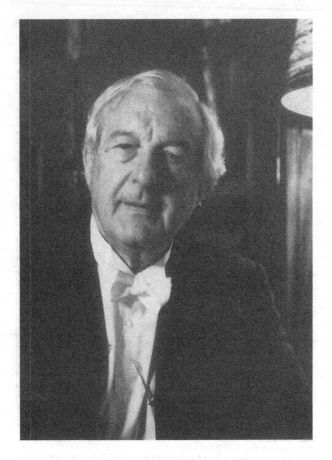

Fig. 56. The Lord Butterfield Kt, O.B.E., D.M., F.R.C.P., Regius
Professor of Physic, 1975–1987.

been acted upon, and the year closed with agreement on a policy for the
visiting of children in hospital by their parents which by today's standards
was draconian in the extreme.

Eighteen months after the commencement of the National Health
Service the medical staff were established and beginning to plan expansion within the limitations of the shortage of beds, supporting medical and
other services, and above all, money and space. The prospect of a new
hospital was the spur which excited clinical and academic staff alike and
influenced decisions on many matters, and it is to look at the early history
of the planning that we turn next.

We have already noted that before the Appointed Day Messrs Easton

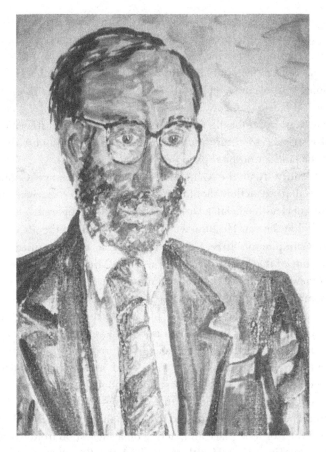

Fig. 57. Professor Keith Peters F.R.C.P., M.D. (Hon) Wales,
Regius Professor of Physic 1987 to present date. From a painting
by Sir Roy Calne F.R.S. (Source of Figs. 54–57 Lord Butterfield.)

and Robertson had been appointed architects for a new hospital to be
built on a site of over 60 acres in Trumpington. By August 1948 the Board
agreed to forward to the Ministry of Health its short-term plans for
Addenbrooke's along with a long-term proposal to acquire what had now
become 92.217 acres at Trumpington. This suggestion apparently gave
rise to difficulties and after what was described in the Board Minutes as 'a
discussion with a Ministry official' the General Purposes and Finance
Committee were told that the Ministry would authorise the purchase of
the freehold of 56 acres at a cost not to exceed £6,250 with the option to
purchase a further 35 acres.

After this promising start things moved more slowly. In June 1949 the consultant staff were pressing the Board of Governors to establish a building committee for the new Hospital, but they were told that the Planning Committee would initially take on this responsibility since both Sir Lionel Whitby and a representative of the consultant staff, Mr A.S.H. Walford, F.R.C.S., an E.N.T. surgeon, sat on it. Drafting of a compulsory purchase order for the site proceeded but by October it seemed that the Ministry of Agriculture and Fisheries had expressed doubts about the use of the land for hospital purposes.

In January 1950 the General Purposes and Finance Committee resolved that no action should be taken on a letter received from a Ministry of Health official, a Dr Maitland, who had apparently expressed the view that the new Hospital would be better built on the site of the old one in Trumpington Street. The letter however clearly caused trouble and in June of that year it was noted that the Ministry had revised their earlier views and now thought that not more than 25 acres were needed. The Board decided that if this was to be the case the site should be nearer to the centre of the City than the proposed site in Trumpington and should be better served by public transport. If less than 25 acres was likely to be available, then the plans should be reduced by omitting the maternity and infectious disease units, and some of the non-clinical University buildings. Only in the last resort should consideration be given to the suggestion that the old site in Trumpington should be rebuilt.

Behind the scenes, discussions led by the Chairman of the Board and the Regius Professor took place and, acting on a suggestion from Mr Knox-Shaw, the Ministry of Health authorised the Board to enter into a contract to acquire 43.895 acres of a site, owned by the Pemberton Trustees, in Hills Road opposite the junction with Fendon Road; this authorisation was on the understanding that a part of the site would be made available to the University. It was not however until December 1951 that authority was given for a cheque to be drawn in the sum of £4,350 being the total purchase price for what became known as 'The Hills Road Site' and at the same time it was agreed to fence the land for a further £550. The proposal to build on the land in Trumpington was abandoned.

Practical work now began in earnest and having completed the purchase of the land the consultant staff were asked by the Board to revise their original requirements for hospital accommodation. In the summer of 1952 a Dr George Godber of the Ministry of Health suggested that the

Board should formulate their plans in stages, a suggestion which was acted upon and which, with the benefit of hindsight, one can now see significantly improved the chances of work starting on site. At the time (1952) the prevailing Ministry view was that the optimum size of teaching hospitals was 800 beds, an opinion which was not based on research findings, but on the general view that such a size was manageable in terms of scale. It did not conflict with opinion in Cambridge and in August of that year the consultant staff agreed that, because the creation of a neurosurgical unit within existing facilities was not feasible, it should form part of the first building on the new site, and they asked that plans should be drawn up without delay.

The Medical Committee made a number of detailed but important recommendations to the Board of Governors in August; all were accepted and it is worth setting them out in full.

1 A Sub-Committee should be established to handle the planning of the new site.
2 A site layout plan should be prepared and a flexible order of priority determined to allow construction of the new Hospital part by part.
3 The Board of Governors should approach the University and ask that the steps necessary to establish a pre-graduate school of clinical teaching be taken.
4 The Board should ask the Regional Hospital Board to nominate a member or members to the New Site Planning Committee.
5 The Neurosurgical Unit and probably other specialist (Regional) units should be given priority.

With these views established as Board policy it was something of a formality that in the following June it was agreed that no further developments be planned on the Trumpington Street site. Hopes clearly ran high that the first stage of building would soon be started and in order to expedite planning it was agreed that the architect's fees should if necessary be met from the Board's Endowment Funds.

At the end of November 1953 a meeting was held between Mr Knox-Shaw, the Regius Professor, Mr Walford (representing the consultant staff) the Secretary-Superintendent, Mr Beardsall, and the architects, Mr Murray Easton and Mr S.E.T. Cusdin. They considered a development plan for a main, five-storey ward block of 750 beds and a parallel block for X-ray and 'other ancillary services'. A nurses' home and a kitchen would form part of the first stage, the total cost of which was to be limited to £500,000. It was thought that a temporary boiler plant would be needed initially as well as workshops and a laundry. A maternity hospital should be planned on the site in the expectation that it would not be built for some time. It was agreed however that a Medical School, a residents' hostel and an isolation unit should all be included in the plans together with an identified 'sports area' for staff. A separate plan for an Out-patient Department on the site was discussed and, despite the enormous pressures on the existing Trumpington Street accommodation, a proposal to extend that department by adding a gallery was not approved.

During the next eighteen months the proposals were discussed by the staff, and the architects worked at more detailed plans. Mr Cusdin attended a meeting of the Board in July 1955 and gave an explanation of his firm's plan for the site development and the detailed proposals for Stage One which were to include an Out-patient Department, a Casualty Department and a unit of 50 surgical beds with an operating theatre suite; it was agreed to forward these proposals to the Ministry of Health and two months later the Board authorised the architect to prepare plans for Stage Two of the development, again suggesting that although ultimately the cost of the new Hospital would be met by the Exchequer, exceptionally these fees might be met from the Endowment Fund.

In November 1955 the General Purposes and Finance Committee received a request from the Vice Chancellor for a generous allocation of space on the New Site for post-graduate teaching purposes. He said that the University believed that a post-graduate school should develop further before pre-graduate clinical teaching should begin; the Board noted these views and suggested that two University representatives should join the New Site Planning Committee.

~ 44 ~

Planning a Clinical School

The protagonists of the Clinical School realised from the outset that an ordered, methodical and informed committee structure was essential. The establishment of the Clinical School Planning Committee in 1969 was notable in a number of ways; it was set up by the General Board of the Faculties of the University in a way which involved the Hospital from the beginning; the experience of other Schools was recognised to be essential; and as a planning committee its remit was clearly stated to be to plan, not to run, the School. The Committee held its first (informal) meeting on 15 November 1969 and its last on 15 December 1975. Throughout most of the intervening time the Committee met at monthly intervals.

Those present at the first meeting were:

Professor Frank G. Young, F.R.S., Professor of Biochemistry – Chairman;

Professor Arnold S.V. Burgen, F.R.S., Professor of Pharmacology;

Professor Frank Hayhoe, M.D., F.R.C.P., Professor of Haematology;

Dr T.M. Chalmers, M.D., F.R.C.P., Consultant Physician; with

Mr Gordon Anderson, Assistant Secretary of the Faculties, as Secretary.

It was decided to invite four 'external members' to join, who were:

Dr J. Badenoch, D.M., F.R.C.P. Consultant Physician, Oxford;

Professor W.J.H. Butterfield, O.B.E., M.D., F.R.C.P. Professor of Medicine, Guy's Hospital London;

Professor A.L.d'Abreu, C.B.E., F.R.C.S., Professor of Surgery, Birmingham;

Sir Brian Windyer, F.R.C.P., F.R.C.S., Professor of Radiotherapeutics, The Middlesex Hospital and lately Vice Chancellor, University of London.

In addition Dr M.F.T. Yealland, F.R.C.P. Consultant Neurologist, was invited as the representative of the consultant staff of Addenbrooke's

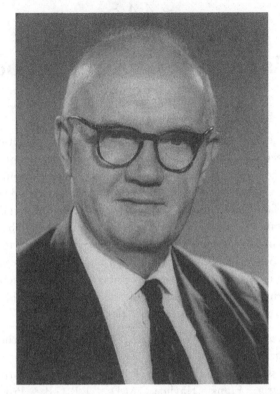

Fig. 58. Sir Frank Young, M.A. (Cantab)., D.Sc.,. Hon. F.R.C.P.,
F.R.S., Chairman of the Clinical School Planning Committee and
Master, Darwin College, where the Committee held its meetings.

Hospital, and the present writer who was House Governor and Secretary
of the Board of Governors was also invited to all meetings.

These formed the nucleus of the Clinical School Planning Committee
which from January 1970 met regularly at Darwin College where
Professor Young, later Sir Frank Young, was Master. The Committee
was joined in later years by others. In 1971 they were joined by C.K.
Philips, Chairman of the Faculty Board of Medicine's Estimates Sub-
Committee and by the Chairman of the Medical Committee of the United
Cambridge Hospitals. At the same time Lord Todd. O.M., F.R.S., Chair-
man of the Board of Governors of the Hospital and Master of Christs
College, and Professor J.S. Mitchell C.B.E., F.R.S., Regius Professor of
Physic also joined. Later in the same year Professor I.H. Mills, M.D.,
F.R.C.P., as Chairman of the Curriculum Sub-Committee together with

Professor R.Y. Calne, F.R.C.S., Professor of Surgery, were added. Finally in 1973 came Sir George Godber after his retirement from the office of Chief Medical Officer of the Department of Health and Social Security, and the Regional Medical Officer, Dr G.D. Duncan. It is also worth stating that, in recognition of the amount and the complexity of the planning that would be involved, early steps were taken to negotiate with the Hospital authority for the release of Dr T.M. Chalmers from some of his Hospital duties to help plan the School; the Board of Governors readily agreed with this suggestion.

On 27 November 1969 an important meeting was held in the offices of the University Grants Committee with its Chairman, Mr K. Berrill, in the Chair. Cambridge was represented by the Vice Chancellor, the Revd Professor W.O. Chadwick, Professors Young, Joslin, and Hayhoe, with Dr T.M. Chalmers and the Secretary General of the Faculties, Mr W.G. Sartain. The main topics under discussion were payments for clinical responsibilities, the financing of a future School, and its starting date and rate of growth. On the subject of payments for clinical responsibility the Cambridge representatives reported that there was a strong body of University opinion against the payment of differential stipends to medical teachers. However it was strongly believed by the planners of the School that without differential payments Cambridge could not hope to attract medical teaching staff of the calibre required. The University Grants Committee (U.G.C.) view as explained by the Chairman was that whereas the duties of the normal university teacher had two components – teaching and research – those of a clinical teacher contained a third, clinical responsibility; he should in their view be compensated for this.

As far as financing, from public funds, the proposed new School, the U.G.C. recognised the exceptional case that was being put to them and unusually agreed to earmark funds for this purpose for a maximum of ten years. It was pointed out that all U.G.C. funds were committed to the task of bringing the number of pre-clinical places up to the required 3700 by 1975 and that there was no chance of money being available to start a clinical course during the remainder of the present quinquennium. They said that the arguments for a Cambridge School were likely to be won on the basis of quality, rather than quantity, and they saw little likelihood of a start being possible before 1973.

In Cambridge it was realised that the design of the curriculum for the new School was going to be central for its success. A Sub-Committee of the Clinical School Planning Committee under the chairmanship of the

Regius Professor of Physic, Professor J.S. Mitchell F.R.S. was established and attention immediately focussed upon the most controversial sugges- tion – namely that the course should be a two-year course followed by a third, pre-registration year. N.H.S. consultant staff as well as academic medical staff were represented on the Curriculum Sub-Committee and many views were debated; Professor Roy Calne for instance submitted a paper arguing strongly in favour of a curriculum which enabled students to learn from the experience of taking personal responsibility for their own patients.

In each of the two years there were to be four elements. In the first year these comprised:

1. a coordinated systematic course based upon the systems of the body and comprising lectures, discussions, seminars, etc.;
2. clinical teaching, for the first eight months in groups of 20 and in the last three attached in groups of 8–10 to clinical 'firms';
3. weekly case conferences, daily pathological demonstrations and group discussions held fortnightly;
4. unallocated time amounting to three full days a week to enable students to pursue their own interests or research.

In the second year priority was to be given to clinical teaching, and students rotated through all specialities during eight months; some of these involved living in, and in the final three months students were attached to a regional hospital. During the year the same pattern of lectures, case conferences and so on continued, and sixteen weeks were allocated for students 'elective' subjects.

It will be seen from the above that the course was a concentrated one and also involved collaboration not only with the N.H.S. staff at Addenbrooke's but also with other hospitals in East Anglia. These regional hospitals were to be called Associate Teaching Hospitals of the University of Cambridge, and officers of the Regional Hospital Board attended meetings of the Clinical School Planning Committee from time to time. As the plans developed so too did the realisation that accurate estimates of cost, and of the numbers of medical teaching staff, academic and N.H.S., were essential; as a rule of thumb it was assumed that N.H.S. staff involved in teaching could be expected to devote about 20% of their time to such activities.

Looking back at the work that was done in these early years one characteristic stands out. This is the extent and the range of external advice that was sought, and very readily given, by experts from other clinical schools, and indeed from other countries. First was of course the help given by the four very senior members of the medical profession who were members of the Committee and who have already been referred to. (Professor Butterfield was later to become Regius Professor at Cambridge and is now Lord Butterfield.) As well as these the Committee met or had correspondence with many experienced medical teachers from the London and the provincial teaching hospitals as well as with others from hospitals, not designated as teaching hospitals, within and outside East Anglia. From abroad much was learnt from the United States, visited by Dr T.M. Chalmers on the Committee's behalf in 1971, from the Netherlands, Scandinavian countries, Turkey and many others; it was as though word had spread that Cambridge University was embarking on an ambitious experiment and others wished to help the enterprise.

During the first twelve months of the Committee's activities it could broadly be said that its attention was focussed upon the planning of the curriculum; upon the need to persuade the University of the need to establish the clinical school and upon the relationship between the academic and N.H.S. components of Addenbrooke's Hospital. By 1970 however it had become clear that planning could not ignore outside events and the Committee began to turn its attention to more mundane matters of administration.

Planning from 1970

In July 1968 the first 'Green Paper' on the Reorganisation of the National Health Service had been published by the then Minister of Health, Kenneth Robinson. In February 1970 his successor, Richard Crossman, who held the office of Secretary of State, published a far more radical Green Paper on the same subject. The Committee studied this carefully because it was clear that widespread changes were impending in the way in which health services were provided. In particular there was to be greater integration in the administration of the various parts of the N.H.S. and much more emphasis placed upon the provision of those services in the community as distinct from services which would have to continue to be based in hospitals.

It was at about this time that the ambitious idea was first mooted that a way might be found to organise all the activities, teaching, research and service provision, as a single integrated entity, called perhaps a Medical Centre and governed by a Medical Council. In the event statutory and other requirements prevented this, but the concept was much debated and led to a paper by Professor Frank Hayhoe and the present writer on a divisional organisation of the Clinical School which mirrored the clinical divisions in the Hospital structure. Considerations of these matters led to the holding of a two-day weekend seminar attended by six representatives of the University and six from the Board of Governors conducted by Professor Elliott Jacques of Brunel University with two of his colleagues, all acknowledged experts in social administration.

The most immediate task facing the Clinical School Planning Committee at the beginning of 1970 was the drafting of a report for the General Board to present to the University. A first draft was considered at the beginning of March which recommended formally the establishment of a course on clinical teaching together with approval for the policy of paying medical teaching staff for clinical responsibility, a topic which of course could not be shelved or hidden. At the same time material prepared by a New Estimates Sub-Committee chaired by C.K. Phillips and which held its first meeting in January was also received. The pace at which work then proceeded can be judged by the fact that the Committee received its third draft only a month after the first; that by February a revised list of additional Chairs had been drawn up totalling fourteen in all and the third draft took account of the Green Paper and stressed the need for team management and the delegation of financial responsibility.

Although the focus of the Committee's work was upon academic issues, and this in turn meant that the Government Department most involved was the University Grants Committee (responsible as it was to the Treasury), service matters, and with them the responsibilities of the Department of Health and Social Service, were also crucial. This is illustrated by the private and confidential meeting held by the Committee with Sir George Godber, then Chief Medical Officer. The notes of this day-long discussion were considered to be so private that they were only sent to members of the Committee and then only after they had been approved by Sir George; after some debate and after clearing with him it was decided that two copies could be sent to the U.G.C. At this distance in time it is difficult to see what was so very sensitive about the matters discussed but the approach indicates how delicate a subject medical education was, and is.

Some of this became apparent at the end of April 1970 when a meeting was held with officers of the U.G.C. It will be recalled the Cambridge supporters of the proposed new School had been much encouraged at the outset by the meeting held at the end of November 1969 when the Chairman of the U.G.C. had told the Vice Chancellor in effect to proceed with planning in the hope that clinical training might start in 1973. In 1970 the officers of the U.G.C. were more guarded. They took the view that the U.G.C. was not committed to the establishment of the School; that if one was started, they foresaw a smaller intake of 40 to 60 as being viable in the national context of student needs. They thought that if a School was started in 1973 it would only be approved if it involved very little by way of capital development.

The planners were not deterred and on 20 May 1970 the General Board discussed the report on the establishment of the Clinical School. With two dissensions it approved the Report which was then placed before the University and it was debated in the Senate House on 9 June 1970. It was approved by 446 votes to 225. Dissent was voiced about the recommendation for enhanced payments for clinical responsibility, but the approval when it came was by a greater margin than the planners had expected and enabled the Clinical School Planning Committee to turn its attention to detailed work: to accommodation needs within the Hospital (embedded accommodation); precise student numbers; relationships with Colleges; the search for, and the timing of the appointment of, a Dean; the numbers of beds available and needed, and so on.

The task was formidable. Some years later in a submission to the Royal Commission on the National Health Service in 1979, The Royal College of Surgeons of England commented:

> Previous attempts to forecast the staffing needs of the N.H.S. have not met with conspicuous success and the most important lesson to be learnt from the past is that the future is unpredictable. (para. 14. 14, Report of the Royal Commission)

The planners of 1970 would have echoed that sentiment, but like the later Royal Commission they 'chanced their arm'.

The matter of embedded accommodation was considered to be so crucial that it too warranted the setting up of a Sub-Committee. It met for the first time in September 1970 and in three meetings had analysed the available space and made wide-ranging recommendations which pressed for the flexible use of accommodation and the avoidance of pre-empting the use of space for particular clinical or academic purposes. This presented difficulties to the Hospital. It should be explained that from the mid 1960s when the plans for Stage Two of Addenbrooke's Hospital were drawn up, on each floor of the main ward block had been included an annexe called a 'Teaching Spur'. The accommodation was planned uniformly on each floor to include offices, discussion rooms and areas large enough for clinical conferences to take place and allowing access for patients in beds. In the L-shaped Pathology Block the same principle had been followed with one arm of the L being earmarked for teaching and research and the other for service needs. By 1970 building was well advanced and, although the building contract which the Hospital had with the contractors, John Mowlem's, was uniquely flexible, decisions on the provision of facilities could not be indefinitely postponed whilst discussions were held about the likely differing needs for teaching the clinical specialities.

The next significant meeting with officers of the U.G.C. took place in January 1971. On this occasion the issue of principle of whether or not there was to be a School was not raised, but argument raged (not too strong a word) on the definition of 'graduate' staff to be employed and for whom the U.G.C. would give approval. The Cambridge planners had assumed that only medically qualified staff were to be so defined, but at this meeting it became clear that the U.G.C. were intending to include all the graduate staff in the Hospital Laboratory Service, a considerable number of whom were not of course medically qualified. The planners agreed to revise their estimates and to prepare papers about the distribution of Chairs, the numbers of academic posts of consultant rank and the costs of payments for teaching which would be made to existing N.H.S. consultant staff.

By June 1971 a measure of agreement had been reached and a letter was received from the U.G.C. to the effect that they would support the establishment of a Cambridge School if the estimates of costs could be brought down to what was described as 'an acceptable level'. They particularly wanted attention to be given to the redeployment of the resources of the Post-graduate Medical School and a re-assessment of the basic teaching needs of the undergraduate clinical course. At the end of that month, agreement was reached with the U.G.C. that consolidated revised estimates would be prepared – that is, estimates for both under-graduate and post-graduate teaching – and that these would be presented to the General Board for consideration at the one meeting that that body held during the coming Long Vacation Term. Finally, at this point, it was decided that a matter which did not have financial implications but which in Cambridge was even more delicate should also be resolved. That was the giving of University status (the degree of M.A.) to all approved N.H.S. staff who would be involved in teaching – a move which was provided for under the Statutes and Ordinances of the University, but which some believed would at a stroke introduce an unbalanced increase in the voting members of Regent House.

Notwithstanding the detailed and, to many, the boring work of planning administrative issues, the Committee held fast to its main objective, so well described in the Report of the Royal Commission on Medical Education (The Todd Report) which had been published in 1968. Its aim was to produce 'not a fully qualified doctor but an educated man who will become fully qualified by post-graduate training'.

Internal and external pressures

The year 1971 was characterised by uncertainty for the planners of the new Clinical School. Externally the U.G.C. held the clues to the answers that were being sought with increasing urgency as the building of Stage Two of the new Hospital proceeded fast and on time. The U.G.C. were themselves in a difficult position; although there was an absolute Government commitment to provide, nationally, 4,100 clinical student places by 1979 (of which 1260 were to be in London), the general financial position was becoming desperate and the Universities of Oxford and London were also waiting for key decisions to be taken about their planned developments.

Internally in Cambridge there were pressures of a different kind. The suggestion had been made that the Clinical School Planning Committee should be disbanded and its place taken by a new Faculty Board of Clinical Medical Studies. The Clinical School Planning Committee were less than enthusiastic about this idea, with some justification since they had amassed a large amount of material, and experience, and were approaching the time when their labours would bear fruit. The suggestion did not proceed because of the length of time and the complexity of the task that would have been needed to revise the Statutes and Ordinances of the University to effect the changes. In order to meet the criticism that the Clinical School Planning Committee was too limited in its membership it agreed to be more relaxed about increasing its size. In the first instance as we have seen, two new members were appointed, the Regius Professor of

Physic, Professor J.S. Mitchell, and the Chairman of the Board of Governors, the Rt Hon. Lord Todd Master of Christ's College.

Pressures of an entirely different kind came from the Hospital. In November 1971 the Clinical School Planning Committee received a detailed report on the outline plans for Stage Three of the new Hospital. It was a key feature of Hospital policy that the momentum of planning and building should not be allowed to fall off as the massive Stage Two development neared completion. The Hospital wished to maintain in being its planning and commissioning teams and by November had a clear idea of the nature and timing of the next and final phase of building. Its general plan was to secure another 10 acres of land and to create a perimeter road; to complete the acute part of the Hospital by providing a further 360 beds and to bring on site mental illness and mental handicap (separate) units, a maternity hospital with all the acute, assessment, and long-stay geriatric beds. With all these went three day hospitals, and the full range of supporting facilities that would be necessary. When completed it was expected that the site would contain over 1530 beds.

The University wished to be involved in the detailed planning that went with these Hospital extensions and arrangements were agreed for their officers to join the Hospital planning groups. An obvious point of interest for them was the need to ensure that facilities were planned to enable 40% of the annual intake of clinical students to be resident on the site, and for this the Clinical School Planning Committee were involved in looking for a nearby property which could be used for this purpose. At the same time, that is early in 1972, the Medical Research Council (M.R.C.) made it known that they hoped to house the Dunn Nutritional Laboratory on the Hills Road site, a laboratory which had been in existence since the early 1920s and which was likely to acquire a greater clinical orientation in the near future; the Clinical School Planning Committee urged the General Board to set up the mechanism to integrate the planning of this Laboratory into the University because they knew of the Hospital's plans for a metabolic unit to be included in Stage Three, the work of which would closely relate to the M.R.C. proposal.

In June 1972 the U.G.C. made known their views on the numbers of staff they would be prepared to finance for the 'consolidated' School – pre- and post-graduate students – and these were as follows, with the Cambridge proposed figures in brackets:

Full-time academic staff: 90 (150)
Externally sponsored research workers: 27 (150)

Honorary academic staff:	15 (45)
Undergraduate clinical students:	300 (300)
Post-graduate research students:	75 (112)

The Cambridge view was that the U.G.C. figures were barely sufficient for intensive teaching and that they left little margin for research, but by December it had become clear that the U.G.C. was not prepared to negotiate on student numbers, even the externally sponsored researchers, presumably on the grounds that space would be needed to house them.

The problem of integrating University building plans with those of the Hospital continued; the Hospital planned to start detailed work on the first element of Stage Three – the psychiatric and geriatric elements and the common services for the whole – in January 1973. Within a year after that a start was to be made on the remainder, dates which with the benefit of hindsight contained a good deal of optimism since they had not been accepted by the officials of the Department of Health.

In mid January 1973 the Vice Chancellor received details of the amounts of the earmarked grant which the U.G.C. would provide to enable 50 clinical students to start in 1976/77, a figure which was to rise to 150 in the following quinquennium. (Note. The figures were: 1975/76 £114,000 and 1976/77 £150,000.) The implications of this decision were that a considerable shift of resources was going to be needed, from the Post-graduate School to pre-graduate training, since the earmarked grant in itself was barely sufficient for the Clinical School. This gave rise to many problems; legislative within the University – the need to seek confirmation from Regent House that, given the U.G.C. grant, the decision to proceed should stand; the urgent need for a Dean to be appointed, notwithstanding the fact that U.G.C. funds were only available from 1975; and finally the mechanism for giving University status to N.H.S. staff had to be confirmed. All these matters were covered in a Report to the University which the Clinical School Planning Committee approved in March 1973.

The Committee next turned its attention to the relationship between clinical students and the Colleges of the University. All students would be reading for Cambridge medical degrees and all would need to be members of Colleges. As they would have limited opportunities to use College facilities, notably residential and dining, it was suggested that Colleges might make only a nominal charge of £5.00 per head per term. The need for long-term residential accommodation for, it was estimated, 300 students, was accepted by the Committee. This need impinged on regional links and Dr Chalmers, with the Regional Medical Officer, Dr Duncan, visited hospitals in Peterborough, Norwich and Ipswich to discuss ways in which collaboration could be sustained.

Despite the many problems the optimism among the planners that the School would begin was maintained and attention again turned in the autumn of 1973 to the future administrative structure. A 'search committee' which included external members of the Committee had been set up with a wide brief to seek candidates for the post of Dean. The view was taken however that, unlike other medical schools, in Cambridge the Regius Professor of Physic must be the Head of the School, with the clinical Dean taking responsibility for day to day administration. The then Regius Professor, Professor J.S. Mitchell was due to retire in 1976 and he was among the first to realise the value of his successor as Regius being in post before the School started and the first students were enrolled. Professor Mitchell therefore offered to resign from the Regius Chair on the understanding that he could resume his previous Chair as Professor of Radiotherapeutics and be accorded the title of Emeritus Regius Professor. This offer was gratefully accepted and at the same time Dr T.M. Chalmers was recommended for appointment as part-time Clinical Dean for three years.

The year 1973 ended, for the planners of the School, on another worrying note. As well as their concerns about the effect of the coming reorganisation of the N.H.S. on their work (the Act to establish the reorganised N.H.S. had been passed and the new Service was due to come into being on 1 April 1974), they were told that the D.H.S.S. had begun to have reservations about the total number of beds that were to be provided on the one site at Hills Road. Whilst understandable, given that the total was approaching 1600, the D.H.S.S. criticisms were unreasonable in that much of the increase had been due to political pressures to associate psychiatric, mental handicap and geriatric units with district hospitals. Be that as it may, the Clinical School Planning Committee found itself debating the implications on teaching and research if the number of beds at Hills Road was reduced to the suggested figure of 1200. They concluded that this would almost certainly mean that student intakes would have to be reduced.

The end of the planning

The Clinical School Planning Committee concluded its work at the end of 1975 and the first clinical students were admitted at the start of the Michaelmas Term, 1976.

This epilogue to the History of Addenbrooke's Hospital ends with the demise of the Board of Governors of the United Cambridge Hospitals on 31 March 1974. The story would not however be complete without reference to the last stages of the planning of the complex arrangements needed to enable Cambridge University and Addenbrooke's Hospital to resume the total training of doctors, arrangements which had lapsed since the beginning of the nineteenth century.

Throughout the deliberations of the Committee its members were concerned that the timetable for the many approvals that were needed should not fall behind schedule. In March 1974 these were all reviewed. University approval of the complex changes to the constitution of the Faculty Board of Medicine was crucial; so too was the need for authority to advertise and select the holders of new Chairs and other academic posts. No less important were the Hospital posts, and at that time the serious economic position of the country was putting in jeopardy the approvals, by the D.H.S.S., for the funding of the new hospital clinical posts. Notwithstanding these difficulties, the Committee were agreed that of overriding importance was the need to start the new School. Even if ideal conditions did not exist in October 1976 they decided that they must perservere with their aim to admit the first students then.

Thanks to financial support from the Cancer Research Campaign, a new Chair in Cancer Research and Oncology had been made possible, but the building of a new department involved detailed and complicated negotiations with the Medical Research Council, as well as with the new Regional and Area Health Authorities. Both these latter were enthusiastic about the development and the Clinical School Planning Committee urged the University to accept the offer with its research potential if links with Dr Sydney Brenner's work in the Molecular Biology Unit were extended. It was finally resolved that Professor Norman Bleehan, the named holder of the Chair, should take up his position as Head of the Department of Radiotherapy from October 1975, Professor Mitchell suggesting that he himself would continue working but as the second

~417~

professor. Both the University and the Hospital expressed their profound appreciation of Professor Mitchell's generosity.

The possibility of creating new clinical academic departments was a subject which most people enjoyed debating. Amongst the disciplines putting forward ideas were community medicine, for which the Department of Health put in a plea; geriatric medicine, an expanding Hospital department for which an academic component was sought; anaesthetics, for which there was hope that external funds might be attracted; radiology, another large and expanding Hospital department; and orthopaedic surgery whose surgeons wrote to the Committee proposing 'closer links' with the Clinical School.

The Committee had to concern itself also with more mundane matters. Much time and energy was spent on the revision of the Statutes, but at a practical level one of the biggest problems was the likely ultimate size of the Hospital. In essence the dilemma arose from the need to provide enough acute beds for teaching, while at the same time satisfying the D.H.S.S. that provision for psychiatry, geriatrics, obstetrics and the young chronic sick at Hills Road, was adequate. The Clinical School Planning Committee concluded that the D.H.S.S. would not be persuaded to change its views, and that in the then existing economic climate the ideal, which was the provision of a second District General Hospital in Cambridge, was not attainable. They concluded that, whilst nothing would persuade them to abandon the timetable, some compromises would have to be made.

It will have been realised that throughout the planning of the new School the links between the University and Addenbrooke's Hospital had been close and constructive. In the later planning stages this collaboration extended to the Region and to the several associated hospitals. The reorganised National Health Service which came into being on 1 April 1974 unleashed a flood of N.H.S. circulars, and the D.H.S.S. pressed for the creation of 'liaison committees' between the several statutory bodies, including Universities, that were concerned with health care. The Clinical School Planning Committee was not impressed with the idea and agreed that the present writer and Dr George Duncan, the Regional Medical Officer, could adequately transmit their views to the new Area and Regional Health Authorities.

The Committee in its final year dealt manfully with the details of planning as well as topics as broad as 'Democracy in the N.H.S.', a Government paper on which they were invited to comment. In January

1975 the Prime Minister's Office announced that Dr W.J.H. Butterfield, then Vice Chancellor of the University of Nottingham, had been appointed to the Regius Chair of Physic. John Butterfield had been one of the four 'external' members of the Clinical School Planning Committee from its inception and his appointment to the Regius Chair was warmly welcomed.

The Committee held its last, the sixty-ninth meeting, at Darwin College on Monday 15 December 1975, and later that evening a dinner was held at Christ's College. Some nine months later under the aegis of a new Faculty Board of Clinical Medicine, the first clinical students began their training on the wards of Addenbrooke's Hospital.

~ 45 ~

The Board of Governors' final years

Strategies and plans

The mid to late 1950s were a period of optimistic planning. The difficulties of the early years of the N.H.S. were past; the economic problems of the sixties and seventies were not anticipated, and as far as Addenbrooke's was concerned it was clear that there was to be a new hospital built at Hills Road, and that given some luck the University would resolve its qualms over the payment of differential salaries to clinicians and join with the Board in creating a Teaching Hospital second to none.

During 1957 the Board decided that an authoritative and objective survey was needed to determine the eventual bed complement that would be needed at the new Hospital bearing in mind its likely regional as well as local role. Under the chairmanship of Professor A.L. Banks, Professor of Human Ecology, a member of the Board of Governors and a part-time adviser to the Ministry of Health, a small committee was established with ample representation from the Region as well as from the consultant staff of the Hospital. Its report was published in 1959 and immediately caused controversy. In total, Banks recommended that the bed complement needed was 680, a figure far below the expectations of the medical staff. At a meeting of the Medical Committee in October 1959 the view was expressed that the figure should be revised to 806 and the committee expressed concern that it had not had an opportunity to 'bring to notice factors which in their view were omitted from consideration by the survey committee'.

Planning for the future was the subject of endless debate and heated argument. The process of decision making on major matters was more complex and most important decisions were in the main taken in Whitehall following representations, often at great length, from those locally involved and informed; there is little evidence about the extent to which local views were influential. One method of consultation at local level was the Planning Liaison Committee with a high-powered membership including the Chairmen of the Board of Governors and the Regional Hospital Board, and the Regius Professor of Physic. This Committee, at one meeting in October 1959, considered not only the report from Professor Banks' Survey Committee, but the Development Plan for the Addenbrooke's Site, the future expansion of geriatric services in Cambridge, the establishment of an orthodontic service and the need for a liaison committee for the Hospital and community maternity services.

The Board of Governors held fast to its preoccupation with building at Hills Road and in October reaffirmed its objectives. These were:

1 to transfer all the Board's Hospitals to Hills Road in the following order: Addenbrooke's, Brookfields, Maternity, Chesterton;
2 that once work had started on Stage One at Hills Road, then building should continue as rapidly as possible 'until the whole new Hospital is completed';
3 that Stage Two of Addenbrooke's should have a mainly surgical emphasis with probably about 300 beds;
4 that Stage Two should include a unit for patients suffering from infectious diseases;
5 that Douglas House should close as an annexe of Addenbrooke's and together with the workload of Brookfields Hospital should move to Hills Road with the completion of Stage Two.

These major strategic issues did not prevent the resolution of more immediate planning matters. In November 1959 work started on planting trees around the whole perimeter of the Hills Road site and discussions were begun with the City, County and Bus authorities about the responsibility for providing a roundabout and a bus terminus at the entrance to the new Hospital site. The probable date for an official opening was given as the spring or early summer of 1962 and the Chairman of the Board, Mr Roger Parker, who was also Lord Lieutenant of the County 'was asked to make provisional enquiries'.

Plans not only for the departments which would comprise Stage One but also overall development for the whole site, were also occupying the New Site Special Committee. The consultant staff became increasingly interested and in December 1959 arranged for a member of the architect's staff to meet with them regularly. The need for a new and senior administrative appointment became apparent and the Board approached

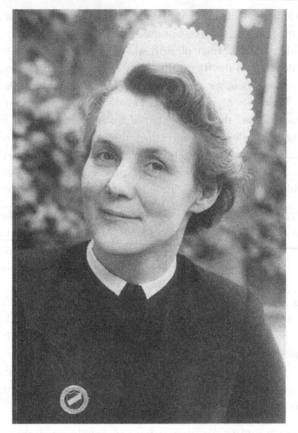

Fig. 59. Miss M.M. Puddicombe, O.B.E., S.R.N., S.C.M., Matron
Addenbrooke's Hospital, 1957–1970. (Photo Ramsay & Muspratt.
Source M.M.P.)

the Ministry for approval to establish this post. When the seniority
proposed was questioned by the Ministry officials, the Board resolved to
seek a meeting with the Minister and by 1960 had won that battle. In the
meantime detailed leasing arrangements were agreed between the Board
of Governors and the University for leasing at a peppercorn rent the area
at Hills Road to be used for University teaching and research purposes.

It was one of the characteristics of this time that, whilst debate and
discussion took place on future plans, the work of the old Addenbrooke's
Hospital, was maintained and expanded. The then Senior Anaesthetist,
Dr Harold Youngman and Matron, Miss M.M. Puddicombe (Fig. 59),
wrote to the Chairman of the Medical Committee at the end of 1959 about

the problems of nursing patients needing intensive care, and particularly those with tracheostomies. They pointed out that during 1959, 21 patients had required intensive treatment and that there were never less than three, and sometimes as many as six, needing such care simultaneously. Each patient needed six nurses per week to carry out specialised techniques, but this number could be halved if all the patients could be nursed in the same area. They pointed too to the disadvantages of the present system whereby clinical control was exercised by different medical 'firms'. The Medical Committee recommended the conversion of a room formerly used as Matron's office to a mixed sex unit, plus the adjacent side rooms of Hatton and Griffiths Wards to form the first intensive care unit of six beds. (This was later appropriately to become known as 'The Blue Room' from the original colour of the wallpaper.)

In November 1959 the first consultant geriatrician, Dr William Davison, was appointed, jointly with the Regional Board, and with beds at Chesterton Hospital. It was not until many years later when Stage Two was completed that he fulfilled his ambition to have beds on the Hills Road site.

With all these clinical changes taking place there was continuous concern about the rising costs of drugs. Annual meetings between the Medical Committee and the Chief Pharmacist were held and in February 1960 the Finance Officer, Mr P.A. Hollings, also attended. The officers' concern was that the limited amount of money available for new developments, such as the geriatric service, and intensive care, was in danger of being whittled away by the unrestrained freedom of doctors to prescribe drugs, the costs of which were rising dramatically. The problem was not solved and the medical staff considered that the drug expenditure was justified; they agreed to regular reviews and made some minor changes in, for example, the control of the use of methylated spirits.

The Medical Committee was more enthusiastic in its support of a proposal from the Regius Professor that funds be sought to establish a Chair in Investigative Medicine. This support was passed to the University in May 1960 and the planners were asked to ensure that provision of at least 25 beds would be made in Stage Two for the holder of this Chair. The Committee did not only concern itself with matters of policy but, for example, debated matters such as the age at which medical records should be destroyed. (They decided that, notwithstanding advice from the Ministry of Health that such records could mostly be destroyed after 40 years, 70 years was the period for which the local records should be retained.) The Committee was closely involved too in the planning of the experimental centralised sterilising services which were soon to replace the individual sterilisers on wards and departments. This switch from water boiling, mostly carried out by nurses, to autoclaving centrally dressings and instruments, was a major change financed in part by the Nuffield Provincial Hospitals Trust. The experiment, for such it was, was particularly significant because it was realised that the lessons learnt at Trumpington Street could be, and were, incorporated in the plans for the new Hospital.

Mainly about planning

Towards the end of 1960 the Board received a long report from its architect, S.E.T. Cusdin, about the implications of major building on the scale being considered. He made a very strong recommendation that the conventional procedures involving the drawing up of detailed, and virtually final, drawings and bills of quantities *before* inviting building and engineering tenders competitively, were inappropriate. He argued this on two grounds; first the speed with which medical and technical changes were taking place meant that it would be to the Hospital's advantage to extend the point at which final decisions were taken on plans for new buildings to the latest moment. Secondly, he pointed to the immense advantage in involving the contractors in the planning processes. These meant that a competitive process for selecting and appointing the main contractor before bills of quantities and working drawings were drawn up, had to be devised.

Cusdin also advocated the setting up of a Stage Two Planning Team immediately and urged the need to persuade the Ministry of Health to authorise a start on Stage Two as soon as Stage One was complete. He illustrated these advantages dramatically by showing that using conventional methods the likely conclusion of Stage Two could not be until 12 or 13 years hence; by using the new procedures, this interval could be reduced to $6\frac{1}{2}$–7 years.

Not surprisingly the Ministry was unmoved. It took until 1966 for the Board to convince suspicious civil servants that procedures which were novel for the public service (although not unknown, if unusual, in the private sector) would not create 'unfortunate precedents'. By that time of course the advantages of continuous building had been lost, but the

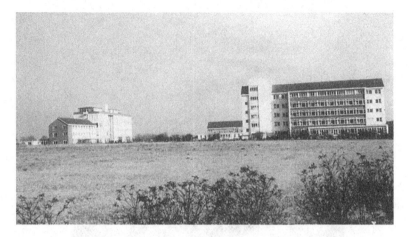

Fig. 60. Stage one of the New Hospital in 1964 showing on the
right the ward block of 100 beds for Neurology and Neurosurgery
and Orthopaedics; on the left the M.R.C. building and the
University Department of Radiotherapeutics. In front is the small
residency and dining room and just visible is part of the Out-
patient Department. (Photo W.G.C.)

immense advantage to the Hospital of having the skills of the contractor
available during the planning, were demonstrated time and time again.

Before going forward to those days we must conclude the story of the
building of the first stage of the new Hospital. In June 1961 the Board was
told that the contractors, Messrs Kerridge of Cambridge, had handed
over the ward block on the date agreed for completion and that the
remaining buildings, the Out-patient Department, the Casualty Department, the X-Ray Department and the small residency would be completed by September. A phased opening of these buildings was decided
upon, largely dictated by the shortage of nursing staff at the time. Patients
were admitted to the first neurosurgical ward on 2 October 1961 and by
the following April all the wards and departments were operating (Fig.
60).

We have already seen that some of the new ideas incorporated in the
new buildings had been tested in the old Hospital. Stage One was no less
important because it incorporated many of the principles to be carried
forward to later building. For instance, there was to be circulation of
goods and services, the general public and staff, and patients, on three
levels; as far as possible 'free ends' were to be left to allow for future
extension and development. Amongst the features in the Stage One

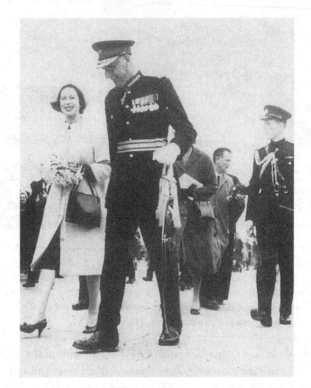

Fig. 61. Her Majesty the Queen with the Chairman of the Board
of Governors, Mr R.H. Parker, C.B.E., M.C., M.A., in his
capacity as Lord Lieutenant of the County.

buildings which the Board regarded as particularly significant was the
emphasis on good communications. For the first time the internal and
external telephone system was combined; a radio-controlled paging
system was included and a mechanical system for conveying medical
records and documents between all wards and departments (the Lamson
Tube system) was installed.

One of the most attractive features of the interior of the first buildings
was the extensive use made of natural wood, still in good condition 30
years later. Emphasis was placed on ease of maintenance but colour (in
the floor tiles and furnishings) were also carefully planned. Reference has
already been made to the external landscaping; inside, troughs and pots
for plants were provided and an anonymous donor gave a sum of money
for the provision of pictures, which were subsequently chosen by the Vice
Chairman of the Board, Mrs E.W. Parsons.

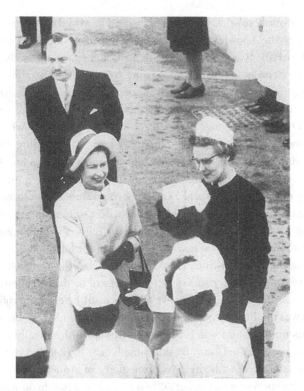

Fig. 62. Her Majesty the Queen with the Matron of
Addenbrooke's Hospital, Miss M.M. Puddicombe, greeting nurses
outside the Out-Patient Department. Behind is the then Minister
of Health, the Rt Hon. Enoch Powell.

The New Hospital was opened by Her Majesty Queen Elizabeth II on
28 May 1962. The Chairman of the Board of Governors, Roger Parker
Esq., C.B.E., M.C., M.A., was also Lord Lieutenant of the County of
Cambridgeshire, and it was in that capacity that he received the Queen in
the forecourt of the Out-patient Department and subsequently entertained her at luncheon at Trinity College (Figs 61 and 62).

Whilst the commissioning of the new buildings was proceeding, and the
time-consuming arrangements for the Royal opening and the subsequent
volume of professional and other visitors were made, other matters
engaged the Board's attention. In June 1960 Addenbrooke's Hospital was
designated as the Regional Centre for radiotherapy, and plans for the first
linear accelerator to be installed at Trumpington Street were made; sadly
no beds for the specialty could be provided at Hills Road until Stage Two.

The grossly over-crowded Maternity Hospital in Mill Road also received attention in the knowledge that the time when its facilities could be provided at Hills Road were, it was then thought, at least twelve years away. An extensive programme aimed at 'humanising' the services and upgrading the facilities was embarked upon. At Trumpington Street, 'the Old Addenbrooke's', there remained the bulk of the acute hospital facilities and with the move of orthopaedic surgery and the whole out-patient and casualty services, there was scope for extending into the accommodation vacated. The Orthopaedic Clinic which was housed in a concrete building in the forecourt and which had been built at the beginning of the Second World War as a decontamination centre in the event of gas attacks, was adapted for work with radioisotopes.

In March 1964 the Board was told that the officers were hopeful that approval to embark on the task of finding a contractor for Stage Two would soon be received from the Ministry of Health; a year later the House Governor had to report that there was still no decision despite the strongest possible representations. It was not until 1 February 1965 that approval was finally given, the news was telephoned whilst the Board was holding its meeting and was conveyed somewhat dramatically to Lady Adrian who was in the Chair. By that time Roger Parker had retired; he had been associated with the governing body of Addenbrooke's since 1921, having succeeded his father. When he retired a luncheon was given in his honour and later the Board were pleased that his son Mr Edmund Parker had been appointed by the Minister to the Board.

The contract with John Mowlem and Co., for building Stage Two was signed on behalf of the Board of Governors by the Chairman, Lady Hester Adrian, and by the House Governor and Secretary, the present writer, on 15 March 1966 (Fig. 63). A small ceremony to commemorate the event was held to mark this milestone in the presence of the Lord Lieutenant, the Vice Chancellor and members and staff of the Board of Governors. The building contract was for over £9 million and it was estimated at the time that the total cost including equipment would exceed £12 million. Very sadly on 20 May 1966 came the news of the sudden and unexpected death of the Chairman, Lady Hester Adrian.

Lady Adrian, the wife of the Master of Trinity College, had been a member of the Board since 1949; she had also been a member of the East Anglian Regional Hospital Board and from 1951 to 1957 Chairman of Fulbourn Hospital Management Committee. She had taken a prominent part in the process that led to the Mental Health Act 1959, having been a

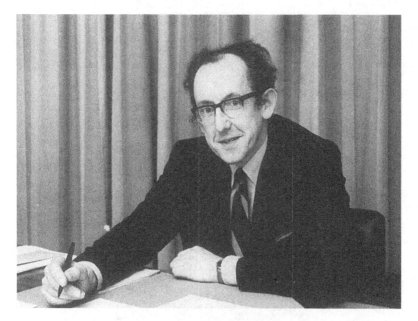

Fig. 63. W. Graham Cannon, M.A., F.H.S.M., House Governor of
Addenbrooke's Hospital and Secretary to the Board of Governors,
the United Cambridge Hospitals, 1962–1974. (Photo Leonard
Beard, Source W.G.C.)

member of the Royal Commission on the Law Relating to Mental Illness
which reported in 1959. She had been appointed a Dame Commander of
the British Empire in 1965.

The appointment of Mr Roy Calne as Professor of Surgery in 1965
marked a definitive step towards, not only the Clinical School, but also the
establishment of a Renal Unit, housed at Douglas House, and the
beginning of transplant surgery in Cambridge (Fig. 64). The first patient
was admitted to the Unit in February and at that time it was expected
that some 20 to 30 kidney transplant operations would be carried out
annually.

The pace of change was such that in 1965 the Board accepted the House
Governor's recommendations for a revision of the administrative and
committee structure controlling its operations. Emphasis was placed on a
clear and logical chain of communication and of responsibility. History
was not entirely neglected and October 1966 saw the 200th anniversary of
the admission of the first patient to Addenbrooke's Hospital, an event
commemorated by a service at St Botoloph's Church when the address

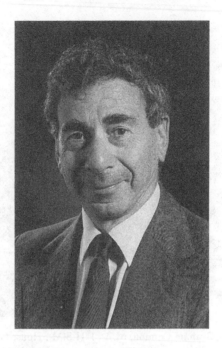

Fig. 64. Sir Roy Calne, F.R.S., M.S., F.R.C.S., Professor of
Surgery and pioneer in the field of transplantation surgery.
(Source R.Y.C.)

was given by the Bishop of Ely. By this time Mrs E.W. Parsons had been
appointed Chairman of the Board, having been a member since 1948. At
the same time Sir Frank Lee, Master of Corpus Christi College, and
previously Permanent Secretary to the Treasury, was elected Vice
Chairman (Fig. 65).

By now the building of Stage Two was well under way. Planning was
handled by three closely related teams. The original planning team with
its medical, administrative and nursing members, and chaired by Dr
Gleeson-White, University Bacteriologist who had been seconded for
the purpose, had always included the representatives of the architect,
consulting engineer, and quantity surveyor; now it was augmented by the
contractor's representative and met regularly in London and in Cambridge. Working in parallel was the construction team on which the
Hospital was represented by Alan Bullwinkle, its Assistant Secretary,
Planning, and which was made up of representatives of all the main
contractors and sub-contractors. Finally there was the Commissioning

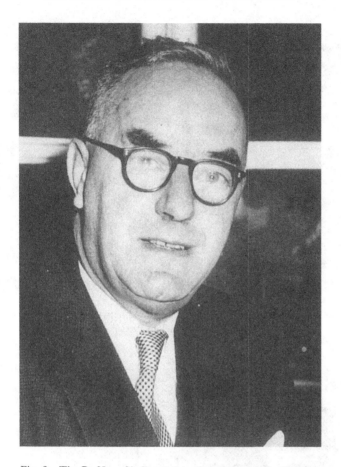

Fig. 65. The Rt Hon. Sir Frank Lee, P.C., G.C.M.G., K.C.B.,
M.A., Vice Chairman of the Board of Governors from 1967 to
1971. Sir Frank was Master of Corpus Christi College and had
previously been Permanent Secretary at H.M. Treasury. (Source
Lady Kathleen Lee).

Team with its full-time medical, administrative and nursing members,
chaired by Dr Tony Hargreaves, a community physician. This Team was
established as soon as the Stage Two contract had been signed and had the
responsibility for bringing the new buildings into use.

Two examples of the practical effect of close collaboration with the
contractor are worth recording. In constructing the central supplies,
laundry, kitchen and engineering area in the centre of the site, an area of
some 4 acres had to be excavated, in parts to a depth of 25 feet. The

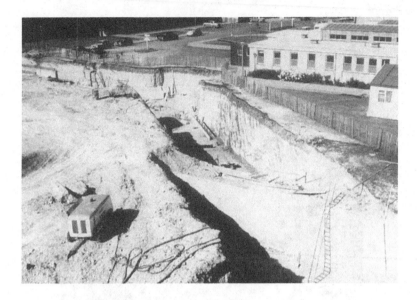

Fig. 66. Excavation for the underground network of walkways.
(Source Mowlem PLC.)

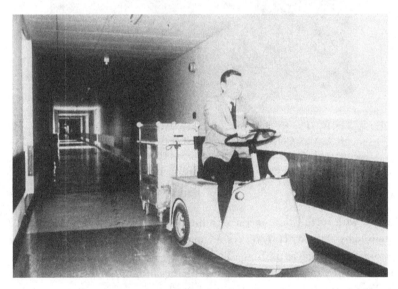

Fig. 67. The completed underground walkway with a motorised
trolley in use. (Source Mowlem PLC.)

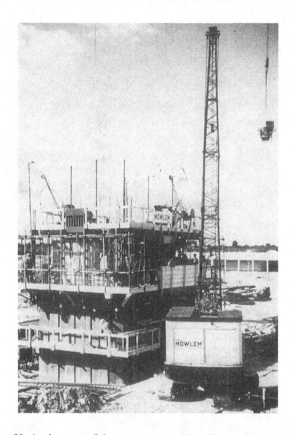

Fig. 68. At the start of the construction of the Tower chimneys for the new Hospital. The method used involved the continuous pouring of cement into a mould which slowly moved upwards; the whole chimney was built in twelve days, work proceeding day and night.

immense amount of spoil from this vast digging had to be disposed of and at Mowlem's instigation an agreement was entered into with the land-owner of the adjacent field, the Pemberton Trustees, for spreading the excavated soil over 25 acres and raising the level of that field by some 6 feet; the work was completed in nine weeks (Figs 66 and 67). The other feat was the construction of the tower chimneys, 220 feet high, an exercise which was accomplished in two weeks by use of a Swedish technique of continuous day and night working (Figs 68, 69 and 70).

As the skyline changed and the number of buildings increased so it was realised that a whole community was being created at Hills Road. The

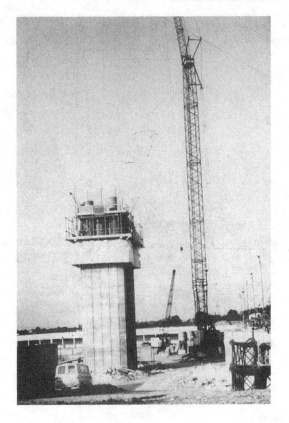

Fig. 69. The work on the chimney near to the half-way stage.

year 1968 closed with an ominous reference in the Board's Annual Report to 'an atmosphere of financial apprehension' as it was realised that the Board's original estimates of the cost of maintaining the vast enterprise were if anything understated, whilst the Department of Health remained intent upon reducing the amount of the funds that would be made available for this purpose. It was at this time that there began in earnest the struggle to match the endless series of needs with the very limited resources – people as well as money – that were available.

The final chapter

Mrs E.W. Parsons retired in 1968 and was appointed a Commander of the Order of the British Empire for her long service both to Addenbrooke's

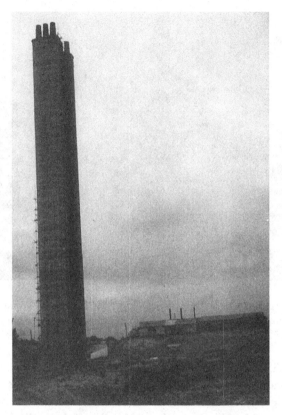

Fig. 70. The completed Tower. (Photos 68–70 W.G.C.)

and to public services in Cambridge over many years. At Addenbrooke's she was succeeded by The Rt Hon. Lord Todd, O.M., then Master of Christ's College (Fig. 71).

It will be evident from the history of the Hospital so far that by 1968 it was a major organisation; one of the largest employers of staff in Cambridge and one which was increasing in size and complexity year by year. In an attempt to inform staff of all aspects of the change that was going on around them but in which at any one time only some were involved, a house journal, *Addenbrooke's News* was started in December 1968. Forty-five editions were produced, the last appearing in February 1976, and its circulation had risen to over 1000 after five editions. It proved to be a much sought-after source of news for the staff and was entirely produced by voluntary effort, originating from the Senior Physicist, Dr John Haybittle who was the first editor. Another source of

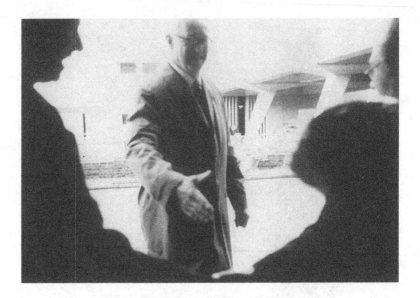

Fig. 71. The Rt Hon, the Lord Todd, O.M., F.R.S., Chairman of
the Board of Governors, 1969–1974, and Master, Christ's College.
(Photo W.G.C.)

information, though more formally produced were the annual reports.
These had appeared in one form or another in an unbroken series since
1766. Since 1948 these recorded the activities of new or expanded
departments of the Hospital and provided lists of the medical and other
professional staff. In the 1948 Report the work of fifteen clinical departments is referred to; by the time of the Final Report in 1974 this had
increased to 36 such departments.

One new department was the Computer Department, set up in 1969
following a detailed computer study. The original plan had been to
develop a computer system in tandem with Charing Cross and other
London teaching hospitals, each developing a particular part of the whole
system; the hope was that after the initial development period the whole
could be integrated into a common and integrated service used similarly
by all five participating hospitals. In the event this ambitious proposal did
not succeed and at the end of the pilot period each hospital, including
Addenbrooke's, developed its own department.

Not everything was smooth running. During the winter of 1969 an
influenza epidemic hit Cambridge and the resulting sickness, amongst
staff and patients indiscriminately, caused immense strain. Wards were

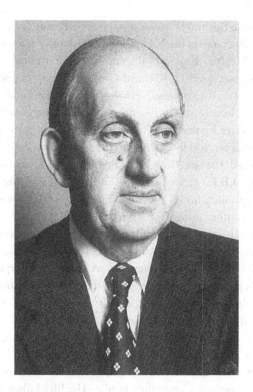

Fig. 72. Sir Francis Pemberton, C.B.E., D.L., Chairman of the
Addenbrooke's Hospital Development Trust which financed the
staff recreation centre (the Frank Lee Centre) and the residence
for relatives of patients which is named after his family. (Photo
Universal Pictorial Press. Source Sir Francis Pemberton)

closed due to lack of staff, this at a time of immense activity and with a bed
complement which was still markedly below what was needed for the
catchment area served by the Hospital. In April 1970 one of Addenbrooke's most distinguished governors, Sir Frank Lee, died. In the
relatively short time he had been associated with the Board Sir Frank had
contributed much from his vast knowledge of management in the public
service. Happily his name is perpetuated in the staff recreational centre,
the inspiration for which came from him. Having identified the need for
such a centre he persuaded the landowner, then Mr, now Sir, Francis
Pemberton (Fig. 72), of the adjacent land to donate over 2 acres for the
purpose of building a centre, and drew up a constitution which ensured its
independence.

In 1968 came the hint of major organisational change. The first Green Paper on the structure of the N.H.S. was published in this year by the then Minister of Health, Kenneth Robinson. More radical proposals for change were to come from Richard Crossman in 1970 and the present writer and other senior officers were increasingly occupied in discussions nationally and locally about the effects of these changes on the provision of hospital service by teaching hospitals. Changes in the organisation of hospital nursing services following a national review had already begun to be implemented; the last Matron of Addenbrooke's Hospital, Miss M.M. Puddicombe O.B.E., retired in 1970 and a Chief Nursing Officer with overall responsibility for all the Board's nursing services was appointed.

The organisation of medical services was not exempt from change at this time. The Hospital had already moved to a divisional system outlined in two national reports of working parties set up by Sir George Godber, then Chief Medical Officer. These reports, known colloquially as 'The Cogwheel Reports' – from the design on the cover – were much discussed by the Consultant Staff Council, the body to which all consultant medical staff belonged, as well as by the Medical Advisory Committee. Nearer to home was the reorganisation in June 1969 of the Cambridge Laboratory Service. This comprised the University Departments of Pathology and Biochemistry administered and financed jointly by the University and the Board of Governors, and the Public Health Laboratory Service (P.H.L.S.). These were all amalgamated and the P.H.L.S. moved to some of the first accommodation to be completed at Hills Road as part of Stage Two.

At Hills Road building proceeded fast; the main ward block was 'topped out' in October 1970 by the present writer on behalf of the Chairman of the Board, Lord Todd (Fig. 73), and, even better, the Department of Health had approved funding for a further stage of building after Stage Two, although with lower cost limits than the Board would have liked. Planning momentum was however maintained, although the Board had as its major concern the problems which it knew would develop as a result of the under-funding of the costs for running the new services that were being built.

There was no stopping development. One of the most important areas for growth was in the training fields and in these there was much activity in Cambridge. The establishment of the Clinical School has already been recorded; in nursing, where a vigorous nursing school had existed for many years, new curricula were developed and in 1970 a new syllabus,

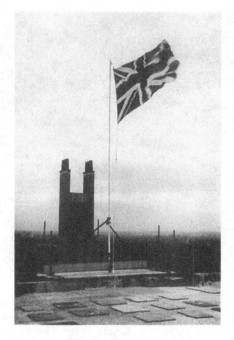

Fig. 73. The 'topping out' of the new Hospital in October 1970.
This occasion marks the moment when the roof of a new building
is completed; beer is drunk and the Union Jack flown from the
highest point. (Photo W.G.C.)

known as the 'two plus one' was introduced. This introduced a pre-registration year for the trained nurse and allowed for a better marriage of classroom learning and practical experience. Training was given in the Education Centre, built as part of Stage Two, and where by 1970 the School of Physiotherapy was inducting its second annual intake of students. The School of Radiography, also in the Centre, was in its sixth year training in both radiography and radiotherapy.

The penultimate report of the Board of Governors includes a request for any items of historical interest relating to the Trumpington Street Hospital. The centre of gravity of Addenbrooke's had moved from the centre of Cambridge, where it had been since 1766, to Hills Road in January 1972. On 31 March 1972 the formal completion of Stage Two was announced which was the date set when the contract had been signed in 1966 (Fig. 74). The Final Report of the Board records the names of members of the Board and of its committees, since 1948; it lists all the

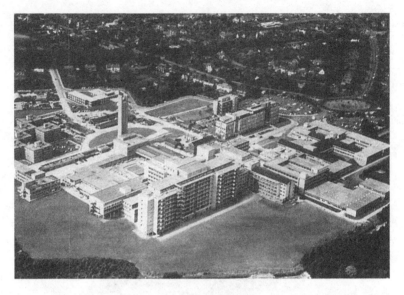

Fig. 74. Aerial photograph of the Hospital as it was in 1972 when
Stage Two of the building had been completed. (Photo Leonard
Beard).

senior officers since that date as well as the names of all the members of the
Consultant Staff Council since its inception. The whole report is prefaced
by a long quotation from an article in *The Lancet* about Addenbrooke's
Hospital as it was in 1873. Part of this is worth repeating because it holds
true today. 'Enough has been said to show that Addenbrooke's Hospital
presents in itself great capabilities as a clinical school, and that it affords a
valuable field of instruction and experience for the medical students of the
University.'

The buildings at Hills Road bear little physical resemblance to those of
the original Hospital from where the last patient was moved to the new
environment in October 1984. The Hospital, however, continues today to
provide a service to the residents of Cambridge as well as to many from
further afield, as it has done since the beginning.

The illustrations which follow (Figs. 75 to 81) show aspects of Addenbrooke's Hospital in recent times.

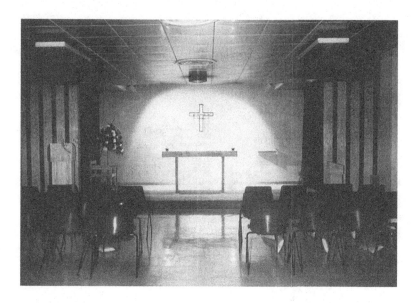

Fig. 75. The Hospital Chapel in 1972. (Photo W.G.C.)

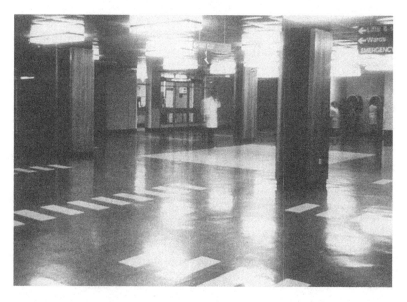

Fig. 76. The main concourse in 1972. (Photo W.G.C.)

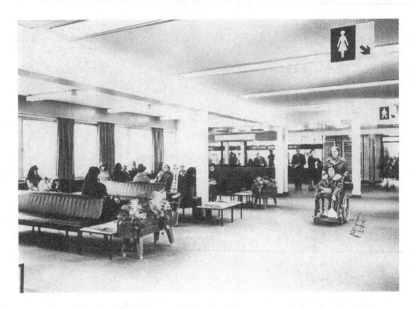

Fig. 77. The Out-patient Hall in 1972. (Photo W.G.C.)

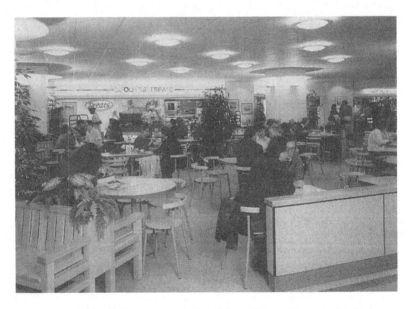

Fig. 78. The main concourse today. (Photo Reeve Photography for
B.A.S.)

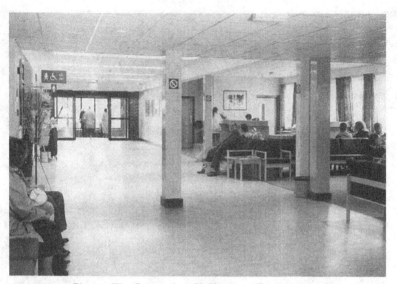

Fig. 79. The Out-patient Hall today. (Department of
Photography and Medical Illustration, Addenbrooke's.)

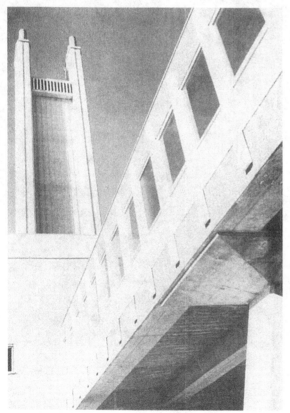

Fig. 80. The Tower
and the Bridge.
(Photo Mowlem's
P.L.C.)

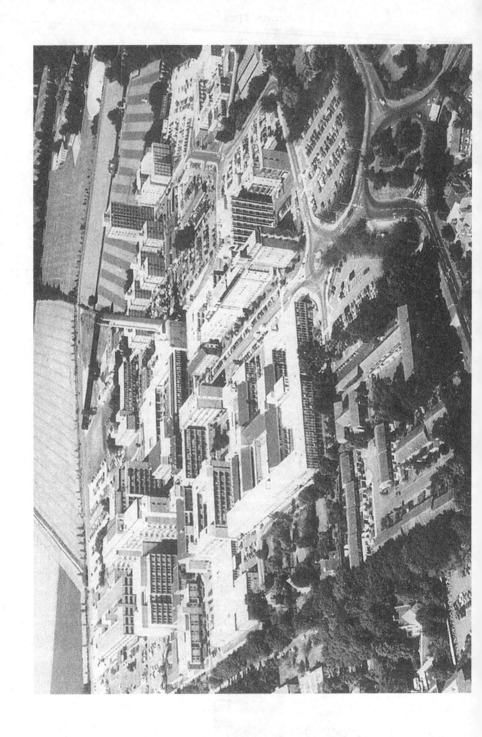

Appendices

Appendices

Appendix I: District nursing in Cambridge

The Cambridge District Nursing Association[1] ran for many years side by side with Addenbrooke's but nursing the sick poor in their homes.

District nursing actually began in England in 1859 in Liverpool when a Mr Rathbone paid a nurse to look after the sick in the community for three months. His family had previously benefited from the services of a nurse and he wanted to extend this privilege to the poor. Although at first the nurse, a Mrs Robinson, found her work heartrending she eventually asked 'that it might continue permanently' and by 1862 Liverpool had been divided up into districts each with a nurse.

The Cambridge Home and Training School for Nurses was set up in 1873 after Addenbrooke's Quarterly Court[2] gave permission to the Ladies Association for Training Nurses for the admission of probationers to the wards to be trained as nurses 'for a period of six months or longer if desirable'. This institution was to 'improve the Religious, Moral and Professional Qualifications of Nurses' and to provide attendants for, among others, the poor. A Miss Henslow was to be superintendent after spending a year at King's College Hospital, London. The Home was organised by a committee of prominent ladies advised by a Council of prominent men.

In 1875 £1,400 was left by a Miss Hutton for a permanent home for the Institution and the lease of no. 13 Fitzwilliam Street was purchased. One provision to the bequest was that '"one Nurse be constantly devoted to gratuitous service among the Poor in Cambridge" – be in fact Cambridge's first District Nurse'.

The Institution also provided attendants for the sick in hospitals and its nurses appear from the Minutes to have often been hired for Addenbrooke's.[3]

The district nursing side of the association expanded, although its fortunes fell to a low ebb during the First World War, and it was subsidised for a period by the Workers Hospital Fund. When this ended in 1932 it was supported by a contributory scheme and then taken over by the State in 1945. The Evelyn Nursing Home had already taken over the private nursing side.

Appendix II: Statistics on patients, 1766 to 1947

The figures below are the statistics for in-patients and out-patients admitted 1766–1947[1] and, as far as can be ascertained, do not include the numbers left on the books at the beginning of each year. Since the numbers of patients left on the books at the beginning and end of the year are usually similar, however, these figures should represent the approximate number of patients treated to a conclusion each year.

Patient admissions, 1766–1948

Year	In-patients admitted	Out-patients admitted	Out-patient attendances	Daily average in Hospital	Average stay of in-patients (days)	Beds available	Private patients admitted
1766	*Hospital opened Monday 13 October 1766*					20	
1767	106	157					
1777	284	309					
1787	350	301					
1797	364	425					
1807	318	354					
1817	428	378		43			
1827	652	1,256		55			
1837	657	984		75			
1847	862	1,150		75			
1857	638	1,700		81			
1867	694	1,920		70.8			
1877	855	2,583		95			
1887	915	3,838		88			
1888	1,013	5,266[a]		99	35		
1897	1,343	6,304		108	28		
1907	1,742	5,422		107	22.3		
1914	1,759	9,903	32,723	111	23	190	
1915	2,259	9,137		130	21		
1916	2,284	8,085		155	24		
1917	2,069	7,563		196.4	30		
1918	2,406	7,351		205	30.8		
1927	3,102	10,979		162	19.16		

Patient admissions, 1766–1948 (cont.)

Year	In-patients admitted	Out-patients admitted	Out-patient attendances	Daily average in Hospital	Average stay of in-patients (days)	Beds available	Private patients admitted
1937	6,041	14,607	72,465	274	16.5	315	
1938	5,777	16,055		281	17.78	316	
1939[b]	7,506	19,945		281	17	316	
1940	6,316	17,784		326	19	465	
1941	9,228	24,432		492	20	650	
1942	10,427	25,358		572.9	20.1	811	
1943	11,613	23,741		598.2	18.8	811	854
1944	11,166	23,385	113,619	576.1	18.9	811	737
1945[c]	9,532	20,052		488.7	18.3	760	
1946[d]	7,466	19,177		315.1	15.3	370	
1947	7,713	24,096	109,511	313.7	14.9	356	
1948	*Taken over by the National Health Service*						

[a] First-year dental patients included.
[b] Over 15 month period.
[c] Statistics affected by gradual closing down of Leys School annexe which was finally vacated on 8 November 1945.
[d] Statistics affected by closing down of University Examination Hall which was finally vacated 28 February 1946.

Appendix III: Addenbrooke's financial position over the years

The Governors were very concerned about the finances of the Hospital and frequently issued appeals for more money. However, the published accounts[1] show that Addenbrooke's investments rose steadily from 1766 when the Hospital was opened until 1823.

After a slight setback (the statement of property invested in the public funds drops from £27,150 in 1823 to £23,699 in 1824) the stock owned again rose almost continuously year after year until 1863 when the Hospital had £47,905 invested. The exact worth of these reserves is unknown, the figures can only be an indication, since the amount shown may not be the current worth of the stock, and there may also be cash in hand, debts, creditors, etc.

Some building work was paid out of the general fund in 1865 and 1867 and there was a run of debit balances between 1881 and 1901 when the new system of accounts was instituted, but at the end of 1901 the balance of the capital account, which would show an accurate picture, was still £46,285.

Under the new system the credit or deficit balance of the general account was settled each year and not carried forward to the next year's income and expenditure account as had often been the case. Even so, Addenbrooke's had mostly deficits until the beginning of the contributory scheme in 1932, and then again from 1936 until the Health Service took over in 1948. Notwithstanding, the balance of the capital account in 1942 was nearly £51,000, though it fell steadily subsequently and, when the Health Service took over, the capital account was in the red to the extent of over £33,000 even though nine properties had been sold to another Hospital account, the Endowment Capital account. (The Hospital owned many accounts, dedicated to different purposes, and some owning stock.)

Over the years legacies and benefactions were sometimes paid into the general account and so counted towards a credit balance, or reducing the debit balance, at the end of the year. But sometimes they were kept separate from the general account and were used to buy stock.

Similarly, stock was sometimes bought and sold out of the general fund and sometimes transactions were kept separate from it. For these reasons the investments of the Hospital seem to be the best guide to its financial position, at least until after 1900 when the capital account was kept separately. However, in spite of the fact that the Hospital's expenditure each year sometimes included the purchase of stock or payments for building and repairs (which at other times may have been paid for out of special funds) it does show how the commitments of the Hospital increased over the years. The figures given here are the total of ordinary and extraordinary expenditure where these are distinguished; when the Governors talked of a deficit they were often referring to the ordinary expenditure alone.

The contribution of the Workers' Hospital Fund towards the maintenance of the Hospital started at quite a modest level – £421 for 1911 which was 4% of total expenditure – but it grew, to £9,267 in 1931, the last year it was operative, which was 27% of total expenditure. Then the Maintenance Fund took over and in its last full year was contributing £64,409 of the total expenditure of £179,856 which was 36%. Unfortunately it was not enough and the Hospital still had a massive deficit. It was rescued by the Health Service.

The Hospital's financial position

(From Hospital statements and report books)

| Year | General income and expenditure | | | |
	Total expenditure (£)	Debit balance on account (£)	Credit balance on account (£)	Investments (£)
1766	*Hospital opened*			1,600
	legacies included			
1767	1,417	—	277	1,600
1768	1,128	—	622	1,600
1769	1,038	—	1,006	1,600
1770	1,593	—	565	2,200
1771	1,767	—	317	2,500
1772	1,467	—	314	2,500

The Hospital's financial position (cont.)

| | General income and expenditure | | | |
| | Total expenditure (£) | Debit balance on account (£) | Credit balance on account (£) | Investments (£) |
Year				
1773	864	—	332	2,500
1774	888	—	268	2,500
1775	1,208	—	517	2,500
1776	(missing)			2,500
1777	(missing)			2,500
1778	(missing)			3,000
1779	1,483	—	293	4,000
1780	1,559	—	493	4,000
1781	1,125	—	209	4,000
1782	1,550	—	224	4,000
1783	1,029	—	426	4,000
1784	1,071	—	213	4,300
1785	1,498	—	100	4,300
1786	892	—	132	4,300
1787	1,073	—	76	4,340
1788	1,311	—	518	4,340
1789	696	—	910	4,340
1790	1,954	—	560	5,800
1791	772	—	752	5,800
1792	1,995	—	412	5,800
1793	853	—	826	6,500
1794	1,153	—	554	7,000
1795	1,222	—	310	7,000
1796	989	—	198	7,000
1797	969	—	274	7,000
1798	1,003	—	161	7,000
1799	975	—	148	7,000
1800	1,077	6 legacies not included	—	7,000
1801	1,189	310	—	7,000
1802	1,123	—	24	7,900
1803	1,303	104	—	10,700
1804	1,152	—	29	10,800
1805	1,227	—	140	11,800
1806	1,136	—	151	12,300
1807	1,218	—	31	13,300
1808	1,303	—	19	13,300
1809	1,591	82	—	13,900
1810	1,583	90	—	14,400
1811	1,509	—	82	14,800
1812	1,638	49	—	15,000
1813	1,609	12	—	15,000

The Hospital's financial position (cont.)

Year	General income and expenditure Total expenditure (£)	Debit balance on account (£)	Credit balance on account (£)	Investments (£)
1814	1,608	—	52	21,500
1815	1,538	—	193	22,300
1816	1,484	—	136	22,800
1817	1,787	—	42	23,250
1818	1,692	—	151	24,000
1819	1,840	—	46	24,600
1820	1,804	—	96	25,400
1821	1,683	—	137	26,000
1822	1,813	—	12	26,650
1823	1,632	—	193	27,150
1824	2,139	251	—	23,699
1825	2,204	330	—	23,699
1826	2,259	385	—	23,699
1827	2,357	414	—	23,850
1828	2,268	—	81	23,850
1829	2,381	182	—	26,150
1830	2,203	43	—	26,600
1831	2,098	—	82	26,600
1832	2,374	272	—	29,000
1833	2,170	—	139	28,100
1834	3,016	1,220	—	29,848
1835	2,526	—	224	29,848
		legacies included		
1836	2,190	—	164	29,848
1837	2,396	—	135	29,948
1838	2,588	74	—	29,948
1839	2,484	223	—	30,746
1840	3,930	43	—	31,978
1841	2,827	227	—	31,978
1842	3,152	—	16	30,534
1843	2,545	—	265	32,634
1844	4,041	—	277	32,890
1845	3,185	—	495	32,240
1846	5,321	—	148	32,740
1847	3,777	—	73	33,321
1848	3,942	—	257	34,519
1849	4,639	—	345	36,660
1850	2,699	—	979	36,965
1851	3,514	—	1,070	38,767
1852	4,422	—	329	40,813
1853	3,303	96	—	40,973
1854	3,330	510	—	41,043

The Hospital's financial position (cont.)

	General income and expenditure			
Year	Total expenditure (£)	Debit balance on account (£)	Credit balance on account (£)	Investments (£)
1855	3,945	351	—	41,658
1856	4,002	276	—	42,216
1857	3,773	404	—	42,504
1858	3,598	351	—	42,501
1859	4,455	—	108	43,674
1860	3,160	—	37	43,755
1861	4,063	182	—	43,443
1862	6,826	246	—	46,453
1863	4,581	116	—	47,905
1864	6,340	—	530	45,310
1865	7,578	—	1,310	43,228
1866	5,543	—	1,205	45,270
1867	8,065	341	—	44,411
1868	4,314	—	348	44,805
1869	4,102	—	566	45,281
1870	3,888	—	839	45,497
1871	(missing)	—	311	46,252
1872	5,338	— *legacies not included*	335	45,765
1873	4,736	— *legacies not included*	351	45,935
1874	6,348	—	212	47,648
1875	5,135	—	777	46,873
1876	6,322	—	153	47,699
1877	6,567	56	—	48,655
1878	6,221	—	346	46,467
1879	6,432	—	331	47,315
1880	5,958	—	432	47,722
1881[a]	7,184	1,290	—	47,772
1882	7,372	1,134	—	48,181
1883	7,071	771	—	48,182
1884	7,001	1,106	—	48,380
1885	7,474	836	—	47,870
1886	7,372	794	—	48,009
1887	7,907	474	—	49,283
1888	7,713	653	—	50,431
1889	7,730	667	—	51,344
1890	7,659	981	—	51,746
1891	8,016	1,108	—	52,330
1892	8,546	1,350	—	52,917
1893	8,083	1,642 *legacies not included*	—	51,738

The Hospital's financial position (cont.)

| | General income and expenditure | | | |
Year	Total expenditure (£)	Debit balance on account (£)	Credit balance on account (£)	Investments (£)
1894	8,262	1,079	—	51,550
1895	9,304	514	—	52,323
1896	8,331	—	994	48,730
1897	8,857	1,521	—	50,786
1898	9,006	513	—	49,098
1899	8,360	1,300	—	41,887
1900	9,285	2,373	—	42,876

New system of accounts: 'Uniform' system

Year	Total expenditure (£)	Debit balance on account (£)	Credit balance on account (£)	Capital account balance (£)	Workers' Hospital Fund contribution (established June 1910) (£)
		legacies not included			
1901	10,216[b]	1,307	—	46,285	
1902	9,569	2,101	—	46,285	
1903	10,567	1,522	—	43,834	
1904	9,999	2,107	—	43,476	
1905	8,999	1,452	—	46,481	
1906	9,286	—	61	45,318	
1907	10,525	1,307	—	43,080	
1908	10,295	824	—	43,649	
1909	10,013	—	287	43,465	
1910	9,932	—	134	41,802	
1911	10,051	—	550	47,432	421
1912	10,216	259	—	46,438	477
1913	10,374	898	—	42,944	420
1914	9,995	—	128	45,373	460
1915	12,300	892	—	46,882	470
1916	15,716	1,500	—	41,224	375
1917	18,577	130	—	42,812	386
1918	21,796	1,450	—	44,815	433
1919	21,318	1,068	—	49,710	500
		legacies included		new method	
1920	25,516	492	—	41,035	800
1921	28,663	1,031	—	42,327	1,250
1922	24,952	30	—	47,757	1,691
1923	25,183	66	—	49,086	1,748
1924	24,377	—	1,306	47,667	2,177
1925	25,598	407	—	43,763	2,341
1926	26,475	125	—	41,766	2,648

New system of accounts: 'Uniform' system

Year	Total expenditure (£)	Debit balance on account (£)	Credit balance on account (£)	Capital account balance (£)	Workers' Hospital Fund contribution (established June 1910) (£)
1927	28,511	—	403	35,969	3,048
1928	31,708	3,044	—	30,071	3,885
1929	32,377	1,146	—	26,039	5,724
1930	32,670	876	—	25,436	7,000
1931	34,021	816	—	31,058	9,267
					Contributory Scheme from 1 October 1931
1932	39,040	—	5,818	39,871	28,185[c]
					Maintenance Fund from 1 October 1932
1933	43,887	—	9,592	55,738	29,000[d]
1934	47,677	—	8,122	54,400	29,688[e]
1935	47,387	—	7,498	58,938	30,720
1936	52,355	2,053	—	50,855	31,226
1937	52,847	1,116	—	42,546	31,655
1938	54,905	—	2,699	41,637	33,910
1939	76,048[f]	3,521[f]	—	40,945[f]	36,587[g]
1940	70,561	—	3,180	50,611	35,736
			legacies not included		
1941	114,404	2,357	—	50,032	45,325
1942	129,969	181[h]	—	50,255	50,842
1943	139,476	7,229[h]	—	43,285	50,488
1944	155,938	14,948[h]	—	42,478	58,590
1945	144,418	—	8,824	30,934	65,672
1946	141,457	32,200	—	−9,392	61,871
1947	179,856	34,267	—	−34,941	64,409
1948[i]	103,053	15,693	—	−33,194[j]	47,047

On 5 July 1948 Addenbrooke's Hospital passed into State ownership.

Notes:

[a] Five-quarters' expenditure and four-quarters' receipts. Previous year's credit carried forward.

[h] Twelve and a half months covered.

[c] Including £380 from March Workers' Hospital Fund.

[d] Plus £443 balance from Contributory Fund accounts.

[e] Plus £539 balance of 1933 accounts.

[f] For 15 months.

[g] For 12 months.

[h] Further payments for the year expected from the Ministry of Health.

[i] To 4 July.

[j] This account had sold nine properties to the Endowment Capital Account and was still in deficit.

Appendix IV: Legacies, 1766 to 1947

The Hospital received a massive amount in subscriptions, donations and legacies over the years,[1] as can be seen from the list of the annual expenses which until later years were virtually all paid out of the money received from private contributors.

Legacies received were almost invariably published in the annual reports, as were the other amounts received, and between 1766 and 1947 they totalled between £230,000 and £240,000,* mostly in small sums. This was considerably less than the amount left by one man, Thomas Guy, founder of Guy's Hospital, when he died in 1724 leaving an estate valued at £335,000.[2]

* Totals for years 1774, 1776–1778 and 1873 not included as not known.

Notes and references

FOREWORD

1 London: Wellcome Institute of the History of Medicine, 1971.
2 Cambridge Medical Society, 1980.

CHAPTER I

1 STEVENSON, L. G., 1953, A note on the Relation of Military Service
   to Licensing in the History of British Surgery, *Bulletin of the History of
   Medicine*, **27**, 420. A clause in Brougham's Act of 1825 enabled Army
   and Navy surgeons to practise as apothecaries. They had enjoyed this
   privilege since Cromwell's ordinance on the matter in 1654.
2 MAPOTHER, E. D., 1868, *The Medical Profession: and its Educational and
   Licensing Bodies*, Fannin & Co, Dublin, p. 13.
3 RIVINGTON, W., 1879, *The Medical Profession*, Fannin, Dublin, p. 31.
4 LANGLEY, B., 1867, *Vita Medica*, Hardwicke, London, p. 19.
5 McMENEMEY, W. H., 1959, *The Life and Times of Sir Charles Hastings*,
   Livingstone, Edinburgh, passim. This biography provides an
   admirable account of the diversity of reforming influences during the
   30 years before 1858.
6 POYNTER, F. N. L., 1858, The Centenary of the General Medical
   Council, *British Medical Journal*, **2**, 1245.
7 Langley, op. cit., passim.
8 LAFFAN, T., 1879, *The Medical Profession in the Three Kingdoms in 1879*,
   Fannin & Co, Dublin.
9 Langley, op. cit., p. 74.
10 Cope, V.Z., 1951, *The General Practitioners*, Clinical Journal, pp. 80–1.
11 GOSDEN, P.H.J.H., 1961, *The Friendly Societies in England, 1815–1875*,
   Manchester University Press.
12 REANEY, M.F., 1905, *The Medical Profession*, Browne & Nolan,
   Dublin.
13 DAVIS, J., 1974, *David Lloyd George and the Medical Insurance Act of 1911
   in Wales and Medicine*, ed. J. Cule, British Society for the History of
   Medicine, London.
14 ECKSTEIN, H., 1959, *The English Health Service*, Harvard University
   Press.

CHAPTER 2

1   The birthplace of Addenbrooke is recorded on his tomb, the registration of his birth has not been traced despite extensive enquiries.
2   Personal communication from Revd S.B. Coley, Vicar of Rowley Regis, dated 15.11.1961.
3   Worcester Wills, Birmingham Probate Registry, dated 22.7.1550.
4   Personal communication from the Revd F.C. Addenbrooke.
5   H. COLL., 29.4.1795.
6   LANGFORD, A.W., 1934, The Life of John Addenbrooke, Thesis for the degree of M.D., University of Cambridge. Dr Langford's thesis has been of great assistance in compiling this short account of Addenbrooke.
7   ROOK, A. and MARTIN, L., 1982, John Addenbrooke MD. 1680–1719, Medical History, 26 (1), April, 169–78.
8   A survey of the University Grace books.
9   STUKELY, W., 1882, The family memoirs and the antiquarian and other correspondence, Surtees Society, Whittaker & Co, Bernard Quaritch, London, William Blackwood & Sons, Edinburgh, pp. 20–43.
10 SAVILLE PECK, E., 1953, Three early materia medica cabinets in Cambridge, Med. Illust. 7, 122–9.
11 JONES, W.H.S., 1936, A History of St Catharine's College, once Catharine Hall, Cambridge, Cambridge University Press, pp. 101–111.
12 JOHN ADDENBROOKE, Dean of Lichfield, quoted by W.A. Langford in John Addenbrooke, Pensioner, Fellow, Lecturer and Bursar of Catharine Hall and Doctor of Medicine, St Catharine's Society magazine, September 1935, pp. 43–51, September 1936, pp. 36–45, September 1937, pp. 61–6.
13 COLE, W., British Library Add. MS 6402. 72.
14 P.R.O. C11/2206/5.

CHAPTER 3

1   A Description of the University, Town and County of Cambridge, 1796. Printed by J. Burges for J. Deighton, Cambridge, p. 152. The population in April 1794 is given as 9868 including 805 members of the University and 121 University servants.
2   GRAY, A., 1925, The Town of Cambridge, Heffer, Cambridge, p. 166.
3   A History of the County of Cambridge and the Isle of Ely, 1959, Vol. 3, The City and University of Cambridge, ed. R.B. Pugh, The Victoria History of the Counties of England, Oxford University Press, p. 111.
4   Deighton, op. cit. n. 1, prefacing page.
5   GUNNING, H., 1854, Reminiscences of the University, Town and County of Cambridge from the year 1780, Bell, London, Vol. 1, p. 40.

6   Gray, op. cit. n. 2, p. 167

7   Gunning, op. cit. n. 5, p. 319.

8   Pugh, op. cit. n. 3, p. 104.

9   Gray, op. cit. n. 2, p. 74.

10 BUSHELL, W.D., 1938, *Hobson's Conduit: The River at Cambridge commonly called Hobson's River*, Cambridge at the University Press.

11 *Cantabrigia Depicta*, 1763, printed for W. Thurlbourn & J. Woodyer, and T. and J. Merril in Cambridge, pp. 112–17.

12 Deighton, op. cit. n. 1, pp. 159–64.

13 Addenbrooke's Hospital Minute Book, Weekly Meeting 30.3.1767.

14 In 1926 the Charity Commissioners agreed to amend the Scheme for the Management of the Hospital to provide for the appointment by the General Committee of six co-optative members to represent the bodies which collected or supplied funds for the Hospital (Report of the General Committee to the Quarterly Court to be held 23.11.1926). The allocation for the present was to be: Auxiliary Association, one member; Cambridge and District Workers' Hospital Fund, two members; The County Organisation Fund, one member; and The Friendly Societies Council (representing the organisers of Friendly Societies' Parades), two members (Report of the General Committee to the Quarterly Court to be held 8.2.1927).

15 WINSTANLY, D.A., 1935, *Unreformed Cambridge*, Cambridge University Press.

16 WORDSWORTH, C., 1874, *Social Life in the English Universities in the Eighteenth Century*, Deighton Bell, Cambridge, p. 275.

17 STOKES, H.P., 1927, *Ceremonies of the University of Cambridge*, Cambridge University Press, p. 36.

18 Gunning, op. cit. n. 5, p. 26.

19 Pugh, op, cit. n. 3, pp. 20–3.

20 MOTTRAM, P.W. and TUKE, A.W., 1926, *History of Barclays Bank*, Blades, East & Blades, London.

CHAPTER 4

1 JONES, W.H.S., 1936, *A History of St Catharine's College*, Cambridge University Press, p. 186.

2 P.R.O. C11/2206/5.

3 P.R.O., Chancery Court Records, 1728–1763.

4 'The State of Dr Addenbrooke's Hospital', 9.4.1766, Cambridge Collection, Cambridge Central Library, C.21.4.

CHAPTER 5

1 Addenbrooke's Hospital Rules and Orders, 1770.

2 Addenbrooke's Hospital Minute Book, General Board 4.8.1766.

3 Addenbrooke's Hospital Minute Book, Weekly Board 15.9.1766.
4 Addenbrooke's Hospital Minute Book, Weekly Board 8.9.1766. Under Rule 43 the purchase of drugs was the responsibility of the Physicians and Surgeons and such local apothecaries as were subscribers. Any three had power to act provided that one of the three was an apothecary.

CHAPTER 6

1 The 1770 Rules are quoted (Rules and Orders of the Public Hospital in the Town of Cambridge founded by Dr Addenbrooke, and Supported by Voluntary Subscriptions). They differed in no important particular from the Rules of 1766, but were more detailed.
2 Rule 50.
3 Rule 53.
4 Rules 56 and 57.
5 Rule 55.
6 Rule 58.
7 Rule 66.
8 Rule 64.
9 Rule 51.
10 Rule 60.
11 Rule 107.
12 Rule 108.
13 Rule 67.
14 Rule 68.
15 Addenbrooke's Hospital Minute Book, Weekly Meeting 19.1.1767.
16 Addenbrooke's Hospital Minute Book, Weekly Board 27.10.1766.
17 Addenbrooke's Hospital Minute Book, Weekly Meeting 23.3.1767.
18 Addenbrooke's Hospital Minute Book, General Board 4.8.1766.

CHAPTER 7

1 HEASMAN, K., 1962, *Evangelicals in Action*, Bles, London, p. 11.
2 Addenbrooke's Hospital Minute Book, Weekly Meeting 22.12.1766.
3 Addenbrooke's Hospital Minute Book, Special General Court 30.10.1769.
4 Addenbrooke's Hospital Minute Book, Weekly Meeting 20.4.1767.
5 Addenbrooke's Hospital Minute Book, General Quarterly Council 26.12.1774.
6 Addenbrooke's Hospital Statement, 1828.

CHAPTER 8

1 Rule 69.
2 Rule 70.
3 Rule 71.
4 Rule 72.
5 Rule 73.
6 ROOK, A., 1969, Robert Glynn (1719–1800), Physician at Cambridge, *Medical History*, **13**, 251.
7 ROOK, A., 1979, Charles Collignon (1725–1785), Cambridge Physician, Anatomist and Moralist, *Medical History*, **23**, 339–45.
8 DUNCAN, A., 1786, *Medical Commentaries*, **10**, 332. Cambridge University Library, Add. 4403, 101.
9 NEWBOLD, M., MS notes 'The Biographies of Cambridge Surgeons up to the year 1815'. We are greatly indebted to the late Mr Maurice Newbold for his researches into the lives of medical practitioners in Cambridge before 1815. Copies of his manuscript notes are in the Cambridge University Library and in the libraries of the Royal College of Physicians of London and the Royal College of Surgeons of England.
10 PRYME, J.T. and BAYNE, A., 1879, *Memorials of the Thackeray Family*. Privately printed.
11 ROOK, A., 1971, The Thackerays and Medicine, *Medical History*, **15**, 12–22.
12 Addenbrooke's Hospital Minute Book, Weekly Meeting 14.11.1768.
13 Addenbrooke's Hospital Minute Book, Special General Court 15.5.1769.
14 *Philosophical Transactions*, 1777, **67**, 15.
15 This brief account of Debraz's association with the Benthams and of his two years in Russia has been compiled from I.R. Christie (ed.), *The Correspondence of Jeremy Bentham*, Vol. 3, 1971, Athlone Press, London. References in letters and a biographical footnote p. 497.
16 Addenbrooke's Hospital Minute Book, Weekly Meeting 9.7.1770.
17 Addenbrooke's Hospital Minute Book, Special Court 24.4.1775.
18 *Cambridge Chronicle* 21.3.1776.
19 A brief report in the *Cambridge Chronicle* of 28.3.1766 states that he had 'avowed himself the author of it'.
20 Addenbrooke's Hospital Minute Book, Weekly Meeting 26.10.1778.
21 Addenbrooke's Hospital Minute Book, Weekly Meeting 15.11.1778.
22 Addenbrooke's Hospital Minute Book, Special General Court 17.12.1781.
23 Addenbrooke's Hospital Minute Book, Special General Court 4.10.1784.
24 Addenbrooke's Hospital Minute Book, General Quarterly Court 30.6.1794.
25 Addenbrooke's Hospital Minute Book, Special General Court 14.6.1802.
26 *Cambridge Chronicle*, 19.3.1808.

CHAPTER 9

1 For example, 25.1.1773: 35.
2 Addenbrooke's Hospital Minute Book, Weekly Meeting 11.11.1771.
3 Addenbrooke's Hospital Minute Book, Weekly Meeting, 15.5.1772.
4 Addenbrooke's Hospital Minute Book, Weekly Meetings 4.3.1771.
5 Addenbrooke's Hospital Minute Book, General Court 8.2.1768.
6 Addenbrooke's Hospital Minute Book, Special General Court 24.4.1768.
7 Addenbrooke's Hospital Minute Book, General Court 12.8.1767.
8 Addenbrooke's Hospital Minute Book, General Court 4.7.1768.
9 Addenbrooke's Hospital Minute Book, General Quarterly Court
   26.6.1769.
10 Addenbrooke's Hospital Minute Book, Weekly Meeting 25.2.1771.
11 Addenbrooke's Hospital Minute Book, Weekly Meeting 24.3.1777.
12 Addenbrooke's Hospital Minute Book, Quarterly Court 27.6.1774.
13 Addenbrooke's Hospital Minute Book, Weekly Meeting 2.6.1781.
14 Addenbrooke's Hospital Minute Book, Weekly Meeting 19.10.1781.
15 Addenbrooke's Hospital Minute Book, Weekly Meeting 31.3.1783.
16 Addenbrooke's Hospital Minute Book, Weekly Meeting 22.1.1798.
17 Addenbrooke's Hospital Minute Book, Weekly Meeting 29.1.1798.
18 Addenbrooke's Hospital Minute Book, Weekly Meeting 26.11.1770.
19 Addenbrooke's Hospital Minute Book, Weekly Meeting 26.3.1770.
20 Addenbrooke's Hospital Minute Book, Weekly Meeting 20.4.1774.
21 Addenbrooke's Hospital Minute Book, Weekly Meeting 20.12.1779.
22 Addenbrooke's Hospital Minute Book, General Quarterly Court,
   October, 1794.
23 Addenbrooke's Hospital Minute Book, Special Court 6.1.1775.
24 Addenbrooke's Hospital Minute Book, General Court 17.1.1775.
25 Addenbrooke's Hospital Minute Book, General Court 14.2.1778.
26 Addenbrooke's Hospital Minute Book, Special General Court 2.11.1778.
27 Addenbrooke's Hospital Minute Book, Special General Court 15.1.1787.
28 Addenbrooke's Hospital Minute Book, Special General Court 14.6.1802.

CHAPTER 10

1 *Cambridge Chronicle* 17.4.1802, 24.4.1802 and 1.5.1802.
2 *Cambridge Chronicle* 24.4.1802.
3 Addenbrooke's Hospital Minute Book, Special General Court 10.5.1802.
4 Addenbrooke's Hospital Annual Report 1802.
5 *Cambridge Chronicle* 11.12.1802.
6 Addenbrooke's Hospital Annual Report 1803.
7 *Cambridge Chronicle* 24.12.1803.
8 *Cambridge Chronicle* 21.7.1804.
9 Addenbrooke's Hospital Minute Book, Weekly Meetings 21.1.1805 and
   11.2.1805.

10   Addenbrooke's Hospital Minute Book, Weekly Meeting 18.2.1805.

11   Addenbrooke's Hospital Minute Book, Weekly Meeting 25.2.1805.

12   Addenbrooke's Hospital Minute Book, General Quarterly Court
     30.3.1807.

13   Addenbrooke's Hospital Minute Book, Weekly Meeting 27.9.1813.

14   Addenbrooke's Hospital Minute Book, Weekly Meeting 24.1.1814.

15   Addenbrooke's Hospital Minute Book, Weekly Meeting 27.7.1818.

16   Addenbrooke's Hospital Minute Book, Weekly Meeting 22.2.1808.

17   Addenbrooke's Hospital Annual Report 1809.

18   Addenbrooke's Hospital Annual Report 1920.

19   GRAY, A.D., 1907, A Biography of John Bowtell, *Proceedings of the
     Cambridge Antiquarian Society*, **47**, 346.

20   Addenbrooke's Hospital Minute Book, General Quarterly Court
     14.6.1802.

21   Addenbrooke's Hospital Rules, 1802, Rule 79.

22   Addenbrooke's Hospital Minute Book, General Quarterly Court
     1.4.1805.

23   Addenbrooke's Hospital Minute Book, Weekly Meeting 2.8.1813.

24   Addenbrooke's Hospital Minute Book, Special General Court
     13.12.1814.

25   PAGET, G.E., 1898, in *A Biographical History of Gonville and Caius
     College, 1349–1897*, ed. J. Venn, vol. 2, Cambridge University Press, p.
     134.

26   *The Lancet*, 1826–7, **12**, 665.

27   Addenbrooke's Hospital Minute Book, Special General Court 3.3.1817.

28   MUNK, W., 1878, *The Roll of the Royal College of Physicians of London*,
     Vol. 3, 1801–1825, published by the College, London, p. 183.

29   Addenbrooke's Hospital Minute Book, Special General Court 3.5.1813.

30   BUSHELL, W.D., 1936, 'The Two Charles Lestourgeons', privately
     printed, Cambridge, Cambridge University Library.

31   Addenbrooke's Hospital Minute Book, Weekly Meeting 5.5.1817.

32   The Annual Reports for 1810–1812 show that five nurses were employed
     during these three years.

33   *Cambridge Chronicle* 23.2.1805.

34   Addenbrooke's Hospital Minute Book, General Quarterly Court
     30.6.1817.

35   From an annotated copy of Rules and Orders of the Public Hospital in
     the Town of Cambridge founded by Dr Addenbrooke and supported
     by voluntary subscriptions, 1802, Cambridge, printed at the
     University Press. The book was bound and labelled 'For the Use of
     the Board'.

36   Personal communication, December, 1988, from Ms Valerie Beamish,
     S.R.D., of the Cambridge Health Authority, who says it should be
     noted that twentieth-century food tables were used in the analysis
     whereas the foods consumed in the nineteenth century were probably
     quite different.

37   Recommended Daily Amount of Food Energy and Nutrient for Groups

of People in the United Kingdom, 1979, Department of Health and
Social Security, H.M.S.O.

[38] Addenbrooke's Hospital Minute Book, General Quarterly Court
6.10.1817.

[39] Addenbrooke's Hospital Minute Book, Special General Court 10.1.1820.

[40] Addenbrooke's Hospital Minute Book, General Quarterly Court
1.1.1821.

[41] Addenbrooke's Hospital Minute Book, General Quarterly Court
6.10.1817.

[42] *Cambridge Chronicle* 17.12.1813, p. 3.

[43] Addenbrooke's Hospital Minute Book, Special General Court 28.4.1823.

[44] Addenbrooke's Hospital Minute Book, Special General Court 26.5.1823.

[45] Addenbrooke's Hospital Minute Book, General Quarterly Court
30.6.1823.

[46] Addenbrooke's Hospital Minute Book, General Quarterly Court
6.10.1823.

[47] Addenbrooke's Hospital Minute Book, Special General Court
18.11.1824.

[48] Addenbrooke's Hospital Minute Book, General Quarterly Court
28.3.1825.

CHAPTER 11

[1] Addenbrooke's Hospital Minute Book, Special General Courts
28.10.1824 and 18.11.24.

[2] Addenbrooke's Hospital Minute Book, Weekly Meeting 8.12.1824.

[3] Addenbrooke's Hospital Minute Book, General Quarterly Court
24.1.1825.

[4] Addenbrooke's Hospital Minute Book, Weekly Meeting 23.10.1839.

[5] Addenbrooke's Hospital Minute Book, General Quarterly Court
1.10.1838.

[6] Addenbrooke's Hospital Minute Book, General Quarterly Court
24.6.1840.

[7] Addenbrooke's Hospital Minute Book, General Quarterly Court
8.10.1840.

[8] Addenbrooke's Hospital Minute Book, General Quarterly Court
1.7.1844.

[9] Addenbrooke's Hospital Minute Book, Weekly Meeting 14.4.1847.

[10] Addenbrooke's Hospital Minute Book, General Quarterly Court
27.12.1847.

[11] Addenbrooke's Hospital Minute Book, General Quarterly Court
1.1.1849.

[12] Addenbrooke's Hospital Minute Book, General Quarterly Court
3.10.1859.

[13] Addenbrooke's Hospital Minute Book, General Quarterly Court
8.10.1840.

14   Addenbrooke's Hospital Minute Book, Weekly Meeting 10.3.1869.
15   ROOK, A., 1971, The Thackerays and Medicine, *Medical History*, **15**, 12.
16   WINSTANLY, D.A., 1955, *Early Victorian Cambridge*, Cambridge University Press.
17   Addenbrooke's Hospital Minute Book, Weekly Meeting 23.2.1828.
18   Addenbrooke's Hospital Minute Book, Special General Court 10.11.1828.
19   Addenbrooke's Hospital Minute Book, General Quarterly Court 4.10.1834.
20   ROLLESTON, SIR H.D., 1932, *The Cambridge Medical School*, Cambridge University Press, p. 172.
21   LANGDON-BROWN, SIR W., 1946, *Some Chapters in Cambridge Medical History*, Cambridge University Press.
22   Addenbrooke's Hospital Minute Book, Weekly Meeting 24.8.1842.
23   Addenbrooke's Hospital Minute Book, Special General Court 29.4.1845.

CHAPTER 12

1   LANGDON-BROWN, SIR W., 1946, The Great Triumvirate and the Rise of the Medical School, in *Some Chapters in Cambridge Medical History*, Cambridge University Press.
2   ROLLESTON, SIR H.D., 1932, *The Cambridge Medical School*, Cambridge University Press.
3   *Munk's Roll*, 1955, vol. 4, *Lives of the Fellows of the Royal College of Physicians of London 1826–1925*, compiled by G.H. Brown, Published by the College, London.
4   PAGET, C.E., 1893, *Some Lectures by Sir George E. Paget with a Memoir*, MacMillan and Bowes, Cambridge.
5   University Papers, 1835–1840, Cambridge University Archives, Cambridge University Library.
6   LANGDON-BROWN, SIR W., 1944, Some Chapters in Cambridge Medical History IV, The Early Nineteenth Century from Pennington to Paget, in Section of the History of Medicine, *Proceedings of the Royal Society of Medicine*, vol. 37.
7   PAGET, G.E., 1864, The President's Address at the Thirty-Second Annual Meeting of the British Medical Association held in Cambridge, August 1864, T. Richards, London.
8   *Dictionary of National Biography*, 1895, ed. Sidney Lee, vol. 63, Smith Elder & Co, London.
9   ACHESON, R.M., 1986, Three Regius Professors, Sanitary Science and State Medicine: the birth of an academic discipline, *British Medical Journal*, **293**, 1602–6.

CHAPTER 13

[1] ROLLESTON, SIR H.D., 1927, Sir George Murray Humphry, M.D., F.R.S., *Annals of Medical History*, **9** (1), 1–11.

[2] *Dictionary of National Biography*, 1908, ed. Sidney Lee, Supplement vol. 10, Smith, Elder & Co., London.

[3] *Plarr's Lives of the Fellows of the Royal College of Surgeons of England, 1930*, revised by Sir D'Arcy Power with the assistance of W.G. Spencer and Prof. G.E.G. Gask, John Wright & Sons Ltd, Bristol.

[4] ROLLESTON, SIR H.D., 1932, *The Cambridge Medical School*, Cambridge University Press.

[5] *The Royal Hospital of Saint Bartholomew 1123–1973*, 1974, ed. Victor Cornelius Medvei and John L. Thornton, W.S. Cowell Ltd, Ipswich, chapters 3 (From its Origins to the End of the Nineteenth Century by John L. Thornton) and 8 (Surgery in the Eighteenth and Nineteenth Centuries by Harvey White).

[6] *The Evolution of Hospitals in Britain*, 1964, ed. F.N.L. Poynter, Pitman Medical Publishing Co., Ltd, p. 64.

[7] *Cambridge Chronicle* 8.10.1842, p. 2.

[8] FAIRFAX FOZZARD, J.A., undated, Professors of Anatomy in the University of Cambridge, Fossla, 31 Beaumont Road, Cambridge.

[9] Medvei and Thornton, op. cit. n. 5, chapter 8.

[10] *Dictionary of National Biography*, 1901, ed. Sidney Lee, Supplement vol. 3, Smith, Elder & Co, London.

[11] ROOK, A., 1971, Haviland, Paget and Humphry: The Introduction of Clinical Teaching at Cambridge, in *Cambridge and its Contribution to Medicine*, ed. Arthur Rook, Wellcome Institute of the History of Medicine, London.

[12] ROOK, A., 1980, *Cambridge Medical Society 1880–1980: A Centennial History*, Cambridge Medical Society.

[13] 'Professorship of Zoology, etc. 1865–66', a collection of University papers in the University Archives, Cambridge University Library.

[14] 'Professor of Surgery, Cambridge University Registry, 1883–1922', University Archives, Cambridge University Library.

[15] *The Times* 30.1.1891, in 'Regius Professor of Physic Guard Book', University Archives, Cambridge University Library.

CHAPTER 14

[1] Addenbrooke's Hospital Minute Book, General Quarterly Court 1.4.1833.

[2] Addenbrooke's Hospital Minute Book, General Quarterly Court 13.5.1833.

[3] Addenbrooke's Hospital Minute Book, Building Committee 22.7.1833.

⁴ Addenbrooke's Hospital Minute Book, General Quarterly Court 27.3.1837.
⁵ Addenbrooke's Hospital Minute Book, Weekly Meeting 5.6.1839.
⁶ Addenbrooke's Hospital Minute Book, Special General Court 4.12.1843.
⁷ Addenbrooke's Hospital Minute Book, Committee 9.2.1849.
⁸ Addenbrooke's Hospital Minute Book, Committee 10.3.1849.
⁹ Addenbrooke's Hospital Minute Book, General Quarterly Court 16.3.1853.
¹⁰ Addenbrooke's Hospital Minute Book, General Quarterly Court 7.6.1853.
¹¹ Proposal of Dr Webster to General Quarterly Court 27.12.1852.
¹² The owners of the plots of land concerned were Westfield's Charity, Corpus Christi College and Dr J.T. Baumgartner.
¹³ Addenbrooke's Hospital Minute Book, General Quarterly Court 1.10.1855.
¹⁴ Addenbrooke's Hospital Minute Book, General Quarterly Court 30.12.1839.
¹⁵ Addenbrooke's Hospital Minute Book, Adjourned General Quarterly Court 10.5.1847.
¹⁶ Addenbrooke's Hospital Minute Book, Weekly Meeting 22.1.1851.
¹⁷ Addenbrooke's Hospital Minute Book, Weekly Meeting 19.3.1851.
¹⁸ Addenbrooke's Hospital Minute Book, Weekly Meeting 5.3.1851.
¹⁹ Addenbrooke's Hospital Minute Book, Weekly Meeting 28.3.1851.
²⁰ Addenbrooke's Hospital Minute Book, Weekly Meeting 23.4.1856.

CHAPTER 15

¹ Addenbrooke's Hospital Minute Book, Weekly Meeting 27.3.1843.
² Addenbrooke's Hospital Minute Book, Weekly Meeting 23.4.1851.
³ Addenbrooke's Hospital Minute Book, Weekly Meeting 28.3.1859.
⁴ Addenbrooke's Hospital Minute Book, Weekly Meeting 25.10.1854.
⁵ ALLEN, C.J., 1961, The Great Eastern Railway, 3rd edition, Allen, London.
⁶ DARBY, H.C., 1938, Cambridgeshire in the Nineteenth Century, in The Cambridge Region, ed. H.C. Darby, Cambridge University Press, pp. 116–34.
⁷ GORDON, D.I., 1968, A Regional History of the Railways of Great Britain, vol. 5, The Eastern Counties, David & Charles, Newton Abbott.
⁸ Addenbrooke's Hospital Minute Book, Weekly Meeting 14.12.1844.
⁹ Addenbrooke's Hospital Minute Book, Weekly Meeting 14.5.1845.
¹⁰ COLEMAN, T., 1968, The Railway Navvies, Harmsworth, Penguin Books.
¹¹ Addenbrooke's Hospital Minute Book, General Quarterly Court 28.6.1847.
¹² Addenbrooke's Hospital Minute Book, Weekly Meeting 29.10.1847.

CHAPTER 16

1 Addenbrooke's Hospital Minute Book, Weekly Meeting 14.6.1818.
2 BURY, J.P.T., 1967, *Romilly's Cambridge Diary 1832–1842*, Cambridge University Press, p. 14.
3 HUMPHRY, G.M., 1851, *Lectures on Surgery: Delivered in the Medical School of Cambridge* (reprinted from the *Provincial Medical and Surgical Journal*), Deighton & Co., Worcester, p. 39.
4 A full account of the introduction of anaesthesia in Cambridge, Wisbech and Bury St Edmunds is given by ROOK, A., The First Experiences with Ether Anaesthesia in Cambridgeshire and West Suffolk, *Anaesthesia*, **30**, 677.
5 *Cambridge Chronicle* 13.3.1847.
6 *Cambridge Chronicle* 20.3.1847.
7 HUMPHRY, G.M., 1856, A Report of some cases of operation: (Division of stricture of the urethra and rectum; amputation at the hip joint; excision of the condyle of the lower jaw; excision of the knee; ovariotomy; encysted urinary calculus; tracheotomy). Treated for the most part in Addenbrooke's Hospital, Cambridge and in the year 1855. T. Richards, 37 Great Queen Street, London.
8 RAINS, A.J.H. and RITCHIE H.D., 1977, *Bailey and Love's Short Practice of Surgery*, 17th edition, H.K. Lewis and Co. Ltd, London.
9 SQUIRE, P., 1864, *A Companion to the British Pharmacopeia*, John Churchill & Sons, New Burlington Street, London.
10 SQUIRE, P., 1882, *Companion to the Latest Edition of the British Pharmacopoeia*, 13th edition, J. & A. Churchill, New Burlington Street, London.

CHAPTER 17

1 Report by Dr John Syer Bristow and Mr Timothy Holmes on the Hospitals of the United Kingdom, Appendix No. 15 to Sixth Report of the Medical Officer of the Privy Council, 1863, Parliamentary Papers, 1864, vol. 28, H.M.S.O.
2 RICHARDSON, B.W., 1864, The Medical History of Cambridge, *Medical Times and Gazette*, **2**, 599, 628 and 657.
3 DUNCUM, B.W., 1947, *The Development of Inhalation Anaesthesia*, Oxford University Press, pp. 247–8.
4 BUCKLE, F., 1865, *Vital and Economical Statistics of the Hospitals, Infirmaries etc of England and Wales for the Year 1863*, Churchill, London. See also discussion of these figures by WOODWARD, J., 1974, *To Do the Sick No Harm*, Routledge and Kegan Paul, London.

CHAPTER 18

[1] Addenbrooke's Hospital Minute Book, General Quarterly Court 26.3.1860.
[2] Addenbrooke's Hospital Minute Book, General Quarterly Court 6.10.1862.
[3] Addenbrooke's Hospital Minute Book, New Building Committee, 31.10.1862.
[4] Addenbrooke's Hospital Minute Book, General Quarterly Court 30.3.1863.
[5] PARKER, A., 1986, 'The Enlargement of Addenbrooke's Hospital in the 1860's', Cambridge Collection, Cambridge Central Library, C.21.4.
[6] Addenbrooke's Hospital Minute Book, General Quarterly Court 5.10.1863.
[7] Addenbrooke's Hospital Minute Book, General Quarterly Court 28.3.1864.
[8] Addenbrooke's Hospital Minute Book, Special General Court 2.5.1864.
[9] Addenbrooke's Hospital Minute Book, General Quarterly Court 27.6.1864.
[10] Addenbrooke's Hospital Minute Book, General Quarterly Court 26.6.1865.
[11] Addenbrooke's Hospital Minute Book, Building Committee 20.12.1865.
[12] Addenbrooke's Hospital Minute Book, Building Committee 28.12.1865.
[13] Addenbrooke's Hospital Minute Book, General Quarterly Court 1.1.1866.
[14] House Surgeon's Report to the Governors 30.5.1866.
[15] PEVSNER, N., 1956, *Matthew Digby Wyatt*, Cambridge University Press.
[16] Editorial, 1866, Addenbrooke's Hospital, Cambridge, *The Lancet*, **1**, 464.
[17] Report by Dr John Syer Bristow and Mr Timothy Holmes on the Hospitals of the United Kingdom, Appendix No. 15 to Sixth Report of the Medical Officer of the Privy Council, 1863, Parliamentary Papers, 1864, vol. 28, H.M.S.O.

CHAPTER 19

[1] Addenbrooke's Hospital Minute Book, General Quarterly Court, 26.3.1866,.
[2] Addenbrooke's Hospital Minute Book, Weekly Meeting 10.1.1866.
[3] Addenbrooke's Hospital Minute Book, General Quarterly Court 26.3.1866.
[4] FRAZER, W.M., 1950, *A History of English Public Health*, Bailliere Tindall & Cox, London, p. 288.

5   Addenbrooke's Hospital Minute Book, Weekly Meetings 1871.
6   Addenbrooke's Hospital Minute Book, Weekly Meeting 22.2.1871.
7   Addenbrooke's Hospital Minute Book, Weekly Meeting 27.3.1871.
8   Addenbrooke's Hospital Minute Book, Weekly Meeting 5.4.1871.
9   Addenbrooke's Hospital Minute Book, Medical Staff Meeting 11.8.1883.
10 Addenbrooke's Hospital Minute Book, Committee 27.1.1886.
11 Addenbrooke's Hospital Minute Book, Weekly Meeting 10.3.1886.
12 Addenbrooke's Hospital Minute Book, Weekly Meeting 16.6.1886.
13 Addenbrooke's Hospital Minute Book, Weekly Meeting 13.5.1885.
14 Addenbrooke's Hospital Minute Book, Weekly Meeting 17.11.1886.
15 Addenbrooke's Hospital Minute Book, Weekly Meeting 22.12.1886.
16 Addenbrooke's Hospital Minute Book, Weekly Meeting 18.1.1888.
17 Addenbrooke's Hospital Minute Book, Weekly Meeting 28.3.1888.
18 Addenbrooke's Hospital Minute Book, Weekly Meeting 5.11.1890.
19 Addenbrooke's Hospital Minute Book, Weekly Meeting 2.10.1889.
20 Addenbrooke's Hospital Minute Book, Weekly Meeting 10.6.1891.
21 Addenbrooke's Hospital Minute Book, Committee 21.4.1891.
22 Addenbrooke's Hospital Minute Book, Weekly Meeting 13.4.1892.
23 Addenbrooke's Hospital Minute Book, Weekly Meeting 16.1.1895.
24 Addenbrooke's Hospital Minute Book, Weekly Meeting 23.1.1893.
25 Addenbrooke's Hospital Minute Book, Weekly Meeting 27.2.1895.
26 Addenbrooke's Hospital Minute Book, Weekly Meeting 26.5.1875.
27 GROVE, R., 1976, *The Cambridgeshire Coprolite Riding Rush*, Oleander Press, Cambridge.
28 WHERRY, G., 1925, unpublished reminiscences. Addenbrooke's Hospital Archives.
29 Addenbrooke's Hospital Minute Book, Weekly Meeting 14.3.1883.
30 Addenbrooke's Hospital Minute Book, Committee on Out-patients 9.4.1883.
31 Addenbrooke's Hospital Minute Book, Weekly Meeting 31.12.1890.
32 Addenbrooke's Hospital Minute Book, Committee 29.1.1891.
33 Addenbrooke's Hospital Minute Book, Committee on Out-patients 6.3.1890.
34 Addenbrooke's Hospital Minute Book, Weekly Meeting 10.5.1893.
35 Addenbrooke's Hospital Minute Book, Weekly Meeting 12.7.1893.
36 Addenbrooke's Hospital Minute Book, Weekly Meeting 18.12.1895.
37 Addenbrooke's Hospital Minute Book, Weekly Meeting 13.2.1889.
38 Addenbrooke's Hospital Minute Book, Weekly Meeting 4.3.1896.
39 Addenbrooke's Hospital Minute Book, Weekly Meeting 1.3.1891.
40 Addenbrooke's Hospital Minute Book, Weekly Meeting 30.8.1899.

CHAPTER 20

1   There is slight overlap between some of these categories.
2   SQUIRE, P., 1882, *Companion to the latest edition of the British*

Pharmacopoeia, 13th edition, J. & A. Churchill, New Burlington Street, London.

3   SQUIRE, P., 1899, *Companion to the Latest Edition of the British Pharmacopoeia*, 17th edition, J. & A. Churchill, 7 Great Marlborough Street, London.

4   BEASLEY, H., 1892, *The Book of Prescriptions*, John Churchill, London.

5   Personal communication, December, 1988, from Ms Valerie Beamish, S.R.D., of the Cambridge Health Authority, who says it should be noted that twentieth-century food tables were used in this analysis and the foods consumed earlier in the century were probably quite different.

6   PANTON, P., 1951, *Leaves from a Doctor's Life*, William Heineman.

7   MARTINDALE, W. and WESTCOTT, W., 1898, *The Extra Pharmacopoeia*, 9th edition, H.K. Lewis, 136 Gower Street, London W.C.

8   HOBLYN, R.D., 1887, *A Dictionary of Terms used in Medicine and the Collateral Sciences*, 11th edition, revised by John A.P. Price, Whittaker & Co., London.

CHAPTER 21

1   Addenbrooke's Hospital Minute Book, Special General Court 25.11.1867.

2   Addenbrooke's Hospital Minute Book, Weekly Meeting 14.10.1868.

3   Addenbrooke's Hospital Minute Book, Weekly Meeting 27.9.1871.

4   Addenbrooke's Hospital Minute Book, Weekly Meeting, 11.9.1872.

5   Addenbrooke's Hospital Minute Book, Weekly Meeting 26.6.1872.

6   Addenbrooke's Hospital Minute Book, General Quarterly Court 30.9.1872.

7   Addenbrooke's Hospital Minute Book, Weekly Meeting 4.12.1872.

8   Addenbrooke's Hospital Minute Book, Weekly Meeting 18.2.1874.

9   Addenbrooke's Hospital Minute Book, General Quarterly Court 23.2.1874.

10 Addenbrooke's Hospital Minute Book, General Quarterly Court 30.3.1874.

11 Addenbrooke's Hospital Minute Book, General Quarterly Court, 27.12.1875.

12 Addenbrooke's Hospital Minute Book, Weekly Meeting 30.5.1877.

13 WHERRY, G., 1925, unpublished reminiscences. Addenbrooke's Hospital Archives.

14 Addenbrooke's Hospital Minute Book, Weekly Meeting 2.1.1889.

15 Editorial, 1912, Dr Latham of Cambridge, *British Medical Journal*, 1, 694.

16 *Munk's Roll*, vol 4, *Lives of the Fellows of the Royal College of Physicians of London 1826–1925*, compiled by G.H. Brown, published by the College, London, p. 153.

17 PAGET, C.E., 1893, *Some Lectures of the late Sir George Paget, Edited with a Memoir*, MacMillan and Bowes, Cambridge.
18 Addenbrooke's Hospital Minute Book, Weekly Meeting 6.11.1867.
19 Addenbrooke's Hospital Minute Book, Special General Court 26.7.1869.
20 Addenbrooke's Hospital Minute Book, Weekly Meeting 10.4.1872.
21 Addenbrooke's Hospital Minute Book, General Quarterly Court 3.10.1870.
22 Addenbrooke's Hospital Minute Book, Special General Court 31.10.1870.
23 Addenbrooke's Hospital Minute Book, Weekly Meeting 12.5.1875.
24 Addenbrooke's Hospital Minute Book, Weekly Meeting 16.6.1875.
25 Addenbrooke's Hospital Minute Book, Weekly Meeting 21.6.1875.
26 Addenbrooke's Hospital Minute Book, Weekly Meeting 22.3.1876.
27 Addenbrooke's Hospital Minute Book, Committee 23.3.1876.
28 Addenbrooke's Hospital Minute Book, General Quarterly Court 27.3.1876.
29 Addenbrooke's Hospital Minute Book, Weekly Meeting 10.9.1879.
30 Addenbrooke's Hospital Minute Book, Weekly Meeting 1.10.1879.
31 Addenbrooke's Hospital Minute Book, General Quarterly Court 6.10.1879.
32 Addenbrooke's Hospital Minute Book, General Quarterly Court 31.12.1877.
33 Addenbrooke's Hospital Minute Book, Weekly Meeting 7.2.1878.
34 Addenbrooke's Hospital Minute Book, Special General Court 24.11.1879.
35 Addenbrooke's Hospital Minute Book, Weekly Meeting 30.4.1884.
36 Addenbrooke's Hospital Minute Book, Weekly Meeting 22.3.1889.
37 Addenbrooke's Hospital Minute Book, General Quarterly Court 30.6.1884.
38 MACALISTER, LADY E.F.B., 1935, *Sir Donald MacAlister of Tarbert by his wife, with chapters by Sir R. Rait and Sir N. Walker*, Macmillan & Co., London.
39 Addenbrooke's Hospital Minute Book, Weekly Meeting 7.8.1889.
40 Addenbrooke's Hospital Minute Book, General Quarterly Court 5.10.1891 and Adjourned Quarterly Court 16.10.1891.
41 Addenbrooke's Hospital Minute Book, Special General Court 18.11.1891.

CHAPTER 22

1 Addenbrooke's Hospital Minute Book, General Quarterly Court 26.6.1865.
2 Addenbrooke's Hospital Minute Book, General Quarterly Court 2.10.1865.
3 Addenbrooke's Hospital Minute Book, Weekly Meeting 3.1.1866.

4   Addenbrooke's Hospital Minute Book, Weekly Meeting 10.1.1866.

5   Addenbrooke's Hospital Minute Book, Weekly Meeting 17.1.1866.

6   Addenbrooke's Hospital Minute Book, Weekly Meeting 1.8.1866.

7   Addenbrooke's Hospital Minute Book, Weekly Meeting 15.8.1866.

8   Addenbrooke's Hospital Minute Book, Weekly Meeting 26.12.1866.

9   Addenbrooke's Hospital Minute Book, General Quarterly Court
1.7.1867.

10   Addenbrooke's Hospital Minute Book, Financial Committee 31.7.1867.

11   Addenbrooke's Hospital Minute Book, Weekly Meeting 25.9.1867.

12   Addenbrooke's Hospital Minute Book, Financial Committee 4.12.1867.

13   Addenbrooke's Hospital Minute Book, Financial Committee 22.1.1868.

14   Addenbrooke's Hospital Minute Book, General Quarterly Court
30.3.1868.

15   Addenbrooke's Hospital Minute Book, Adjourned Quarterly Court
25.5.1868.

16   CHARLES CARDALE BABINGTON (1808–1895), Professor of
Botany.

17   Addenbrooke's Hospital Minute Book, General Quarterly Court
29.6.1868.

18   Addenbrooke's Hospital Minute Book, Weekly Meeting 21.10.1868.

19   Addenbrooke's Hospital Minute Book, Weekly Meeting 28.10.1868.

20   Addenbrooke's Hospital Minute Book, Weekly Meeting 11.12.1872.

21   Addenbrooke's Hospital Minute Book, Weekly Meeting 18.12.1872.

22   Addenbrooke's Hospital Minute Book, Weekly Meeting 27.8.1873.

23   Addenbrooke's Hospital Minute Book, Weekly Meeting 15.4.1874.

24   Addenbrooke's Hospital Minute Book, Weekly Meeting 29.4.1874.

25   See, for example, Weekly Meeting 16.2.1876.

26   Addenbrooke's Hospital Minute Book, Special General Court 26.7.1874.

27   Addenbrooke's Hospital Minute Book, General Quarterly Court
26.3.1877.

28   Addenbrooke's Hospital Minute Book, Select Committee 6.4.1877.

29   Addenbrooke's Hospital Minute Book, General Quarterly Court
9.4.1877.

30   Addenbrooke's Hospital Minute Book, Select Committee 2.4.1877.

31   Addenbrooke's Hospital Minute Book, General Quarterly Court
(adjourned) 14.5.1877.

32   COPE, Z., 1961, *Six Disciples of Florence Nightingale*, Pitman Medical,
London, pp. 57 ff.

33   WHERRY, G., 1925, unpublished reminiscences. Addenbrooke's
Hospital Archives.

34   Addenbrooke's Hospital Minute Book, Weekly Meeting 13.6.1877.

35   Addenbrooke's Hospital Minute Book, Weekly Meeting 11.7.1877.

36   Addenbrooke's Hospital Minute Book, Weekly Meeting 4.8.1877.

37   Addenbrooke's Hospital Minute Book, Weekly Meeting 15.8.1877.

38   Addenbrooke's Hospital Minute Book, Weekly Meeting 19.9.1877.

39   Addenbrooke's Hospital Minute Book, Weekly Meeting 5.9.1877.

40   Addenbrooke's Hospital Minute Book, Committee 11.12.1877.
41   Addenbrooke's Hospital Minute Book, Weekly Meeting 6.3.1878.
42   Addenbrooke's Hospital Minute Book, Weekly Meeting 13.3.1878.
43   Addenbrooke's Hospital Minute Book, Weekly Meeting 15.5.1878.
44   Addenbrooke's Hospital Minute Book, Weekly Meeting 11.2.1880.
45   Addenbrooke's Hospital Minute Book, Weekly Meeting 25.2.1880.
46   Addenbrooke's Hospital Minute Book, General Quarterly Court
      27.3.1882.
47   Addenbrooke's Hospital Minute Book, Weekly Meeting 27.7.1886.
48   Addenbrooke's Hospital Minute Book, Weekly Meeting 6.8.1884.
49   Addenbrooke's Hospital Minute Book, Committee 3.2.1886.
50   Addenbrooke's Hospital Minute Book, Weekly Meeting 24.2.1886.
51   Addenbrooke's Hospital Minute Book, Adjourned Committee
      26.10.1886.
52   Addenbrooke's Hospital Minute Book, Weekly Meeting 16.3.1887.
53   Addenbrooke's Hospital Minute Book, Weekly Meeting 11.5.1887.

CHAPTER 23

1   Addenbrooke's Hospital Minute Book, General Quarterly Court
     15.7.1867.
2   Addenbrooke's Hospital Minute Book, Weekly Meeting 25.9.1867.
3   Addenbrooke's Hospital Minute Book, General Quarterly Court
     15.7.1867.
4   Addenbrooke's Hospital Minute Book, General Quarterly Court
     30.9.1867.
5   Addenbrooke's Hospital Minute Book, General Quarterly Court
     30.12.1867.
6   Addenbrooke's Hospital Minute Book, Improvement of Funds
     Committee 26.6.1868.
7   Addenbrooke's Hospital Minute Book, General Quarterly Court
     26.6.1871.
8   Addenbrooke's Hospital Minute Book, Improvement Committee
     20.12.1872.
9   Addenbrooke's Hospital Minute Book, Improvement Committee
     16.1.1873.
10   Addenbrooke's Hospital Minute Book, General Quarterly Court
     7.5.1875.
11   Addenbrooke's Hospital Minute Book, Improvement Committee
     20.12.1875.
12   Addenbrooke's Hospital Minute Book, General Quarterly Court
     1.1.1877.
13   Addenbrooke's Hospital Minute Book, Expenditure Committee 7.3.1877.
14   Addenbrooke's Hospital Minute Book, General Quarterly Court
     26.3.1877.

15 Addenbrooke's Hospital Minute Book, General Quarterly Court 31.12.1877.

16 Addenbrooke's Hospital Minute Book, Finance Committee 12.3.1879.

17 Addenbrooke's Hospital Minute Book, Finance Committee 24.3.1880.

18 Addenbrooke's Hospital Minute Book, Finance Committees 2.10.1880 and 24.12.1880.

19 Addenbrooke's Hospital Minute Book, Finance Committee 30.9.1881.

20 Addenbrooke's Hospital Minute Book, Finance Committee 24.3.1882.

21 Addenbrooke's Hospital Minute Book, Finance Committee 22.6.1883.

22 Addenbrooke's Hospital Minute Book, General Quarterly Court 6.10.1884.

23 Addenbrooke's Hospital Minute Book, Finance Committee 28.1.1885.

24 Addenbrooke's Hospital Minute Book, General Quarterly Court 4.10.1897.

25 Addenbrooke's Hospital Minute Book, Special Finance Committee 30.9.1898.

26 BURDETT, SIR H.C., 1898, Addenbrooke's Hospital, Cambridge. Report on Certain Proposed Changes in its Constitutional, Financial, Nursing, Administrative, and Structural Arrangements. Cambridge Collection, Cambridge Central Library, C.21.4.

27 Addenbrooke's Hospital Minute Book, General Quarterly Court 19.5.1899.

28 Addenbrooke's Hospital Minute Book, Finance Committee 22.1.1899.

29 Addenbrooke's Hospital Minute Book, General Quarterly Court 27.3.1899.

30 Addenbrooke's Hospital Minute Book, Finance Committee 16.5.1899.

31 Addenbrooke's Hospital Minute Book, General Quarterly Court 19.5.1899.

CHAPTER 24

1 Addenbrooke's Hospital Minute Book, Select Governors 16.6.1887.

2 Addenbrooke's Hospital Minute Book, Weekly Meeting 2.1.1889.

3 Addenbrooke's Hospital Minute Book, General Quarterly Court 1.7.1888.

4 Addenbrooke's Hospital Minute Book, Weekly Meeting 20.12.1893.

5 Addenbrooke's Hospital Minute Book, Weekly Meeting 4.7.1894.

6 Addenbrooke's Hospital Minute Book, Weekly Meeting 15.3.1893.

7 Report of Committee on Probationers' Accommodation, inserted in Minute Book 17.12.1894.

8 Addenbrooke's Hospital Minute Book, General Quarterly Court 31.12.1894.

9 Addenbrooke's Hospital Minute Book, Committee 10.3.1895.

10 Addenbrooke's Hospital Minute Book, Weekly Meeting 8.1.1896.

11 Addenbrooke's Hospital Minute Book, Weekly Meeting 28.3.1896.

[12] Addenbrooke's Hospital Minute Book, Weekly Meeting 16.2.1898.
[13] Addenbrooke's Hospital Minute Book, Weekly Meeting 23.2.1898.
[14] Addenbrooke's Hospital Minute Book, Weekly Meeting 29.11.1899.
[15] Addenbrooke's Hospital Minute Book, Weekly Meeting 13.12.1899.
[16] Addenbrooke's Hospital Minute Book, Weekly Meeting 17.1.1900.
[17] Addenbrooke's Hospital Minute Book, Weekly Meeting 19.2.1900.
[18] Addenbrooke's Hospital Minute Book, Weekly Meeting 14.3.1900.
[19] Addenbrooke's Hospital Minute Book, Finance Committee 23.3.1900.
[20] Addenbrooke's Hospital Minute Book, Weekly Meeting 6.6.1901.
[21] Addenbrooke's Hospital Minute Book, General Quarterly Court 2.7.1901.
[22] Addenbrooke's Hospital Minute Book, Weekly Meeting 6.3.1901.
[23] Addenbrooke's Hospital Minute Book, Weekly Meeting 17.7.1901.

CHAPTER 25

[1]   Addenbrooke's Hospital Minute Book, Repairing Committee 20.2.1867.
[2]   Addenbrooke's Hospital Minute Book, General Quarterly Court 25.3.1872.
[3]   Addenbrooke's Hospital Minute Book, General Quarterly Court 5.10.1874.
[4]   Addenbrooke's Hospital Minute Book, Building Committee 19.3.1878.
[5]   Addenbrooke's Hospital Minute Book, Weekly Meeting 4.12.1878.
[6]   Addenbrooke's Hospital Minute Book, Weekly Meeting 9.2.1881.
[7]   Addenbrooke's Hospital Minute Book, Weekly Meeting 13.10.1882.
[8]   Addenbrooke's Hospital Minute Book, Weekly Meeting 21.2.1883.
[9]   Addenbrooke's Hospital Minute Book, Weekly Meeting 22.2.1884.
[10] Addenbrooke's Hospital Minute Book, Building Committee 18.4.1884.
[11] Addenbrooke's Hospital Minute Book, Building Committee 21.4.1891.
[12] Addenbrooke's Hospital Minute Book, Building Committee 22.4.1892.
[13] Addenbrooke's Hospital Minute Book, General Quarterly Court 13.7.1892.
[14] Addenbrooke's Hospital Minute Book, Committee on Drainage 5.9.1892.
[15] Addenbrooke's Hospital Minute Book, Committee on Drainage 7.9.1892.
[16] Addenbrooke's Hospital Minute Book, General Quarterly Court 3.10.1892.
[17] Addenbrooke's Hospital Minute Book, Weekly Board 30.11.1892.
[18] Addenbrooke's Hospital Minute Book, General Quarterly Court 6.2.1893.
[19] Addenbrooke's Hospital Minute Book, Committee on Drainage 24.3.1893.
[20] Addenbrooke's Hospital Minute Book, Weekly Board 19.4.1893.
[21] Addenbrooke's Hospital Minute Book, Committee on Drainage 19.4.1893.
[22] Addenbrooke's Hospital Minute Book, Weekly Meeting 13.10.1894.

23 Addenbrooke's Hospital Minute Book, Weekly Meeting 18.3.1895.
24 Addenbrooke's Hospital Minute Book, Special General Court 10.6.1895.
25 Addenbrooke's Hospital Minute Book, Weekly Meeting 5.2.1896.
26 Addenbrooke's Hospital Minute Book, Weekly Meeting 12.2.1896.
27 Addenbrooke's Hospital Minute Book, General Quarterly Court
   18.5.1896.
28 Addenbrooke's Hospital Minute Book, Weekly Meeting 11.3.1896.
29 Addenbrooke's Hospital Minute Book, Weekly Meeting 17.6.1896.
30 Addenbrooke's Hospital Minute Book, Weekly Meeting 10.5.1896.
31 Addenbrooke's Hospital Minute Book, General Quarterly Court
   29.6.1896.
32 Addenbrooke's Hospital Minute Book, General Quarterly Court
   10.8.1896.
33 Addenbrooke's Hospital Minute Book, Special General Court
   16.11.1896.
34 Addenbrooke's Hospital Minute Book, Weekly Meeting 10.3.1897.
35 Addenbrooke's Hospital Minute Book, Steam Laundry Committee
   2.11.1897.
36 Addenbrooke's Hospital Minute Book, Weekly Meeting 4.8.1897.
37 Addenbrooke's Hospital Minute Book, Weekly Meeting 8.12.1897.
38 Addenbrooke's Hospital Minute Book, General Quarterly Court
   25.2.1898.
39 Addenbrooke's Hospital Minute Book, General Quarterly Court
   28.3.1898.
40 Addenbrooke's Hospital Minute Book, General Quarterly Court
   31.12.1900.
41 Addenbrooke's Hospital Minute Book, Weekly Meeting 6.2.1901.
42 Addenbrooke's Hospital Minute Book, Hot Water Committee 5.6.1902.
43 Addenbrooke's Hospital Minute Book, General Quarterly Court
   30.6.1902.
44 Addenbrooke's Hospital Minute Book, Weekly Meeting 13.8.1902.
45 Addenbrooke's Hospital Minute Book, Hot Water Committee 14.8.1902.
46 Addenbrooke's Hospital Minute Book, Weekly Meeting 20.8.1902.
47 Addenbrooke's Hospital Minute Book, Weekly Meeting 5.11.1902.
48 Addenbrooke's Hospital Minute Book, Advisory Council 3.10.1902.
49 Addenbrooke's Hospital Minute Book, General Quarterly Court
   6.10.1902.
50 Addenbrooke's Hospital Minute Book, Weekly Meeting 8.10.1902.
51 Addenbrooke's Hospital Minute Book, Meeting of the Committee re the
   Origin of the Fire 5.11.1902.
52 Addenbrooke's Hospital Minute Book, General Quarterly Court
   11.11.1902.
53 Addenbrooke's Hospital Minute Book, Weekly Meeting 6.5.1903.
54 Addenbrooke's Hospital Minute Book, Works Sub-Committee
   16.12.1903.

55 Addenbrooke's Hospital Minute Book, General Quarterly Court
    11.4.1904.
56 Addenbrooke's Hospital Minute Book, General Quarterly Court
    6.3.1905.
57 General Committee Minute Book, Special Committee 17.3.1905.
58 Addenbrooke's Hospital Minute Book, General Committee 6.3.1905.
59 Addenbrooke's Hospital Minute Book, General Committee 17.12.1906.
60 Addenbrooke's Hospital Minute Book, General Committee 14.12.1903.
61 Addenbrooke's Hospital Minute Book, House Sub-Committee 4.1.1904.
62 Addenbrooke's Hospital Minute Book, General Committee 14.11.1904.
63 Addenbrooke's Hospital Minute Book, General Committee 28.11.1904.
64 Addenbrooke's Hospital Minute Book, House Sub-Committee 8.1.1906.
65 Addenbrooke's Hospital Minute Book, General Committee 17.4.1906.
66 PANTON, P., 1951, *Leaves from a Doctor's Life*, Heinemann, p. 61.

CHAPTER 26

1   ROLLESTON, SIR H.D., 1932, *The Cambridge Medical School*,
    Cambridge University Press.
2   LANGDON-BROWN, SIR W., 1946, *Some Chapters in Cambridge
    Medical History*, Cambridge University Press.
3   ROOK, A., 1979, Charles Collignon (1725–1785): Cambridge
    Physician, Anatomist and Moralist, *Medical History*, **23**, 339–45.
4   Addenbrooke's Hospital Minute Book, Committee Report, Relations
    with the University, General Quarterly Court 7.5.1895.
5   Addenbrooke's Hospital Minute Book, General Quarterly Court
    5.10.1840.
6   Addenbrooke's Hospital Minute Book, Committee for the Improvement
    of the Funds 29.2.1860.
7   Addenbrooke's Hospital Minute Book, Weekly Meeting 20.10.1869.
8   Addenbrooke's Hospital Minute Book, Weekly Meeting 8.10.1879.
9   Addenbrooke's Hospital Minute Book, Weekly Meeting 17.12.1890.
10 Addenbrooke's Hospital Minute Book, Committee Meeting of Medical
    Officers and Deputation from the Weekly Board 20.12.1890.
11 Addenbrooke's Hospital Minute Book, Weekly Meeting 24.12.1890.
12 Addenbrooke's Hospital Minute Book, Weekly Meeting 20.2.1895.
13 Addenbrooke's Hospital Minute Book, General Quarterly Court
    25.3.1895.
14 Letter from Mr G.B. Finch on behalf of the Hospital Investigation
    Committee, Minutes of the Special Board for Medicine, 8.12.1899,
    University Archives, Cambridge University Library, Min.V.33.
15 ROLLESTON, SIR H.D., 1929, *The Right Honourable Sir Clifford Allbutt,
    K.C.B., A Memoir*, Macmillan & Co. Ltd, London.
16 COLE, L., 1971, Cambridge Medicine and the Medical School in the

Twentieth Century, in *Cambridge and its Contribution to Medicine*, ed.
Arthur Rook, Wellcome Institute of the History of Medicine, London.
17   Addenbrooke's Hospital Minute Book, Weekly Meeting 14.8.1901.
18   *Cambridge Daily News* 14.2.1914.
19   Addenbrooke's Hospital Minute Book, Weekly Meeting 28.8.1901.
20   *Cambridge Chronicle* 20.2.1914.

CHAPTER 27

1   Addenbrooke's Hospital Minute Book, Weekly Meeting 9.5.1894.
2   Addenbrooke's Hospital Minute Book, Weekly Meeting 11.7.1894.
3   Addenbrooke's Hospital Minute Book, Weekly Meeting 12.2.1896.
4   Addenbrooke's Hospital Minute Book, Weekly Meeting 3.6.1896.
5   Addenbrooke's Hospital Minute Book, General Quarterly Court
    29.6.1896.
6   Addenbrooke's Hospital Minute Book, Select Governors and Medical
    Officers 4.6.1895.
7   Addenbrooke's Hospital Minute Book, General Quarterly Court
    27.6.1898.
8   Addenbrooke's Hospital Minute Book, Select Governors and Medical
    Officers 7.12.1898.
9   Addenbrooke's Hospital Minute Book, Weekly Meeting 5.7.1899.
10   Addenbrooke's Hospital Minute Book, Advisory Council 27.12.1901.
11   Addenbrooke's Hospital Minute Book, General Committee 28.3.1904.
12   Addenbrooke's Hospital Minute Book, Weekly Meeting 12.9.1904.
13   Addenbrooke's Hospital Minute Book, General Committee 25.9.1905.
14   Addenbrooke's Hospital Minute Book, Weekly Meeting 9.10.1905.
15   Addenbrooke's Hospital Minute Book, General Committee 15.12.1905.
16   Addenbrooke's Hospital Minute Book, Weekly Meeting 5.2.1906.
17   Addenbrooke's Hospital Minute Book, General Committee 4.11.1907.
18   Addenbrooke's Hospital Minute Book, General Committee 9.6.1908.
19   Addenbrooke's Hospital Minute Book, General Committee 5.7.1909.
20   Addenbrooke's Hospital Minute Book, General Committee 17.1.1910.
21   Addenbrooke's Hospital Minute Book, General Committee 28.8.1910.
22   Addenbrooke's Hospital Minute Book, General Committee 17.10.1910.
23   Addenbrooke's Hospital Minute Book, General Committee 28.11.1910.
24   Addenbrooke's Hospital Minute Book, General Committee 28.12.1910.
25   Addenbrooke's Hospital General Committee Minute Book, Selection
    Committee 27.10.1911.
26   Addenbrooke's Hospital General Committee Minute Book, Selection
    Committee 12.4.1913.
27   Addenbrooke's Hospital Minute Book, General Committee 27.4.1914.
28   ROLLESTON, SIR H.D., 1932, *The Cambridge Medical School*,
    Cambridge University Press.

29 MACALISTER, LADY E.F.B., 1935, *Sir Donald MacAlister of Tarbert by his wife, with chapters by Sir R. Rait and Sir N. Walker*, Macmillan & Co., London, p. 120.

30 Addenbrooke's Hospital Minute Book, Weekly Meeting 5.10.1892.

31 ROLLESTON, SIR H.D., 1929, *The Right Honourable Sir Clifford Allbutt, K.C.B., A Memoir*, Macmillan & Co., Ltd, London, p. 111.

32 Addenbrooke's Hospital Minute Book, Weekly Meeting 5.7.1896.

33 Addenbrooke's Hospital Minute Book, Weekly Meeting 30.6.1897.

34 Addenbrooke's Hospital Minute Book, Adjourned General Quarterly Court 6.2.1899.

35 Senate, Grace 3, 15.3.1900. University Archives, Cambridge University Library.

36 Addenbrooke's Hospital Minute Book, Adjourned General Quarterly Court 23.4.1900.

37 Addenbrooke's Hospital Minute Book, Special General Court 29.10.1894.

38 Addenbrooke's Hospital Minute Book, Special General Court 26.11.1894.

39 Addenbrooke's Hospital Minute Book, General Quarterly Court 1.7.1895.

40 Addenbrooke's Hospital Minute Book, General Quarterly Court 27.3.1899.

41 Addenbrooke's Hospital Minute Book, General Quarterly Court 31.3.1902.

42 Addenbrooke's Hospital Minute Book, Advisory Council 9.6.1902.

43 Addenbrooke's Hospital Minute Book, General Quarterly Court 5.10.1903.

44 MARSH, V.S., 1921, *A Memoir of Howard Marsh*, Murray, London, pp. 62ff.

45 WHITE H., 1974, in *The Royal Hospital of Saint Bartholomew 1123–1973*, ed. Victor Cornelius Medvei and John L. Thornton, W.S. Cowell Ltd, Ipswich, p. 217.

46 Addenbrooke's Hospital Minute Book, General Committee 17.4.1905.

47 Addenbrooke's Hospital Minute Book, General Committee 26.6.1911.

48 Addenbrooke's Hospital Minute Book, House Committee 9.10.1906.

49 Addenbrooke's Hospital Minute Book, House Committee 18.9.1906.

50 Addenbrooke's Hospital Minute Book, General Committee 30.10.1906.

51 Addenbrooke's Hospital Minute Book, General Committee 23.3.1908.

52 Addenbrooke's Hospital Minute Book, General Committee 23.3.1909.

53 Addenbrooke's Hospital Minute Book, General Committee 5.4.1909.

54 Addenbrooke's Hospital Minute Book, General Committee 7.6.1909.

55 Addenbrooke's Hospital Minute Book, General Committee 2.8.1909.

CHAPTER 28

1 ROOK, A., 1979, Charles Collignon (1725–1785): Cambridge
   Physician, Anatomist and Moralist, *Medical History*, **23**, 339–45.
2 GRAHAM SMITH, W., MS 'History of the Department of Pathology',
   Cambridge University Library, Add. 7328.
3 FOSTER, W.D., 1962, *A Short History of Clinical Pathology*, Livingstone,
   Edinburgh.
4 KING, L.S. and MEEHAM, M.C., 1973, A History of the Autopsy,
   American Journal of Pathology, **73**, 514.
5 Addenbrooke's Hospital Minute Book, Report of Medical Staff to
   General Committee 6.4.1908.
6 Foster, op. cit. n. 3, p. 112.
7 ROOK, A., 1980, *The Cambridge Medical Society, A Centennial History*,
   Cambridge Medical Society.
8 Addenbrooke's Hospital Minute Book, Advisory Council 27.12.1902.
9 Addenbrooke's Hospital Minute Book, General Committee 6.7.1908.
10 Addenbrooke's Hospital Minute Book, General Committee 11.8.1908.
11 Addenbrooke's Hospital Minute Book, General Committee 3.6.1912.
12 Addenbrooke's Hospital Minute Book, General Committee 24.6.1912.
13 Addenbrooke's Hospital Minute Book, Letter from Mrs Bonnett's
   solicitor, General Committee 15.7.1912.
14 Addenbrooke's Hospital Minute Book, General Committee 12.8.1912.
15 Addenbrooke's Hospital Minute Book, Report of the General Committee
   to the Quarterly Court to be held 6.11.1912.
16 Addenbrooke's Hospital Minute Book, General Committee 14.10.1912.
17 Addenbrooke's Hospital Minute Book, General Committee 15.12.1913.
18 Addenbrooke's Hospital Minute Book, General Committee 12.1.1914.
19 *Cambridge Daily News* 14.2.1914. The report of the luncheon was by
   courtesy of the *Medical World*, the journal owned by Malden.

CHAPTER 29

1 Addenbrooke's Hospital Minute Book, General Quarterly Court
   19.3.1900.
2 Addenbrooke's Hospital Minute Book, Advisory Council's Report to the
   Michaelmas Quarterly Court 1903.
3 Addenbrooke's Hospital Minute Book, Advisory Council 19.6.1900.
4 Addenbrooke's Hospital Minute Book, Report of Advisory Council
   17.12.1900.
5 Addenbrooke's Hospital Minute Book, Advisory Council 27.9.1901.
6 Addenbrooke's Hospital Minute Book, Advisory Council 27.12.1902.
7 Addenbrooke's Hospital Minute Book, General Quarterly Court
   29.12.1902.

8   Addenbrooke's Hospital Minute Book, General Quarterly Court
    29.1.1903.
9   Addenbrooke's Hospital Minute Book, General Committee 5.12.1904.
10 Addenbrooke's Hospital Minute Book, Finance Committee 3.4.1905.
11 Addenbrooke's Hospital Minute Book, General Committee 1.11.1905.
12 Addenbrooke's Hospital Minute Book, Advisory Council 7.5.1906.
13 Addenbrooke's Hospital Minute Book, General Committee 1.10.1906.
14 Addenbrooke's Hospital Minute Book, General Committee 2.12.1907.
15 Addenbrooke's Hospital Minute Book, Report of Special Committee
    1.6.1908.
16 Addenbrooke's Hospital Minute Book, General Committee 17.5.1910.
17 Addenbrooke's Hospital Minute Book, General Committee 25.7.1910.
18 Addenbrooke's Hospital Minute Book, General Committee 16.10.1911.
19 Addenbrooke's Hospital Minute Book, General Quarterly Court
    3.8.1910.
20 Addenbrooke's Hospital Minute Book, General Court 22.9.1910.

CHAPTER 30

1   Addenbrooke's Hospital Minute Book, Weekly Meeting 30.5.1910.
2   Addenbrooke's Hospital Minute Book, Advisory Council 19.6.1900.
3   Addenbrooke's Hospital Minute Book, General Committee 28.11.1910.
4   Addenbrooke's Hospital Minute Book, General Committee 27.2.1911.
5   Addenbrooke's Hospital Minute Book, General Committee 14.3.1914.
6   Addenbrooke's Hospital Minute Book, Advisory Council 17.6.1902.
7   Addenbrooke's Hospital Minute Book, General Quarterly Court
    30.6.1902.
8   Addenbrooke's Hospital Minute Book, Weekly Meeting 27.10.1902.
9   Addenbrooke's Hospital Minute Book, Weekly Meeting 11.12.1902.
10 Addenbrooke's Hospital Minute Book, House Committee 29.12.1902.
11 Addenbrooke's Hospital Minute Book, House Sub-Committee 27.4.1907.
12 Addenbrooke's Hospital Minute Book, General Committee 11.11.1908.
13 Addenbrooke's Hospital Minute Book, General Committee 8.3.1909.
14 Addenbrooke's Hospital Minute Book, General Committee 17.11.1910.
15 Addenbrooke's Hospital Minute Book, General Committee 13.7.1914.
16 Addenbrooke's Hospital Minute Book, General Committee 28.11.1904.
17 Addenbrooke's Hospital Minute Book, House Sub-Committee 13.3.1905.
18 Addenbrooke's Hospital Minute Book, General Committee 20.3.1905.
19 Addenbrooke's Hospital Minute Book, General Committee 27.3.1905.
20 Addenbrooke's Hospital Minute Book, General Committee 9.7.1906.

CHAPTER 31

1   Addenbrooke's Hospital Minute Book, Select Governors 27.11.1901.
2   Addenbrooke's Hospital Minute Book, Probationers' Committee
      21.12.1901.
3   Addenbrooke's Hospital Minute Book, Weekly Meeting 2.4.1902.
4   Addenbrooke's Hospital Minute Book, Probationers' Committee
      1.5.1902.
5   Addenbrooke's Hospital Minute Book, Weekly Meeting 11.6.1902.
6   Addenbrooke's Hospital Minute Book, General Quarterly Court
      30.6.1902.
7   Addenbrooke's Hospital Minute Book, Weekly Meeting 2.7.1902.
8   Addenbrooke's Hospital Minute Book, Adjourned Weekly Meeting
      3.7.1902.
9   Addenbrooke's Hospital Minute Book, Adjourned Weekly Meeting
      4.7.1902.
10 Addenbrooke's Hospital Minute Book, Weekly Meeting 16.7.1902.
11 Addenbrooke's Hospital Minute Book, Weekly Meeting 27.8.1902.
12 Addenbrooke's Hospital Minute Book, Weekly Meeting 3.9.1902.
13 Addenbrooke's Hospital Minute Book, General Quarterly Court
      30.3.1903.
14 Addenbrooke's Hospital Minute Book, Weekly Meeting 22.4.1903.
15 Addenbrooke's Hospital Minute Book, Select Governors 25.1.1903.
16 Addenbrooke's Hospital Minute Book, General Quarterly Court
      29.1.1903.
17 Addenbrooke's Hospital Minute Book, General Committee 16.5.1904.
18 Addenbrooke's Hospital Minute Book, General Committee 15.8.1904.
19 Addenbrooke's Hospital Minute Book, General Committee 14.11.1904.
20 Addenbrooke's Hospital Minute Book, General Committee 20.12.1904.
21 Addenbrooke's Hospital Minute Book, Weekly Meeting 16.1.1905.
22 Addenbrooke's Hospital Minute Book, General Committee 10.4.1905.
23 Addenbrooke's Hospital Minute Book, General Committee 1.5.1905.
24 Addenbrooke's Hospital Minute Book, House Sub-Committees 26.6.1905
      and 3.7.1905.
25 Addenbrooke's Hospital Minute Book, Special Meeting of the House
      Committee 11.7.1905.
26 Addenbrooke's Hospital Minute Book, House Sub-Committee 18.7.1905.
27 Addenbrooke's Hospital Minute Book, House Sub-Committee
      22.10.1905.
28 Addenbrooke's Hospital Minute Book, House Sub-Committee
      21.11.1905.
29 Addenbrooke's Hospital Minute Book, General Quarterly Court
      7.2.1906.
30 Addenbrooke's Hospital Minute Book, House Sub-Committee 5.11.1906.

[31] Addenbrooke's Hospital Minute Book, House Sub-Committee
      10.12.1907.
[32] Addenbrooke's Hospital Minute Book, General Committee 3.2.1908.
[33] Addenbrooke's Hospital Minute Book, General Committee 1.6.1908.
[34] Addenbrooke's Hospital Minute Book, General Committee 13.4.1908.
[35] Addenbrooke's Hospital Minute Book, General Committee 24.5.1909.
[36] Addenbrooke's Hospital Minute Book, General Committee 13.12.1909.
[37] Addenbrooke's Hospital Minute Book, General Committee 30.10.1911.
[38] Addenbrooke's Hospital Minute Book, General Committee 28.7.1913.

CHAPTER 32

[1] Addenbrooke's Hospital Minute Book, General Committee 11.6.1906.
[2] Addenbrooke's Hospital Minute Book, General Committee 15.5.1912.
[3] Addenbrooke's Hospital Minute Book, Weekly Meeting 12.6.1901.
[4] Addenbrooke's Hospital Minute Book, General Committee 20.5.1912.
[5] Addenbrooke's Hospital Minute Book, General Committee 3.6.1912.
[6] Addenbrooke's Hospital Minute Book, General Committee 21.4.1913.
[7] Addenbrooke's Hospital Minute Book, General Quarterly Court
     6.5.1913.
[8] Addenbrooke's Hospital Minute Book, General Committee 27.10.1913.

CHAPTER 33

[1] *First Eastern General Hospital Gazette* 13.4.1915, p. 3.
[2] *First Eastern General Hospital Gazette* 27.4.1915, p. 95.
[3] *First Eastern General Hospital Gazette* 6.7.1915, p. 199.
[4] Ibid., p. 247.
[5] *First Eastern General Hospital Gazette* 12.10.1915, p. 269.
[6] Addenbrooke's Hospital Minute Book, House Sub-Committee 17.8.1914.
[7] Addenbrooke's Hospital Minute Book, House Sub-Committee
     11.10.1915.
[8] Addenbrooke's Hospital Minute Book, General Committee 25.9.1916.
[9] Addenbrooke's Hospital Minute Book, House Sub-Committee 30.7.1917.
[10] Addenbrooke's Hospital Minute Book, General Committee 25.3.1918.
[11] Addenbrooke's Hospital Minute Book, House Sub-Committee 27.1.1919.

CHAPTER 34

[1] *The Historical Register of the University of Cambridge*, 1917, ed. J.R. Tanner,
     Cambridge University Press.
[2] Addenbrooke's Hospital Minute Book, General Committee 14.12.1903.
[3] Addenbrooke's Hospital Minute Book, House Sub-Committee 4.1.1904.

4   CONYBEARE, D., 1937, Benefactors of Addenbrooke's, in 'The Cam, a Cambridge Town Magazine', Jan–June, p. 168. The Cambridge Collection, Cambridge Central Library, C.05.

5   Addenbrooke's Hospital Minute Book, General Quarterly Court 6.5.1913.

6   Addenbrooke's Hospital Minute Book, General Quarterly Court 11.11.1902.

7   Addenbrooke's Hospital Minute Book, General Committee 29.5.1911.

8   Addenbrooke's Hospital Minute Book, Special Meeting of the General Committee 21.4.1913.

9   Addenbrooke's Hospital Minute Book, Special Sub Committee Meeting 29.5.1919.

10 Addenbrooke's Hospital Minute Book, General Committee 28.6.1920.

11 Addenbrooke's Hospital Minute Book, General Committee 9.8.1920.

12 Addenbrooke's Hospital Minute Book, General Committee 16.6.1919.

13 Addenbrooke's Hospital Minute Book, General Committee 12.6.1922.

14 Addenbrooke's Hospital Minute Book, General Committee 1.1.1923.

15 Addenbrooke's Hospital Minute Book, Special Meeting of the General Committee 20.11.1922.

16 Addenbrooke's Hospital Minute Book, General Committee 9.4.1923.

17 Addenbrooke's Hospital Minute Book, General Quarterly Court 14.5.1923.

18 Addenbrooke's Hospital Minute Book, Special General Committee 11.12.1922.

19 Addenbrooke's Hospital Minute Book, General Committee 27.10.1924.

20 Addenbrooke's Hospital Minute Book, General Committee 21.4.1925.

21 Addenbrooke's Hospital Minute Book, Special Committee 2.5.1919.

22 Addenbrooke's Hospital Minute Book, General Committee 13.11.1922.

23 Addenbrooke's Hospital Minute Book, General Quarterly Court 11.5.1926.

24 Addenbrooke's Hospital Minute Book, General Quarterly Court 10.5.1927.

25 *Cambridge Chronicle* 10.8.1927.

26 *Cambridge Chronicle* 6.7.1927 and 13.7.1927.

27 Addenbrooke's Hospital Minute Book, General Committee 21.8.1928.

28 *Cambridge Chronicle* 6.6.1928.

29 Addenbrooke's Hospital Minute Book, General Committees 9.4.1923, 3.9.1923, 27.10.1924, 22.3.1926 and 13.7.1926.

30 Addenbrooke's Hospital Minute Book, General Committee 26.6.1928.

31 Addenbrooke's Hospital Minute Book, General Committee 10.7.1928.

32 Addenbrooke's Hospital Minute Book, General Committee 16.10.1928.

33 Addenbrooke's Hospital Minute Book, General Quarterly Court 19.2.1929.

34 Addenbrooke's Hospital Minute Book, General Quarterly Court 19.8.1930.

35 'Table Talk', *Cambridge Daily News* 15.3.1930.

[36]   Addenbrooke's Hospital Annual Report 1934.
[37]   Addenbrooke's Hospital Minute Book, General Quarterly Court
       16.2.1932.
[38]   Addenbrooke's Hospital Minute Book, General Committee 5.6.1932.
[39]   Addenbrooke's Hospital Minute Book, General Committee 12.5.1931.
[40]   *Cambridge Chronicle* 19.8.1931.
[41]   Addenbrooke's Hospital Minute Book, General Quarterly Court
       19.8.1930.
[42]   Addenbrooke's Hospital Minute Book, 15.6.1932.
[43]   Addenbrooke's Hospital Minute Book, General Committee 6.1.1931.
[44]   *Cambridge Chronicle* 13.7.1932.
[45]   'Table Talk', *Cambridge Daily News* 1.10.1932.
[46]   Addenbrooke's Hospital Minute Book, General Committee 2.4.1929.
[47]   Addenbrooke's Hospital Minute Book, General Quarterly Court 16.8.1932.
[48]   Addenbrooke's Hospital Minute Book, General Committee 2.2.1932 and
       15.5.1934.
[49]   Mrs E.A. Goode of Mitchell House, Cottenham, had died in 1933 and
       left a handsome legacy amounting to nearly £32,000 to the Hospital.
       Addenbrooke's Hospital Annual Reports 1933, 1934 and 1935.
[50]   Addenbrooke's Hospital Minute Book, General Committee 15.5.1934.
[51]   Addenbrooke's Hospital Annual Report 1935.
[52]   Numbers 25 and 26 although the Annual Reports say numbers 26 and
       27.
[53]   Addenbrooke's Hospital Minute Book, Special Meeting of the House
       Committee 17.11.1933.
[54]   Addenbrooke's Hospital Annual Report 1936.
[55]   Addenbrooke's Hospital Minute Book, General Quarterly Courts
       25.2.1936 and 26.5.1936.
[56]   Addenbrooke's Hospital Minute Book, General Committee 3.11.1936.
[57]   Addenbrooke's Annual Report 1939.
[58]   Addenbrooke's Annual Report 1940.
[59]   Addenbrooke's Annual Report 1941.
[60]   Addenbrooke's Annual Report 1942.
[61]   Addenbrooke's Hospital General Committee Minute Book, General
       Committee 22.8.1944.
[62]   Addenbrooke's Hospital General Committee Minute Book, General
       Committee 24.4.1945.
[63]   Addenbrooke's Hospital General Committee Minute Book, General
       Committee 26.6.1945.
[64]   Addenbrooke's Hospital General Committee Minute Book, General
       Purposes Committee 20.8.1945.
[65]   Addenbrooke's Hospital General Committee Minute Book, General
       Committee 24.7.1945.
[66]   Addenbrooke's Hospital General Committee Minute Book, General
       Committee 28.8.1945.
[67]   Addenbrooke's Hospital General Committee Minute Book, General
       Purposes Committee 17.9.1945.

68   Addenbrooke's Hospital General Committee Minute Book, General
Committee 18.12.1945.

69   Addenbrooke's Hospital Annual Report 1945.

70   Addenbrooke's Hospital General Committee Minute Book, General
Purposes Committee 18.3.1946.

71   Addenbrooke's Hospital General Committee Minute Book, General
Committee 26.8.1947.

72   Addenbrooke's Hospital General Committee Minute Book, General
Purposes Committee 17.11.1947.

CHAPTER 35

1   Addenbrooke's Hospital Annual Reports.

2   Addenbrooke's Hospital Minute Book, General Quarterly Court
3.2.1915.

3   Addenbrooke's Hospital Minute Book, General Committee 10.7.1928.

4   Addenbrooke's Hospital Minute Book, General Committee 13.11.1928.

5   Addenbrooke's Hospital Minute Book, General Committee 26.11.1929.

6   Addenbrooke's Hospital Minute Book, General Committee 25.10.1930.

7   Addenbrooke's Hospital Minute Book, General Committee 11.11.1930.

8   Addenbrooke's Hospital Minute Book, Conference with Workers'
Hospital Fund held 29.11.1930.

9   Addenbrooke's Hospital Minute Book, Contributory Scheme Sub-
Committee Meeting 10.12.1930.

10   Cambridge & District Workers' Hospital Fund, 'Summary of Receipts
and Payments, June 1, 1920–June 1921'. Cambridge Collection,
Cambridge Central Library.

11   Addenbrooke's Hospital Minute Book, Special Meeting of the General
Committee 16.10.1930.

12   Addenbrooke's Hospital Minute Book, General Committee 24.2.1931.

13   Addenbrooke's Hospital Minute Book, General Committee 12.5.1931.

14   Addenbrooke's Hospital Minute Book, General Committee 23.6.1931,
7.7.1931 and 18.8.1931.

15   Addenbrooke's Hospital Minute Book, General Committee 21.7.1931.

16   Addenbrooke's Hospital Minute Book, General Committees 28.5.1923
and 3.5.1931.

17   Addenbrooke's Hospital Minute Book, General Quarterly Court
24.11.1931.

18   Addenbrooke's Hospital Annual Report 1931.

19   Addenbrooke's Hospital Minute Book, General Committee 19.1.1932.

20   Addenbrooke's Hospital Minute Book, General Committee 2.2.1932.

21   Addenbrooke's Hospital Minute Book, General Committee 1.3.1932.

22   Addenbrooke's Hospital Minute Book, General Committee 15.3.1932.

23   Addenbrooke's Hospital Minute Book, General Committee 5.4.1932.

24   Addenbrooke's Hospital Minute Book, General Committee 19.4.1932.

25   Addenbrooke's Hospital Minute Book, General Committee 3.5.1932.

26   Addenbrooke's Hospital Minute Book, General Committee 19.7.1932.
27   Addenbrooke's Hospital Minute Book, General Committee 16.8.1932.
28   Addenbrooke's Hospital Minute Book, General Committee 21.9.1932.
29   Addenbrooke's Hospital Minute Book, General Committee 27.9.1932.
30   Addenbrooke's Hospital Minute Book, General Committee 25.10.1932.
31   Addenbrooke's Hospital Minute Book, General Committee 11.7.1933.
32   Addenbrooke's Hospital Minute Book, General Committee 24.9.1935.
33   Addenbrooke's Hospital Minute Book, General Committee 14.2.1933.
34   Addenbrooke's Hospital Annual Report 1933.
35   Addenbrooke's Hospital Minute Book, General Committees 23.7.1935
     and 22.10.1935.
36   Addenbrooke's Hospital Minute Book, General Committee 23.11.1937.
37   Addenbrooke's Hospital Minute Book, General Committee 1.12.1936.
38   Addenbrooke's Hospital Minute Book, Finance Committee 18.5.1937.
39   Addenbrooke's Hospital General Committee Minute Book, Special
     Meeting of the General Committee 6.8.1940.
40   Addenbrooke's Hospital General Committee Minute Book, General
     Committee 25.1.1944.
41   Addenbrooke's Hospital General Committee Minute Book, Finance
     Committee 16.6.1947.
42   Addenbrooke's Hospital General Committee Minute Book, General
     Committee 27.4.1948.

CHAPTER 36

1   Addenbrooke's Hospital Annual Report 1914.
2   Addenbrooke's Hospital Minute Book, General Committee 12.4.1915.
3   Addenbrooke's Hospital Minute Book, General Committees 15.4.1915
     and 17.5.1915.
4   Addenbrooke's Hospital Minute Book, General Committee 28.6.1915.
5   Addenbrooke's Hospital Minute Book, General Committee 11.6.1917.
6   Addenbrooke's Hospital Minute Book, General Committee 25.6.1917.
7   Addenbrooke's Hospital Minute Book, General Committee 20.10.1919.
8   Addenbrooke's Hospital Minute Book, General Committee 15.12.1919.
9   Addenbrooke's Hospital Minute Book, Report of the General Committee
     to the Quarterly Court to be held 9.2.1920.
10   Addenbrooke's Hospital Minute Book, Report of the General Committee
     to the Quarterly Court to be held 10.5.1920.
11   Addenbrooke's Hospital Minute Book, Report of the General Committee
     to the Quarterly Court to be held 9.8.1920.
12   Addenbrooke's Hospital Minute Book, General Committee 14.3.1921.
13   Addenbrooke's Hospital Minute Book, General Committee 28.2.1921.
14   Addenbrooke's Hospital Minute Book, Report of the General Committee
     to the Quarterly Court to be held 14.2.1921.
15   Addenbrooke's Hospital Minute Book, General Committee 3.10.1921.

16 Addenbrooke's Hospital Minute Book, General Committee 7.4.1924.
17 Addenbrooke's Hospital Minute Book, General Committee 14.11.1921.
18 Addenbrooke's Hospital Minute Book, General Committee 2.1.1922.
19 Addenbrooke's Hospital Minute Book, Report of the General Committee
    to the Quarterly Court to be held 14.11.1921.
20 Addenbrooke's Hospital Minute Book, General Committee 2.1.1922.
21 Addenbrooke's Hospital Minute Book, Report of the General Committee
    to the Quarterly Court to be held 14.8.1922.
22 Addenbrooke's Hospital Minute Book, Report of the General Committee
    to the Quarterly Court to be held 13.11.1922.
23 Addenbrooke's Hospital Minute Book, Report of the General Committee
    to the Quarterly Court to be held 14.5.1923.
24 Addenbrooke's Hospital Minute Book, Report of the General Committee
    to the Quarterly Court to be held 11.2.1924.
25 Addenbrooke's Hospital Minute Book, Finance Committee 14.4.1924.
26 Addenbrooke's Hospital Minute Book, Report of the General Committee
    to the Quarterly Court to be held 12.5.1924.
27 Addenbrooke's Hospital Minute Book, Report of the General Committee
    to the Quarterly Court to be held 3.8.1923.
28 Addenbrooke's Hospital Minute Book, Report of the General Committee
    to the Quarterly Court to be held 11.8.1924.
29 Addenbrooke's Hospital Minute Book, Report of the General Committee
    to the Quarterly Court to be held 9.2.1925.
30 ROLLESTON, SIR H.D., 1932, *The Cambridge Medical School*,
    Cambridge University Press, p. 186.
31 Addenbrooke's Hospital Minute Book, Report of the General Committee
    to the Quarterly Court to be held 10.11.1925.
32 Addenbrooke's Hospital Minute Book, Report of the General Committee
    for the quarter ended 31.3.1926.
33 Addenbrooke's Hospital Minute Book, Report of the General Committee
    to the Quarterly Court to be held 23.11.1926 and General Committee
    23.11.1926.
34 Addenbrooke's Hospital Minute Book, Report of the General Committee
    to the Quarterly Court to be held 10.5.1927.
35 Addenbrooke's Hospital Minute Book, Report of the General Committee
    to the Quarterly Court to be held 8.2.1927.
36 Addenbrooke's Hospital Minute Book, Reports of the General
    Committee to the Quarterly Courts to be held 8.11.1927 and
    14.2.1928.
37 Addenbrooke's Hospital Minute Book, Report of the General Committee
    to the Quarterly Court to be held 14.2.1928.
38 Addenbrooke's Hospital Minute Book, Report of the General Committee
    to the Quarterly Court to be held 15.5.1928.
39 Addenbrooke's Hospital Minute Book, Report of the General Committee
    to the Quarterly Court to be held 21.8.1928.
40 Addenbrooke's Hospital Minute Book, Reports of the General

Committee to the Quarterly Courts to be held 13.11.1928 and 19.2.1929.

41 Addenbrooke's Hospital Minute Book, General Committee 13.11.1928.
42 Addenbrooke's Hospital Minute Book, Special Selection and Advisory Committee 21.10.1929.
43 Addenbrooke's Hospital Minute Book, General Committee 7.1.1930.
44 Addenbrooke's Hospital Minute Book, Report of the General Committee to the Quarterly Court to be held 18.2.1930.
45 Addenbrooke's Hospital Minute Book, General Committee 15.4.1930.
46 Addenbrooke's Hospital Minute Book, General Committee 1.4.1930.
47 Addenbrooke's Hospital Minute Book, General Committee 7.1.1930.
48 Addenbrooke's Hospital Annual Report 1929.
49 Addenbrooke's Hospital Minute Book, General Committee 18.2.1930.
50 Addenbrooke's Hospital Minute Book, General Committee 4.3.1930.
51 Addenbrooke's Hospital Minute Book, General Committee 27.5.1930.
52 Addenbrooke's Hospital Minute Book, General Committee 8.7.1930.
53 Addenbrooke's Hospital Minute Book, General Committee 22.7.1930.
54 Addenbrooke's Hospital Minute Book, General Committee 27.7.1931.
55 Addenbrooke's Hospital Minute Book, General Committee 8.7.1930.
56 Addenbrooke's Hospital Minute Book, General Committee 15.9.1931.
57 Addenbrooke's Hospital Minute Book, House Committee 11.10.1932.
58 Addenbrooke's Hospital Minute Book, Report of the General Committee to the Quarterly Court to be held 27.11.1934.
59 Addenbrooke's Hospital Minute Book, Report of the General Committee to the Quarterly Court to be held 20.8.1935.
60 Addenbrooke's Hospital Minute Book, Bye-laws Drafting Sub-Committee 7.2.1935.
61 Addenbrooke's Hospital Minute Book, General Committee 2.4.1935.
62 Addenbrooke's Hospital Minute Book, Report of the General Committee to the Quarterly Court to be held 19.11.1935.
63 Addenbrooke's Hospital Minute Book, Report of the General Committee to the Quarterly Court to be held 28.5.1937.
64 Addenbrooke's Hospital Minute Book, General Committee 27.7.1937.
65 Addenbrooke's Hospital Minute Book, John Bonnett Clinical Laboratory Committee 19.7.1937.
66 Addenbrooke's Hospital Minute Book, General Committee 27.10.1937.
67 Addenbrooke's Hospital Minute Book, Report of the General Committee to the Quarterly Court to be held 23.11.1937.
68 Addenbrooke's Hospital Minute Book, General Committee 26.10.1937.
69 Addenbrooke's Hospital Minute Book, Reports of the General Committee to the Quarterly Courts to be held 26.5.1931 and 26.5.1936.
70 Addenbrooke's Hospital Minute Book, Selection Committee 18.11.1937.
71 Addenbrooke's Hospital Minute Book, Report of the General Committee to the Quarterly Court to be held 23.8.1938.
72 Addenbrooke's Hospital Minute Book, Report of the General Committee to the Quarterly Court to be held 22.11.1938.

[73] Addenbrooke's Hospital Minute Book, Standing Selection Committee 21.4.1939.
[74] Addenbrooke's Hospital Minute Book, General Purposes Committee 19.7.1939.
[75] Addenbrooke's Hospital Minute Book, General Committee 28.11.1939.
[76] Addenbrooke's Hospital General Committee Minute Book, General Committee 23.1.1940.
[77] Addenbrooke's Hospital General Committee Minute Book, Report of the General Committee to the Quarterly Court to be held 27.2.1940.
[78] Addenbrooke's Hospital General Committee Minute Book, General Committee 23.7.1940.
[79] Addenbrooke's Hospital General Committee Minute Book, General Committee 24.9.1940.
[80] Addenbrooke's Hospital General Committee Minute Book, General Committee 22.10.1940.
[81] Addenbrooke's Hospital General Committee Minute Book, General Committee 18.12.1940.
[82] Addenbrooke's Hospital General Committee Minute Book, General Committee 28.1.1941.
[83] Addenbrooke's Hospital General Committee Minute Book, General Committee 25.2.1941.
[84] Addenbrooke's Hospital General Committee Minute Book, Report of the General Committee to the Quarterly Court to be held 26.8.1941.
[85] Addenbrooke's Hospital General Committee Minute Book, General Committee 25.11.1941.
[86] Addenbrooke's Hospital General Committee Minute Book, Report of the General Committee for the quarter ended 30.6.1942.
[87] Addenbrooke's Hospital General Committee Minute Book, General Committee 28.7.1942.
[88] Addenbrooke's Hospital General Committee Minute Book, General Committee 22.12.1942.
[89] Addenbrooke's Hospital General Committee Minute Book, Report of the General Committee to the Quarterly Court to be held 25.5.1943.
[90] Addenbrooke's Hospital General Committee Minute Book, General Purposes Committee 15.4.1943.
[91] Addenbrooke's Hospital General Committee Minute Book, Report of the General Committee for the quarter ended 30.6.1943.
[92] Addenbrooke's Hospital General Committee Minute Book, Report of the General Committee to the Quarterly Court to be held 23.11.1943.
[93] Addenbrooke's Hospital General Committee Minute Book, Report of the General Committee to the Quarterly Court to be held 22.2.1944.
[94] Addenbrooke's Hospital General Committee Minute Book, Report of the General Committee to the Quarterly Court to be held 23.5.1944.
[95] Addenbrooke's Hospital General Committee Minute Book, General Committee 23.10.1945.
[96] Addenbrooke's Hospital General Committee Minute Book, Report of the General Committee for the Quarter ended 31.12.1945.

97 Addenbrooke's Hospital General Committee Minute Book, Report of the General Committee to the Quarterly Court to be held 26.11.1946.
98 Addenbrooke's Hospital General Committee Minute Book, General Committee 26.11.1946.
99 Addenbrooke's Hospital General Committee Minute Book, Standing Selection and Advisory Committee 19.11.1946.
100 Addenbrooke's Hospital General Committee Minute Book, Standing Selection and Advisory Committee 9.8.1946.
101 Addenbrooke's Hospital General Committee Minute Book, Standing Selection and Advisory Committee 14.8.1946.
102 Addenbrooke's Hospital General Committee Minute Book, General Committee 20.8.1946.
103 Addenbrooke's Hospital General Committee Minute Book, Reports of the General Committee for the quarters ended 31.12.1946 and 31.3.1947.
104 Addenbrooke's Hospital General Committee Minute Book, Report of the General Committee to the Quarterly Court to be held 20.5.1947.
105 Addenbrooke's Hospital General Committee Minute Book, General Purposes Committee 18.8.1947.
106 Addenbrooke's Hospital General Committee Minute Book, Standing Selection and Advisory Committee 17.11.1947.
107 Addenbrooke's Hospital General Committee Minute Book, Standing Selection and Advisory Committee 9.2.1948.
108 Addenbrooke's Hospital General Committee Minute Book, General Purposes Committee 16.2.1948.
109 Addenbrooke's Hospital General Committee Minute Book, Standing Selection and Advisory Committee 5.5.1948.
110 Addenbrooke's Hospital General Committee Minute Book, General Purposes Committee 18.8.1947.
111 Addenbrooke's Hospital General Committee Minute Book, General Committee 25.11.1947.

CHAPTER 37

1   *Cambridge Chronicle* 30.11.1932.
2   Addenbrooke's Hospital Minute Book, General Committee 28.7.1913.
3   Addenbrooke's Hospital Minute Book, House Committee 16.1.1922.
4   Addenbrooke's Hospital Minute Book, House Committee 30.12.1924.
5   Addenbrooke's Hospital Minute Book, General Committee 27.10.1925.
6   *British Medical Journal* 31.8.1974.
7   Addenbrooke's Hospital Minute Book, General Committee 14.6.1927.
8   Addenbrooke's Hospital Minute Book, General Committee 6.3.1928.
9   Addenbrooke's Hospital Minute Book, General Committee 8.2.1927.
10 Addenbrooke's Hospital Minute Book, House Committee 10.7.1928.
11 Addenbrooke's Hospital Minute Book, General Committee 27.7.1931.

12 Addenbrooke's Hospital Minute Book, Cambridge Chronicle 30.11.1932.
13 Addenbrooke's Hospital Minute Book, General Purposes Committee
    5.7.1937.
14 Addenbrooke's Hospital Minute Book, General Committee 25.1.1938.
15 Addenbrooke's Hospital Minute Book, General Committee 24.5.1938.
16 Addenbrooke's Hospital Minute Book, General Committee 24.10.1939.
17 Addenbrooke's Hospital Minute Book, General Committee 25.7.1939.
18 Addenbrooke's Hospital Minute Book, General Committee 28.11.1939.
19 Addenbrooke's Hospital General Committee Minute Book, Special
    Meeting of the General Committee 17.6.1940.
20 Addenbrooke's Hospital General Committee Minute Book, General
    Committee 25.6.1940.
21 Addenbrooke's Hospital General Committee Minute Book, General
    Committee 27.8.1940.
22 Addenbrooke's Hospital General Committee Minute Book, General
    Committee 22.10.1940.
23 Addenbrooke's Hospital General Committee Minute Book, Special
    Meeting of the General Committee 18.2.1941.
24 Addenbrooke's Hospital General Committee Minute Book, Special
    Meeting of the General Committee 18.2.1941 and General Committee
    25.3.1941.
25 Addenbrooke's Hospital General Committee Minute Book, General
    Committee 29.4.1941.
26 Radiotherapy at Hills Road, The Addenbrooke's News No. 21, April 1972,
    p. 5.
27 Addenbrooke's Hospital Annual Report 1944.
28 Addenbrooke's Hospital General Committee Minute Book, General
    Committee 22.1.1946.

CHAPTER 38

1   Addenbrooke's Hospital Minute Book, Special Meeting of the General
    Committee 11.8.1913, and Report of the General Committee to the
    Quarterly Court to be held 5.11.1913.
2   Addenbrooke's Hospital Annual Report 1914.
3   Addenbrooke's Hospital Minute Book, General Committee 17.8.1914.
4   Addenbrooke's Hospital Minute Book, General Committee 29.6.1914.
5   Addenbrooke's Hospital Minute Book, House Sub-Committee 26.4.1915.
6   Addenbrooke's Hospital Minute Book, House Sub-Committee
    11.10.1915.
7   Addenbrooke's Hospital Minute Book, House Sub-Committee 17.1.1916.
8   Addenbrooke's Hospital Minute Book, House Sub-Committee 31.1.1916.
9   Addenbrooke's Hospital Minute Book, House Sub-Committee
    13.11.1916.
10 Addenbrooke's Hospital Minute Book, House Sub-Committee 14.5.1917.

11 Addenbrooke's Hospital Minute Book, General Committee 14.1.1918.
12 Addenbrooke's Hospital Minute Book, House Sub-Committee 25.2.1918.
13 Addenbrooke's Hospital Minute Book, House Sub-Committee 23.9.1918.
14 Addenbrooke's Hospital Minute Book, Report of the General Committee
    for the quarter ended 31.12.1918.
15 Addenbrooke's Hospital Minute Book, House Committees 24.3.1919,
    28.4.1919, 25.8.1919 and 8.9.1919.
16 Addenbrooke's Hospital Minute Book, House Committee 8.9.1919.
17 Addenbrooke's Hospital Minute Book, House Committee 7.4.1919.
18 Addenbrooke's Hospital Minute Book, General Quarterly Court
    12.5.1919.
19 Addenbrooke's Hospital Minute Book, General Committee 9.8.1920.
20 Addenbrooke's Hospital Minute Book, House Committee 28.7.1919.
21 Addenbrooke's Hospital Minute Book, House Committee 26.5.1919.
22 Addenbrooke's Hospital Minute Book, House Committee 30.6.1919.
23 Addenbrooke's Hospital Minute Book, House Committee 15.12.1919.
24 Addenbrooke's Hospital Minute Book, House Committee 9.8.1920.
25 Addenbrooke's Hospital Minute Book, House Committee 15.11.1920.
26 Addenbrooke's Hospital Minute Book, House Committee 28.2.1921.
27 Addenbrooke's Hospital Minute Book, Nursing Committee 7.7.1921.
28 Addenbrooke's Hospital Minute Book, General Committee 20.6.1921.
29 Addenbrooke's Hospital Minute Book, General Committee 18.7.1921.
30 Addenbrooke's Hospital Minute Book, Nursing Committee 7.7.1921.
31 Addenbrooke's Hospital Minute Book, House Committee 24.7.1922.
32 Addenbrooke's Hospital Minute Book, House Committee 23.10.1922.
33 Addenbrooke's Hospital Minute Book, House Committee 13.11.1922.
34 Addenbrooke's Hospital Minute Book, Joint Meeting of the Nursing
    Committees of Addenbrooke's Hospital and the West Suffolk General
    Hospital, Bury St Edmunds, 15.1.1923.
35 Addenbrooke's Hospital Minute Book, House Committee 13.2.1922.
36 Addenbrooke's Hospital Minute Book, Nursing Committee 23.3.1922.
37 Addenbrooke's Hospital Minute Book, House Committee 25.6.1923.
38 Addenbrooke's Hospital Minute Book, House Committee 7.4.1925.
39 Addenbrooke's Hospital Minute Book, General Committee 5.5.1925.
40 Addenbrooke's Hospital Minute Book, Report of the General Committee
    for the quarter ended 30.6.1925.
41 Addenbrooke's Hospital Minute Book, House Committee 29.12.1925.
42 Addenbrooke's Hospital Minute Book, House Committee 13.4.1926.
43 Addenbrooke's Hospital Minute Book, Nursing Committee 21.5.1926.
44 Addenbrooke's Hospital Minute Book, Nursing Committee 8.5.1926.
45 Addenbrooke's Hospital Minute Book, House Committee 14.12.1926.
46 Addenbrooke's Hospital Minute Book, General Committee 28.12.1926.
47 Addenbrooke's Hospital Minute Book, General Committee 11.1.1927.
48 Addenbrooke's Hospital Minute Book, Nursing Sub-Committee
    16.5.1927.
49 Addenbrooke's Hospital Minute Book, General Committee 31.5.1927.

50   Addenbrooke's Hospital Minute Book, General Committee 6.9.1927.
51   Addenbrooke's Hospital Minute Book, Nursing Committee 3.10.1927.
52   Addenbrooke's Hospital Minute Book, House Committee 10.1.1928 and
     Report of the General Committee for the quarter ended 31.3.1928.
53   Addenbrooke's Hospital Minute Book, House Committee 17.4.1928.
54   Addenbrooke's Hospital Minute Book, House Committee 26.6.1928.
55   Addenbrooke's Hospital Minute Book, House Committee 16.10.1928.
56   Addenbrooke's Hospital Minute Book, House Committee 21.2.1928.
57   Addenbrooke's Hospital Minute Book, House Committee 20.8.1929.
58   Addenbrooke's Hospital Minute Book, House Committee 12.6.1928.
59   Addenbrooke's Hospital Minute Book, House Committee 15.4.1930.
60   Addenbrooke's Hospital Minute Book, House Committee 26.6.1928 and
     Report of the General Committee for the quarter ended 30.6.1928.
61   Addenbrooke's Hospital Minute Book, House Committee 21.8.1928.
62   Addenbrooke's Hospital Minute Book, House Committees 13.11.1928
     and 8.1.1929.
63   Addenbrooke's Hospital Minute Book, Nursing Committees 26.3.1929
     and 13.5.1929.
64   Addenbrooke's Hospital Minute Book, Nursing Committee 10.6.1929.
65   Addenbrooke's Hospital Minute Book, General Committee 11.6.1929.
66   Addenbrooke's Hospital Minute Book, Nursing Committee 19.7.1929.
67   Addenbrooke's Hospital Minute Book, Nursing Committee 27.9.1929.
68   Addenbrooke's Hospital Minute Book, Report of the General Committee
     for the quarter ended 30.9.1929.
69   Addenbrooke's Hospital Minute Book, House Committee 20.8.1929.
70   Addenbrooke's Hospital Minute Book, Nursing Committee 27.9.1929.
71   Addenbrooke's Hospital Minute Book, House Committee 1.10.1929.
72   Addenbrooke's Hospital Minute Book, General Committee 1.10.1929.
73   Addenbrooke's Hospital Minute Book, Nursing Committee 18.10.1929.
74   Addenbrooke's Hospital Minute Book, General Committee 29.10.1929.
75   Addenbrooke's Hospital Minute Book, Report of the General Committee
     for the quarter ended 31.12.1929.
76   Addenbrooke's Hospital Minute Book, House Committee 26.11.1929.
77   Addenbrooke's Hospital Minute Book, General Committee 10.6.1930.
78   Addenbrooke's Hospital Minute Book, House Committee 10.6.1930.
79   Addenbrooke's Hospital Minute Book, Nursing Committee 13.6.1930.
80   Addenbrooke's Hospital Minute Book, Nursing Committee 15.11.1930.
81   Addenbrooke's Hospital Minute Book, House Committees 22.7.1930 and
     19.8.1930.
82   Addenbrooke's Hospital Minute Book, Nursing Committee 19.12.1930.
83   Addenbrooke's Hospital Minute Book, House Committee 3.2.1931.
84   Addenbrooke's Hospital General Committee Minute Book, House
     Committee 24.10.1947.
85   Addenbrooke's Hospital Minute Book, House Committee 20.1.1931.
86   Addenbrooke's Hospital Annual Report 1931.
87   Addenbrooke's Hospital Annual Reports.

88 Addenbrooke's Hospital Minute Book, House Committee 27.10.1931.
89 Addenbrooke's Hospital Annual Report 1938.
90 Addenbrooke's Hospital Minute Book, House Committee 3.2.1931.
91 Addenbrooke's Hospital Minute Book, House Committee 7.1.1930.
92 Addenbrooke's Hospital Minute Book, House Committee 22.1.1930.
93 Addenbrooke's Hospital Minute Book, House Committee 18.8.1931.
94 Addenbrooke's Hospital Minute Book, House Committee 29.9.1931.
95 Addenbrooke's Hospital Minute Book, Nursing Committee 18.5.1932.
96 Addenbrooke's Hospital Minute Book, Nursing Committee 21.11.1932.
97 Addenbrooke's Hospital Minute Book, Report of the General Committe
    to the Quarterly Court to be held 28.5.1935. The Annual Reports say
    Numbers 26 and 27.
98 Addenbrooke's Hospital Minute Book, House Committee 13.11.1934
    and General Committee 8.1.1935.
99 Addenbrooke's Hospital Minute Book, House Committee 8.1.1935.
100 Addenbrooke's Hospital Minute Book, House Committee 7.4.1936.
101 Addenbrooke's Hospital Minute Book, Special Meeting of House
    Committee 28.4.1936.
102 Addenbrooke's Hospital Minute Book, House Committee 26.5.1936.
103 Addenbrooke's Hospital Minute Book, Nursing Committee 3.2.1937.
104 Addenbrooke's Hospital Minute Book, House Committee 13.7.1937.
105 Addenbrooke's Hospital Minute Book, House Committee 25.5.1937.
106 Addenbrooke's Hospital Minute Book, General Committee 26.10.1937.
107 Addenbrooke's Hospital Minute Book, House Committee 9.11.1937.
108 Addenbrooke's Hospital Minute Book, General Committee 25.1.1938.
109 Addenbrooke's Hospital Minute Book, House Committee 8.2.1938.
110 Addenbrooke's Hospital Minute Book, House Committee 8.3.1938.
111 Addenbrooke's Hospital Minute Book, Report of the General Committee
    for the quarter ended 31.3.1938.
112 Addenbrooke's Hospital Minute Book, House Committee and General
    Committee 26.4.1938.
113 Addenbrooke's Hospital Minute Book, General Committee 27.9.1938.
114 Addenbrooke's Hospital Minute Book, Nursing Committee 2.5.1939.
115 Addenbrooke's Hospital Minute Book, General Committee 23.5.1939.
116 Addenbrooke's Hospital Minute Book, House Committee 22.11.1938,
    and Addenbrooke's Hospital Annual Report 1939.
117 Addenbrooke's Hospital Minute Book, House Committee 18.4.1939.
118 Addenbrooke's Hospital Minute Book, House Committee 25.4.1939.
119 Addenbrooke's Hospital Minute Book, General Committee 26.9.1939.
120 Addenbrooke's Hospital General Committee Minute Book, House
    Committee 23.7.1940.
121 Addenbrooke's Hospital General Committee Minute Book, House
    Committee 22.10.1940, and General Committee 26.11.1940.
122 Addenbrooke's Hospital General Committee Minute Book, General
    Committee 27.5.1941.
123 Addenbrooke's Hospital General Committee Minute Book, General
    Committee 22.7.1941.

[124] Addenbrooke's Hospital General Committee Minute Book, General Committee 24.6.1941.
[125] Addenbrooke's Hospital General Committee Minute Book, House Committee 8.8.1941.
[126] Addenbrooke's Hospital General Committee Minute Book, Report of the General Committee to the Quarterly Court to be held 24.2.1942.
[127] Addenbrooke's Hospital General Committee Minute Book, General Committee 26.8.1941.
[128] Addenbrooke's Hospital General Committee Minute Book, Finance Committee 17.5.1943.
[129] Addenbrooke's Hospital General Committee Minute Book, House Committee 25.5.1943, and General Committee 29.5.1943.
[130] Addenbrooke's Hospital General Committee Minute Book, House Committee 25.1.1944.
[131] Addenbrooke's Hospital General Committee Minute Book, House Committee 7.3.1944.
[132] Addenbrooke's Hospital General Committee Minute Book, General Committee 21.3.1944.
[133] Addenbrooke's Hospital General Committee Minute Book, House Committee 26.9.1944.
[134] Addenbrooke's Hospital General Committee Minute Book, House Committee 12.33.1946.
[135] Addenbrooke's Hospital General Committee Minute Book, House Committee 24.7.1945.
[136] Addenbrooke's Hospital General Committee Minute Book, Nursing Committee 24.8.1945.
[137] Addenbrooke's Hospital General Committee Minute Book, General Committee 28.8.1945.
[138] Addenbrooke's Hospital General Committee Minute Book, Report of the General Committee for the quarter ended 31.12.1945.
[139] Addenbrooke's Hospital General Committee Minute Book, House Committee 12.3.1946.
[140] Leader, *The Lancet*, 7.9.1949, p. 301.
[141] Addenbrooke's Hospital Minute Book, House Committee 22.1.1930.
[142] Letter from F.B. Parsons, *British Medical Journal*, 28.9.1940, p. 429.
[143] Letter from R.R. Macintosh, *The Lancet*, 14.9.1940, p. 345.
[144] Letter from the Association of Anaesthetists in Great Britain and Ireland, *The Lancet*, 7.9.1940, p. 307.
[145] Letter from J. Elam, *The Lancet*, 7.9.1940, p. 309.
[146] Personal communication, 8.12.1988, from Mrs P.N. Harris, formerly Sister Kemp.
[147] Addenbrooke's Hospital General Committee Minute Book, Finance Committee 14.1.1946.
[148] Addenbrooke's Hospital General Committee Minute Book, Report of the General Committee for the quarter ended 31.3.1947.
[149] Addenbrooke's Hospital General Committee Minute Book, Report of the General Committee for the quarter ended 31.12.1942.

150 Addenbrooke's Annual Report 1942.
151 Addenbrooke's Hospital General Committee Minute Book, General
      Committee 28.1.1947.

CHAPTER 39

1 HUXLEY, E., 1975, *Florence Nightingale*, Weidenfeld & Nicholson,
    London.
2 ROOK, A., 1972, Alice Fisher – A Great Matron, *The Addenbrooke's
    News*, October. The Cambridge Collection, Cambridge Central
    Library.
3 Addenbrooke's Hospital Annual Report 1888.
4 Addenbrooke's Hospital Annual Report 1889.
5 Addenbrooke's Hospital Annual Report 1891.
6 Addenbrooke's Hospital Annual Report 1893.
7 Addenbrooke's Hospital Annual Report 1894.
8 Addenbrooke's Hospital Annual Report 1895,
9 Addenbrooke's Hospital Annual Report 1897.
10 Addenbrooke's Hospital Annual Report 1896.
11 Addenbrooke's Hospital Annual Report 1898.
12 Addenbrooke's Hospital Annual Report 1906.
13 Addenbrooke's Hospital Annual Report 1915.
14 Addenbrooke's Hospital Annual Report 1921.
15 Addenbrooke's Hospital Annual Report 1922.
16 Addenbrooke's Hospital Annual Report 1923.
17 Addenbrooke's Hospital Annual Report 1926.
18 Addenbrooke's Hospital Minute Book, Nursing Committee 21.11.1932.
19 Addenbrooke's Hospital Minute Book, House Committee Special
      Meeting 17.11.1933.
20 Addenbrooke's Hospital Minute Book, General Committee 19.12.1923.
21 Addenbrooke's Hospital Minute Book, General Committee 1.5.1934.
22 Addenbrooke's Hospital Annual Report 1935.
23 Minute Book, Nursing Committee 16.1.1935.
24 Addenbrooke's Hospital Annual Report 1933.
25 Addenbrooke's Hospital Annual Report 1937.
26 Addenbrooke's Hospital Annual Report 1939.
27 Addenbrooke's Hospital Annual Reports 1939 and 1942.
28 Addenbrooke's Hospital Annual Report 1945.
29 Addenbrooke's Hospital General Committee Minute Book, General
      Committee 27.11.1945 and Addenbrooke's Hospital Annual Report
      1946.

CHAPTER 40

[1] ROOK, A., 1980, *Cambridge Medical Society 1880–1980, A Centennial History*, Cambridge Medical Society.

[2] METTLER, C., 1947, in *History of Medicine*, ed. Fred A. Mettler, The Blakiston Company, Philadelphia, p. 988.

[3] Addenbrooke's Hospital Minute Book, House Sub-Committee 12.11.1917.

[4] Addenbrooke's Hospital Minute Book, House Sub-Committee 26.11.1917.

[5] Addenbrooke's Hospital Minute Book, General Committee 26.5.1919.

[6] Addenbrooke's Hospital Minute Book, General Committee 16.6.1919.

[7] Addenbrooke's Hospital Minute Book, House Committee 21.7.1919.

[8] LINDSAY, L., 1935, The Eastern Counties, *British Dental Journal*, **59**, 121.

[9] Addenbrooke's Hospital Minute Book, Weekly Meeting 1.8.1883.

[10] Obituary, 1918, *British Dental Journal*, **39**, 107.

[11] Addenbrooke's Hospital Minute Book, General Quarterly Court 31.12.1894.

[12] Addenbrooke's Hospital Minute Book, Advisory Council 19.2.1901.

[13] Addenbrooke's Hospital Minute Book, General Committee 12.1.1911.

[14] Addenbrooke's Hospital Minute Book, General Committee 16.6.1919.

[15] Addenbrooke's Hospital Minute Book, General Committee 17.5.1909.

[16] Addenbrooke's Hospital Minute Book, General Committee 5.3.1909.

[17] Addenbrooke's Hospital Minute Book, General Committee 21.6.1909.

[18] Addenbrooke's Hospital Minute Book, General Committee 10.5.1920.

[19] Addenbrooke's Hospital Minute Book, House Committee 10.12.1923.

[20] Addenbrooke's Hospital Minute Book, House Committee 14.1.1924.

[21] Addenbrooke's Hospital Minute Book, General Committee 7.1.1930.

[22] Addenbrooke's Hospital Minute Book, General Committee 10.12.1929.

[23] Addenbrooke's Hospital Minute Book, General Committee 17.1.1910.

[24] Addenbrooke's Hospital Minute Book, General Committee 14.2.1910.

[25] Addenbrooke's Hospital Minute Book, House Committee 26.6.1922.

[26] Addenbrooke's Hospital Minute Book, General Committee 26.11.1940.

[27] Addenbrooke's Hospital Minute Book, General Committee 25.3.1941.

[28] Addenbrooke's Hospital Minute Book, General Committee 30.12.1918.

[29] Addenbrooke's Hospital Minute Book, General Committee 8.9.1919.

[30] Addenbrooke's Hospital Minute Book, General Committee 20.10.1919.

CHAPTER 41

[1] COLE, L., 1971, Cambridge Medicine and the Medical School in the Twentieth Century, in *Cambridge and Its Contribution to Medicine*, ed.

Arthur Rook, Wellcome Institute of the History of Medicine, London, pp. 257–84.

2 Addenbrooke's Hospital Minute Book, General Committee 10.11.1913.

3 Addenbrooke's Hospital Minute Book, General Committee 29.6.1914.

4 ROLLESTON, SIR H.D., 1932, *The Cambridge Medical School*, Cambridge University Press.

5 Addenbrooke's Hospital Minute Book, General Committee 8.7.1918.

6 Addenbrooke's Hospital Minute Book, General Committee 22.7.1918.

7 Addenbrooke's Hospital Minute Book, General Committee 12.8.1918.

8 Addenbrooke's Hospital Minute Book, General Committee 18.12.1934.

9 Addenbrooke's Hospital Minute Book, Bye-laws Drafting Sub-Committee Meeting 15.2.1935.

10 Addenbrooke's Hospital Minute Book, General Committee 27.7.1937.

11 Addenbrooke's Hospital Minute Book, General Committee 23.11.1937.

12 Addenbrooke's Hospital Minute Book, General Committee 22.33.1938.

13 Frank Edward Elmore of Threefields, Boxmore, Herts, died 26.7.1932 leaving his residuary estate on Trust for the provision of scholarships for medical research for male post-graduates of British or Colonial birth, other than Scottish birth, at Cambridge University. The balance of the Fund, after expenses, was to be applied in promoting or assisting generally the provision of medical education at the University. Statutes of the University of Cambridge and Passages from Acts of Parliament Relating to the University, 1985. Published by Authority. Cambridge University Press.

14 Addenbrooke's Hospital Minute Book, General Committee 26.4.1938.

15 Addenbrooke's Hospital Minute Book, General Committee 24.5.1938.

16 Addenbrooke's Hospital Minute Book, General Committee 25.7.1939.

17 Addenbrooke's Hospital General Committee Minute Book, General Committee 24.4.1945.

18 Addenbrooke's Hospital General Committee Minute Book, General Purposes Committee 15.4.1943.

19 Addenbrooke's Hospital General Committee Minute Book, General Committee 20.4.1943.

20 Addenbrooke's Hospital General Committee Minute Book, General Committee 26.10.1943.

21 Addenbrooke's Hospital General Committee Minute Book, General Committee 22.2.1944.

22 Addenbrooke's Hospital General Committee Minute Book, General Committees 21.3.1944 and 25.4.1944.

23 Addenbrooke's Hospital General Committee Minute Book, General Committee 24.4.1945.

24 Addenbrooke's Hospital Annual Report 1946.

25 Addenbrooke's Hospital General Committee Minute Book, General Purposes Committee 18.8.1947.

Appendix I

Kenny, A.M.R., 1952. 'The Cambridge District Nursing Association 1873–1945'. Cambridge Collection, Cambridge Central Library.
Addenbrooke's Hospital Minute Book, Weekly Meeting 18.12.1872 and General Quarterly Court 30.12.1872.
Addenbrooke's Hospital Minute Book, Weekly Meeting 22.4.1903.

Appendix II

Addenbrooke's Hospital Annual Reports and Addenbrooke's Hospital Statements.

Appendix III

Addenbrooke's Hospital Annual Reports and Addenbrooke's Hospital Statements.

Appendix IV

Addenbrooke's Hospital Annual Reports and Addenbrooke's Hospital Statements.
Cameron, H.C., 1954, *Mr Guy's Hospital 1725–1948*, Longmans, Green & Co., London, New York, Toronto.

Index

Harvey, William, (1578–1657), Physician 108

Harwood, Sir Bustik (1745–1814), Professor of Anatomy (1785) 60, 83, 88, 188, 236

Hatton, Miss E.A., benefactor (1846) 150

Haviland, Henry James (1825–1900), Physician (1861) 104, 183

Haviland, John (1785–1851) Physician & Regius Professor of Physic (1815) 83ff, 99ff, 106f, 112f, 120, 122, 235, 255

Haybittle, Dr John, Senior Physicist (1970) 435

Hayhoe, Professor Frank, Professor of Haematology (1969) 405, 407, 410

Hayles, Richard (1714–1781), Surgeon (1766) 32, 44, 57, 59f, 63

Hayles, Mr W.H., Physicist (1896) 332

Haynes, Dr (d.1942), Physician (1919) 312, 316, 318, 321f, 368

Headley, Dr Charles 85f

Hempsons, Solicitors 339

Henslow, Miss S.M., Superintendent, Nurses' Home (1874) 197f, 202, 447

hepatitis 163

Her Majesty Queen Elizabeth II 426

Heberden, William, Physician (1748) 15, 59

hernia, strangulated 175

Hewitt, Cornwallis (1787–1841), Downing Professor of Medicine (q.v.) (1814) 84f

Higgins, Dr Hubert, General Practitioner and Surgeon (1896) 169, 250, 253

Hill, Dr Alex, Master, Downing College (1892) 246

Hills, Dr Hyde, General Practitioner (c.1890) 250

'Hints for Hospital Nurses' by Alice Fisher (q.v.) and Rachel Williams 199

Hobson, Carrier 23

Hoffman, John, Hospital Governor and local chemist (1776) 65

Hole, Miss, Deputy Matron (1886) 204

Hollings, Mr P.A., Finance Officer (1948) 394, 423

Holm, Dr G.F., apprentice to House Surgeon (1855) 98

Holmes, Timothy (1825–1907) Surgeon, St George's Hospital (1863) 143f, 151ff, 237

home care nursing system 397

home for nurses 275

Home Sister, first appointed 1925 346

home nursing 305

Home of Recovery, Hunstanton 298, 305, 393

Hopkins, Allan (d.1775), Surgeon (1766) 32, 44, 57, 60, 63

Hopkins, Mrs Mary, Matron (1778) 75

hospital contributory schemes 10

Hospital for Sick Children, London 252

Hospital Laboratory Service 412

Hospital Saturday Committee 212

Hospital Sunday 207

House Committee 395

House Governor 428

House Surgeon 97: apprentices to 236; as anaesthetist 142; collecting charges 271; duties of 97f, 373; pupils of 98

Housekeeper 357

Hovell, Thomas, Hospital Governor (1833) 120

Human Ecology, Professor of 388

Humfrey, Charles, architect (1823) 93f

Humphry, William Gilson, (1815–1880) Fellow of Trinity College (1837) 103, 110

Humphry, Sir George Murray (1820–1896), Surgeon (1842) 101ff, 107, 109, Chapter 13, 138f, 143, 147f, 166, 183, 188, 191f, 196, 207f, 224ff, 229, 239, 241ff, 248, 252, 256f, 315, 365, 372, 375

Humphry, Dr Laurence (1856–1920), Physician (1884) 189f, 250, 313, 316, 365

Humphry, Lady Mary, wife of Sir George Murray 115

Hunter, John (1728–1793), Surgeon, London 107, 111

Hunter, William (1718–1783), Anatomist, London 107, 191, 256

Huntingdon County Hospital 98, 186, 306f

Hurrell, Smith, Dispenser (1840) 99

Hutton, Miss, benefactor (1875) 447

hysterectomy, abdominal 174

immunology 108

infectious diseases 93, 146; beds at Hills